Learning Disabilities Sourcebook, 3rd Edition
Leukemia Sourcebook
Liver Disorders Sourcebook
Lung Disorders Sourcebook
Medical Tests Sourcebook, 3rd Edition
Men's Health Concerns Sourcebook, 2nd Edition
Mental Health Disorders Sourcebook, 4th Edition
Mental Retardation Sourcebook
Movement Disorders Sourcebook, 2nd Edition
Multiple Sclerosis Sourcebook
Muscular Dystrophy Sourcebook
Obesity Sourcebook
Osteoporosis Sourcebook
Pain Sourcebook, 3rd Edition
Pediatric Cancer Sourcebook
Physical & Mental Issues in Aging Sourcebook
Podiatry Sourcebook, 2nd Edition
Pregnancy & Birth Sourcebook, 2nd Edition
Prostate Cancer Sourcebook
Prostate & Urological Disorders Sourcebook
Reconstructive & Cosmetic Surgery Sourcebook
Rehabilitation Sourcebook
Respiratory Disorders Sourcebook, 2nd Edition
Sexually Transmitted Diseases Sourcebook, 3rd Edition
Sleep Disorders Sourcebook, 2nd Edition
Smoking Concerns Sourcebook
Sports Injuries Sourcebook, 3rd Edition
Stress-Related Disorders Sourcebook, 2nd Edition
Stroke Sourcebook, 2nd Edition
Surgery Sourcebook, 2nd Edition
Thyroid Disorders Sourcebook
Transplantation Sourcebook
Traveler's Health Sourcebook
Urinary Tract & Kidney Diseases & Disorders Sourcebook, 2nd Edition
Vegetarian Sc
Women's Hea
Edition
Workplace He
Worldwide Health Sourcebook

Teen Health Series

Abuse & Violence Information for Teens
Accident & Safety Information for Teens
Alcohol Information for Teens, 2nd Edition
Allergy Information for Teens
Asthma Information for Teens
Body Information for Teens
Cancer Information for Teens
Complementary & Alternative Medicine Information for Teens
Diabetes Information for Teens
Diet Information for Teens, 2nd Edition
Drug Information for Teens, 2nd Edition
Eating Disorders Information for Teens, 2nd Edition
Fitness Information for Teens, 2nd Edition
Learning Disabilities Information for Teens
Mental Health Information for Teens, 2nd Edition
Pregnancy Information for Teens
Sexual Health Information for Teens, 2nd Edition
Skin Health Information for Teens, 2nd Edition
Sleep Information for Teens
Sports Injuries Information for Teens, 2nd Edition
Stress Information for Teens
Suicide Information for Teens
Tobacco Information for Teens

4/1/11

Sexually Transmitted Diseases SOURCEBOOK

Fourth Edition

[redacted]

Health Reference Series

Fourth Edition

Sexually Transmitted Diseases SOURCEBOOK

Basic Consumer Health Information about the Symptoms and Treatment of Chlamydia, Gonorrhea, Hepatitis, Herpes, HIV/AIDS, Human Papillomavirus (HPV), Pelvic Inflammatory Disease, Syphilis, Trichomoniasis, Vaginal Infections, and Other Sexually Transmitted Diseases (STDs), Including Recent Facts about Prevalence, Risk Factors, Diagnosis, Treatment, and Prevention

Along with Tips on Discussing and Living with STDs, Updates on Current Research and Vaccines, a Glossary of Related Terms, and Resources for Additional Help and Information

Edited by
Laura Larsen

Omnigraphics

P.O. Box 31-1640, Detroit, MI 48231

Bibliographic Note
Because this page cannot legibly accommodate all the copyright notices, the Bibliographic Note portion of the Preface constitutes an extension of the copyright notice.

Edited by Laura Larsen

Health Reference Series

Karen Bellenir, *Managing Editor*
David A. Cooke, M.D., *Medical Consultant*
Elizabeth Collins, *Research and Permissions Coordinator*
Cherry Edwards, *Permissions Assistant*
EdIndex, Services for Publishers, *Indexers*

* * *

Omnigraphics, Inc.

Matthew P. Barbour, *Senior Vice President*
Kevin M. Hayes, *Operations Manager*

* * *

Peter E. Ruffner, *Publisher*

ISBN 978-0-7808-1073-0

Library of Congress Cataloging-in-Publication Data

Sexually transmitted diseases sourcebook : basic consumer health information about the symptoms and treatment of chlamydia, gonorrhea, hepatitis, herpes, HIV/Aids, human papillomavirus (HPV), pelvic inflammatory disease, syphilis, trichomoniasis, vaginal infections, and other sexually transmitted diseases (STDs), including recent facts about prevalence, risk factors, diagnosis, treatment, and prevention; along with tips on discussing and living with STDs, updates on current research and vaccines, a glossary of related terms, and resources for additional help and information / edited by Laura Larsen. -- 4th ed.

p. cm. -- (Health reference series)

Includes bibliographical references and index.

Summary: "Provides basic consumer health information about risk factors, symptoms, testing, and treatment of sexually transmitted infections, along with prevention guidelines. Includes index, glossary of related terms, and other resources"--Provided by publisher.

ISBN 978-0-7808-1073-0 (hardcover : alk. paper) 1. Sexually transmitted diseases--Popular works. I. Larsen, Laura.

RC200.2.S387 2009
616.95'1--dc22

2009019867

Table of Contents

Visit www.healthreferenceseries.com to view *A Contents Guide to the Health Reference Series*, a listing of more than 15,000 topics and the volumes in which they are covered.

Part II: Preventing Sexually Transmitted Diseases

Part III: Types of Sexually Transmitted Diseases and Their Treatments

Part V: Discussing and Living with Sexually Transmitted Diseases

Part VI: Sexually Transmitted Disease Vaccines and Research

Part VII: Additional Help and Information

Preface

About This Book

Sexually transmitted diseases are passed through microorganisms that survive on the genital area or through bodily fluids. Many of them do not have clear symptoms, and long-term undiagnosed infections can lead to other health problems such as infertility, cancers, and the continuing spread of disease. Some STDs, such as chlamydia and gonorrhea, are curable with proper treatment, but others are not. Some diseases, such as syphilis, once decreasing in number are on the rise in certain populations. Teenagers are among the most affected. The Centers for Disease Control and Prevention (CDC) estimates that half of the 19 million new STD cases every year occur among teens and young adults and that more than 65 million Americans are currently living with an STD.

Sexually Transmitted Diseases Sourcebook, Fourth Edition provides updated information about STDs, their symptoms and treatments, and their occurrence in specific groups, such as women, teens, seniors, and homosexuals. It explains treatment and testing options, statistical data, and current research about STD prevention, clinical trials, vaccines, and other medical news. It discusses methods of preventing the spread of STDs, tips for living with STDs, guidelines for disclosing that one has an STD, and suggestions about talking to others about STDs. The book concludes with a glossary of related terms, a directory of resources, and suggestions for further reading.

How to Use This Book

This book is divided into parts and chapters. Parts focus on broad areas of interest. Chapters are devoted to single topics within a part.

Part I: Introduction to Sexually Transmitted Diseases (STDs) provides statistics on STDs in the United States and focuses on the incidence of STDs in men, women, children, teens, minorities, the elderly, and drug users. This part also provides information on why certain populations are at increased risk.

Part II: Preventing Sexually Transmitted Diseases discusses how the use of condoms and the employment of other practices helps protect against the spread of STDs. It describes behaviors that are associated with increased risk for spreading infections, and it also discusses the transmission of disease through occupational exposures and from tattooing. The part concludes with a discussion of sex education and how parents can discuss STD prevention with their children.

Part III: Types of Sexually Transmitted Diseases and Their Treatments offers detailed facts about individual STDs, including modes of transmission, symptoms, treatment options, prevention, and incidence for some of the most common STDs, including chlamydia, gonorrhea, hepatitis, herpes, HIV/AIDS, and syphilis.

Part IV: Testing and Diagnosing Sexually Transmitted Diseases provides general information on STD testing. It discusses issues related to privacy, insurance, and sexual assault. It also supplies in-depth information about HIV testing options and the lab tests that are used to detect some of the other most common STDs.

Part V: Discussing and Living with Sexually Transmitted Diseases explains methods to discuss STDs and your sexual history with a partner, concerns about revealing your HIV status, and how to develop a cooperative doctor-patient relationship regarding STDs and sexual health. It concludes with information about caring for someone with HIV/AIDS.

Part VI: Sexually Transmitted Disease Vaccines and Research includes up-to-date facts about current research initiatives on various topics related to STDs, including therapeutic vaccines, new STD testing methods, microbicides, innovations in HIV/AIDS treatment, and clinical trials. This part also provides information on available vaccines for hepatitis A and B, HPV, and the current search for an effective HIV vaccine.

Part VII: Additional Help and Information offers a glossary of relevant terms, a directory with organizations and hotlines offering STD information and advice, and a listing of magazines, journals, and books for further reading.

Bibliographic Note

This volume contains documents and excerpts from publications issued by the following U.S. government agencies: AIDSinfo; Centers for Disease Control and Prevention (CDC); Health Resources and Services Administration (HRSA); National Institute of Allergy and Infectious Diseases (NIAID); National Institute of Diabetes and Digestive and Kidney Diseases (NIDDK); National Institute on Aging (NIA); National Institute on Drug Abuse (NIDA); National Institutes of Health (NIH); National Women's Health Information Center (NWHIC); U.S. Department of Health and Human Services (DHHS); U.S. Department of Justice (DOJ); and the U.S. Food and Drug Administration (FDA).

In addition, this volume contains copyrighted documents from the following organizations: A.D.A.M., Inc.; AIDS InfoNet; AIDS Treatment Data Network – The Network; American Association for Clinical Chemistry; AVERT; Canadian AIDS Society; Center for AIDS Prevention Studies, University of California, San Francisco; Center for the Advancement of Health; City of Houston, TX; Hepatitis B Foundation; Hepatitis C Support Project; HIV InSite, University of California – San Francisco; HIVandHepatitis.com; Immunization Action Coalition; Kaiser Family Foundation; NAM; National Black Caucus of State Legislators; National Cervical Cancer Coalition; Nemours Foundation; Planned Parenthood Federation of America, Inc.; Project Inform; Public Health Agency of Canada; Reproductive Health Technologies Project; Safeguards LGBT Health Resource Center; San Francisco AIDS Foundation; SexInfo, University of California, Santa Barbara; South Dakota Department of Health; Vaccine Education Center, Children's Hospital of Philadelphia; Virginia Comprehensive Health Education Training and Resource Center; and Washtenaw County Public Health.

Full citation information is provided on the first page of each chapter or section. Every effort has been made to secure all necessary rights to reprint the copyrighted material. If any omissions have been made, please contact Omnigraphics to make corrections for future editions.

Acknowledgements

Thanks go to the many organizations, agencies, and individuals who have contributed materials for this *Sourcebook* and to medical consultant Dr. David Cooke and document engineer Bruce Bellenir. Special thanks go to managing editor Karen Bellenir and research and permissions coordinator Liz Collins for their help and support.

About the Health Reference Series

The *Health Reference Series* is designed to provide basic medical information for patients, families, caregivers, and the general public. Each volume takes a particular topic and provides comprehensive coverage. This is especially important for people who may be dealing with a newly diagnosed disease or a chronic disorder in themselves or in a family member. People looking for preventive guidance, information about disease warning signs, medical statistics, and risk factors for health problems will also find answers to their questions in the *Health Reference Series*. The *Series*, however, is not intended to serve as a tool for diagnosing illness, in prescribing treatments, or as a substitute for the physician/patient relationship. All people concerned about medical symptoms or the possibility of disease are encouraged to seek professional care from an appropriate health care provider.

A Note about Spelling and Style

Health Reference Series editors use *Stedman's Medical Dictionary* as an authority for questions related to the spelling of medical terms and the *Chicago Manual of Style* for questions related to grammatical structures, punctuation, and other editorial concerns. Consistent adherence is not always possible, however, because the individual volumes within the *Series* include many documents from a wide variety of different producers and copyright holders, and the editor's primary goal is to present material from each source as accurately as is possible following the terms specified by each document's producer. This sometimes means that information in different chapters or sections may follow other guidelines and alternate spelling authorities.

For example, occasionally a copyright holder may require that eponymous terms be shown in possessive forms (Crohn's disease *vs.* Crohn disease) or that British spelling norms be retained (leukaemia *vs.* leukemia).

Locating Information within the Health Reference Series

The *Health Reference Series* contains a wealth of information about a wide variety of medical topics. Ensuring easy access to all the fact sheets, research reports, in-depth discussions, and other material contained within the individual books of the *Series* remains one of our highest priorities. As the *Series* continues to grow in size and scope, however, locating the precise information needed by a reader may become more challenging.

A Contents Guide to the Health Reference Series was developed to direct readers to the specific volumes that address their concerns. It presents an extensive list of diseases, treatments, and other topics of general interest compiled from the Tables of Contents and major index headings. To access *A Contents Guide to the Health Reference Series*, visit www.healthreferenceseries.com.

Medical Consultant

Medical consultation services are provided to the *Health Reference Series* editors by David A. Cooke, M.D. Dr. Cooke is a graduate of Brandeis University, and he received his M.D. degree from the University of Michigan. He completed residency training at the University of Wisconsin Hospital and Clinics. He is board-certified in Internal Medicine. Dr. Cooke currently works as part of the University of Michigan Health System and practices in Ann Arbor, MI. In his free time, he enjoys writing, science fiction, and spending time with his family.

Our Advisory Board

We would like to thank the following board members for providing guidance to the development of this *Series*:

- Dr. Lynda Baker, Associate Professor of Library and Information Science, Wayne State University, Detroit, MI
- Nancy Bulgarelli, William Beaumont Hospital Library, Royal Oak, MI

- Karen Imarisio, Bloomfield Township Public Library, Bloomfield Township, MI
- Karen Morgan, Mardigian Library, University of Michigan-Dearborn, Dearborn, MI
- Rosemary Orlando, St. Clair Shores Public Library, St. Clair Shores, MI

Health Reference Series *Update Policy*

The inaugural book in the *Health Reference Series* was the first edition of *Cancer Sourcebook* published in 1989. Since then, the *Series* has been enthusiastically received by librarians and in the medical community. In order to maintain the standard of providing high-quality health information for the layperson the editorial staff at Omnigraphics felt it was necessary to implement a policy of updating volumes when warranted.

Medical researchers have been making tremendous strides, and it is the purpose of the *Health Reference Series* to stay current with the most recent advances. Each decision to update a volume is made on an individual basis. Some of the considerations include how much new information is available and the feedback we receive from people who use the books. If there is a topic you would like to see added to the update list, or an area of medical concern you feel has not been adequately addressed, please write to:

Editor
Health Reference Series
Omnigraphics, Inc.
P.O. Box 31-1640
Detroit, MI 48231
E-mail: editorial@omnigraphics.com

Part One

Introduction to Sexually Transmitted Diseases (STDs)

Chapter 1

Frequently Asked Questions about STDs

What does "STD" mean?

STD is short for "sexually transmitted disease." Another term you may have heard is "venereal disease" or VD.

What are sexually transmitted diseases (STDs)?

The term "sexually transmitted diseases" represents a group of more than 25 different diseases that can be passed from one person to another through sexual contact.

What is the difference between "STD" and "STI"?

STD is short for sexually transmitted disease. STI is short for sexually transmitted infection. They are synonymous. STI is the latest accepted terminology.

What is the difference between bacterial and viral STDs?

The main difference between these two categories of sexually transmitted diseases (STDs) is what causes them—bacterial STDs are caused by bacteria and viral STDs are caused by viruses. As a result of being caused by different microorganisms, bacterial and viral STDs vary in their treatment. Bacterial STDs, such as gonorrhea, syphilis,

---

and chlamydia, are often cured with antibiotics. However, viral STDs, (the four *H*s) such as HIV, HPV (genital warts), herpes, and hepatitis (the only STD that can be prevented with a vaccine), have no cure, but their symptoms can be alleviated with treatment.

In addition to bacteria and viruses, STDs can also be caused by protozoa (trichomoniasis) and other organisms (crabs/pubic lice and scabies). These STDs can be cured with antibiotics or topical creams/lotions.

How common are STDs?

STDs are very common in the U.S. With more than 12 million people in the U.S. infected each year, at least one out of four people will be infected with a STD at some point in his or her life. In the U.S., there are approximately 4 million new chlamydia infections each year, over 40 million people have herpes and 30 million have genital warts. Youth are particularly at risk for STDs. Two-thirds of reportable cases of STDs occur in people under 25 years of age.

What are the typical symptoms of STDs?

One of the most common symptoms of an STD is no symptoms. So it's important to go for check-ups. It is believed that around 80% of women and 40% of men diagnosed with chlamydia may not experience any symptoms. STDs need to be diagnosed correctly and be fully treated as soon as possible to avoid complications that could be serious and/or cause permanent damage to the body.

When they do occur, typical STD symptoms for women may include unusual vaginal discharge (flow), sores, bumps, burning when urinating, and redness or itching around the vaginal area. Typical symptoms for men may include discharge from the penis, burning when urinating, and sores, bumps, or redness on or around the penis. If you have any of these symptoms or your sexual partner has been diagnosed with STDs, you should seek treatment.

How can I tell if my partner has an STD?

In most cases, you cannot tell just by looking if someone has an STD. STDs often have no visible signs.

How are STDs transmitted?

STDs can be transmitted through oral, anal, or vaginal sex. They can be transmitted from partner to partner with or without visible signs or symptoms. Many people can pass a STD to a sex partner without even knowing it. Some STDs can be transmitted without having intercourse; they can be passed through skin-to-skin contact in the genital area.

Can herpes be passed when there are no symptoms?

Yes, it is possible to infect someone with herpes, even when you don't have any signs or symptoms. It was once thought to be transmitted only when sores were present, but recent research has shown that herpes simplex virus (HSV) can be passed even when no visible signs are present. Herpes is not curable and is the most common STD in the U.S.

Can I get STDs from a towel or a toilet seat?

Most STDs, such as chlamydia, gonorrhea, syphilis, herpes, and genital warts, are spread only through direct sexual contact with an infected person. However, crabs (pubic lice) or scabies, which are often sexually transmitted, can be passed through contact with infested items like clothes, sheets, or towels.

What should I do if I think I have an STD?

If you think you have an STD or have put yourself at risk, see a health care provider immediately. Getting tested and seeking treatment early will help to minimize long-term effects of most STDs and prevent infecting others. You should always avoid sexual contact until you have been treated and cured.

How should I know if I need treatment?

The best way to answer this is by getting tested and talking to your health care provider. If you are having any of the following symptoms: a discharge from the penis or vagina, burning, itching, a sore or sores (either painless or painful) or your sexual partner has been diagnosed with an STD, you should seek testing and treatment.

Can I get an STD more than once?

You are not "immune" to a STD even if you have had it before. STDs caused by bacteria (chlamydia, gonorrhea, and syphilis) can be treated and cured, but you can get them again if exposed. Viral STDs cannot be cured and may remain in your body forever. Hepatitis A and B are the only STDs that can be prevented with a vaccine at the present time.

Chapter 2

Trends in Reportable STDs

Chapter Contents

Section 2.1

Statistics for the Most Common STDs in the United States

"Trends in Reportable Sexually Transmitted Diseases in the United States, 2006: National Surveillance Data for Chlamydia, Gonorrhea, and Syphilis," Centers for Disease Control and Prevention (www.cdc.gov), November 13, 2007.

Sexually transmitted diseases (STDs) remain a major public health challenge in the United States. While substantial progress has been made in preventing, diagnosing, and treating certain STDs in recent years, CDC estimates that approximately 19 million new infections occur each year, almost half of them among young people ages 15 to 24.[1] In addition to the physical and psychological consequences of STDs, these diseases also exact a tremendous economic toll. Direct medical costs associated with STDs in the United States are estimated at up to $14.7 billion annually in 2006 dollars.[2]

This document summarizes 2006 national data on trends in three notifiable STDs—chlamydia, gonorrhea, and syphilis—that are published in CDC's report, Sexually Transmitted Disease Surveillance 2006. These data, which are useful for examining overall trends and trends among populations at risk, represent only a small proportion of the true national burden of STDs. Many cases of notifiable STDs go undiagnosed, and some highly prevalent viral infections, such as human papillomavirus and genital herpes, are not reported at all.

Chlamydia: Reported Cases Exceed One Million, but Majority of Infections Remain Undiagnosed

Chlamydia remains the most commonly reported infectious disease in the United States. In 2006, 1,030,911 chlamydia diagnoses were reported, up from 976,445 in 2005. Even so, most chlamydia cases go undiagnosed. It is estimated that there are approximately 2.8 million new cases of chlamydia in the United States each year.[1]

The national rate of reported chlamydia in 2006 was 347.8 cases per 100,000 population, an increase of 5.6% from 2005 (329.4). The increases in reported cases and rates likely reflect the continued expansion of screening efforts and increased use of more sensitive diagnostic tests; however, the continued increases may also reflect an actual increase in infections.

Health Consequences of Chlamydia

Chlamydia is a bacterial infection that can easily be cured with antibiotics, but usually occurs without symptoms and often goes undiagnosed. Untreated, it can cause severe health consequences for women, including pelvic inflammatory disease (PID), ectopic pregnancy, and infertility. Up to 40% of females with untreated chlamydia infections develop PID, and 20% of those may become infertile.[3] Complications from chlamydia among men are relatively uncommon, but may include epididymitis and urethritis, which can cause pain, fever, and in rare cases, sterility.

Impact on Women

Women, especially young women, are hit hardest by chlamydia. Studies have found that chlamydia is more common among adolescent

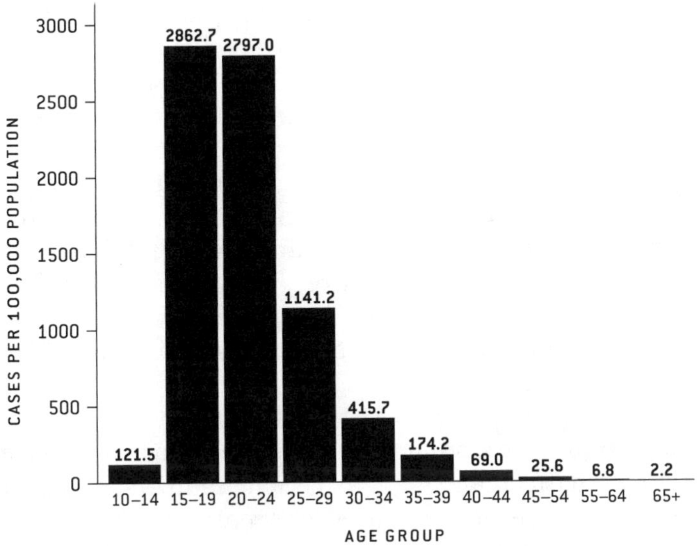

Figure 2.1. *Chlamydia Rates among Females, 2006*

females than adolescent males, and the long-term consequences of untreated disease are much more severe for females. The chlamydia case rate for females in 2006 was three times higher than for males (515.8 vs. 173.0). Much of this difference reflects the fact that females are far more likely to be screened than males. Young females aged 15 to 19 had the highest chlamydia rate (2,862.7), followed by females aged 20 to 24 (2,797.0).

Chlamydia is common among all races and ethnic groups; however, African American women are disproportionately affected. In 2006, the rate of reported chlamydia per 100,000 black females (1,760.9) was more than seven times that of white females (237.0) and more than twice that of Hispanic females (761.3). The rate among American Indian/Alaska Native females was the second highest, at 1,262.3, and the rate among Asian/Pacific Islander females was the lowest, at 201.2.

Because case reports do not provide a complete account of the burden of disease, researchers also evaluate chlamydia prevalence in subgroups of the population to better estimate the true extent of the disease. For example, data from chlamydia screening in family planning clinics across the United States indicate that approximately 7% of 15- to 24-year-old females in these settings are infected.

Importance of Screening

Because chlamydia is most common among young women, CDC recommends annual chlamydia screening for all sexually active women under age 26, as well as older women with risk factors such as new or multiple sex partners.[4] Data from one study in a managed care setting suggest that chlamydia screening and treatment can reduce the incidence of pelvic inflammatory disease by over 50%.[5] Unfortunately, many sexually active young women are not being tested for chlamydia, in part reflecting a lack of awareness among some providers and limited resources for screening.[6] Research has shown that simple changes in clinical procedures, such as coupling chlamydia tests with routine Pap testing, can sharply increase the proportion of sexually active young women screened.[7] Increased prevention screening efforts are critical to preventing the serious health consequences of this infection, particularly infertility.

Recent studies have also shown that many young women who have been diagnosed with chlamydia may become re-infected by male partners who have not been diagnosed or treated.[8,9] CDC's 2006 STD Treatment Guidelines recommend that women be retested for chlamydia approximately three months after treatment, and also recommend the delivery of antibiotic therapy by heterosexual patients to their partners, if other strategies for reaching and treating partners are not likely to succeed.[4] The availability of urine tests for chlamydia is likely contributing to increased detection of the disease in men, and consequently the rising rates of reported chlamydia among males in recent years (from 126.8 in 2002 to 173.0 in 2006).

Gonorrhea: Disease Stable with Slight Increases in Recent Years

Gonorrhea is the second most commonly reported infectious disease in the United States, with 358,366 cases reported in 2006. Following a 74% decline in the rate of reported gonorrhea from 1975 through 1997, overall gonorrhea rates plateaued, then increased for the past two years. In 2006, the gonorrhea rate was 120.9 cases per 100,000 population, an increase of 5.5% since 2005 and an increase for the second consecutive year. Like chlamydia, gonorrhea is substantially under-diagnosed and under-reported, and approximately twice as many new infections are estimated to occur each year as are reported.[1]

Increasing Rates in Southern and Western United States

As in previous years, the South had the highest gonorrhea rate among the four regions of the country. Additionally, rates rose in the South for the first time in eight years, increasing 12.3% between 2005 and 2006 from 141.8 to 159.2 per 100,000 population.

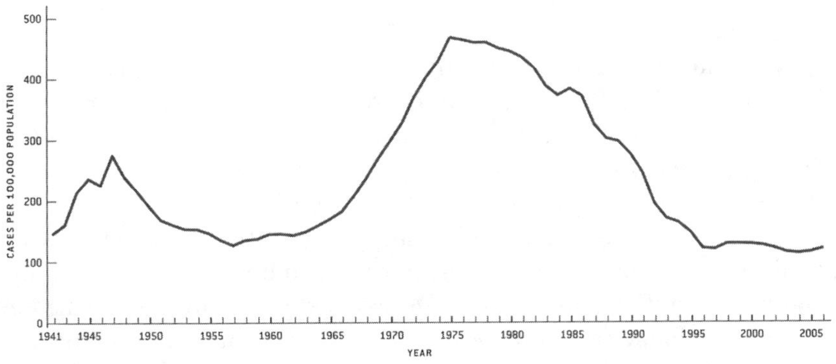

Figure 2.2. *Gonorrhea Rates, 1941–2006*

While the impact is greatest in the South, researchers are also concerned about continued increases in the West, where the rate of reported gonorrhea cases rose 2.9% between 2005 and 2006 (from 80.5 to 82.8 per 100,000) and increased by 31.8% between 2002 and 2006.

Between 2002 and 2006, the rate in the South declined slightly (from 161.8 to 159.2), the Northeast declined 21.2% (from 93.6 to 73.8) and the rate in the Midwest showed minimal change (from 142.2 in 2002 to 136.9 in 2006).

Health Consequences of Gonorrhea

While gonorrhea is easily cured, untreated cases can lead to serious health problems. Among women, gonorrhea is a major cause of PID, which can lead to chronic pelvic pain, ectopic pregnancy, and infertility. In men, untreated gonorrhea can cause epididymitis, a painful infection in the tissue surrounding the testicles that can result in infertility. In addition, studies suggest that presence of gonorrhea infection makes an individual three to five times more likely to acquire HIV, if exposed.[12]

Increased Drug Resistance Leads to New CDC Treatment Guidelines

Drug resistance is an increasingly important concern in the treatment and prevention of gonorrhea.[10] CDC monitors trends in gonorrhea drug resistance through the Gonococcal Isolate Surveillance Project (GISP), which tests gonorrhea samples ("isolates") from the first 25 men with urethral gonorrhea attending STD clinics each month in sentinel clinics across the United States (28 cities in 2006).[11]

Overall, 13.8% of gonorrhea isolates tested through GISP in 2006 demonstrated resistance to fluoroquinolones, a leading class of antibiotics previously recommended to treat the disease, compared to 9.4% in 2005 and 6.8% in 2004. Resistance to the fluoroquinolones has been highest among men who have sex with men (MSM). From 2005 to 2006, resistance among heterosexuals nearly doubled from 3.8 to 7% and continued to increase among MSM from 29 to 39%.

In April 2007, based on preliminary 2006 data that showed widespread fluoroquinolone-resistance among both heterosexuals and men who have sex with men (MSM), CDC revised its gonorrhea treatment guidelines, no longer recommending that this class of antibiotics be used to treat any cases of gonorrhea in the United States.[13] CDC had previously announced that fluoroquinolones were no longer recommended as treatment for gonorrhea among MSM, as well as anyone in California, Hawaii, and other areas where fluoroquinolone-resistant cases were widespread.[4,10]

With the loss of fluoroquinolones, recommended gonorrhea treatments are limited to a single class of antibiotics, cephalosporins. Although 2006 data show no indication of cephalosporin resistance, increased monitoring for emerging resistance and accelerated research into new treatments are needed to continue the nation's progress in controlling this common sexually transmitted disease.

Syphilis: Cases Increase for Sixth Consecutive Year

The rate of primary and secondary (P&S) syphilis—the most infectious stages of the disease—decreased throughout the 1990s, and in 2000 reached an all-time low. However, over the past six years, the syphilis rate in the United States has been increasing. Between 2005 and 2006, the national P&S syphilis rate increased 13.8%, from 2.9 to 3.3 cases per 100,000 population, and the number of cases increased from 8,724 to 9,756.

The overall increase in syphilis rates from 2005 to 2006 was driven primarily by increases among males, with the rate increasing by 11.8% (from 5.1 per 100,000 population in 2005 to 5.7 in 2006) in that group. However, the rate among females increased for the second year in a row, following a decade of declines (from 0.9 per 100,000 in 2005 to 1.0 in 2006, an increase of 11.1%). Additionally, the rate of congenital syphilis (i.e., transmission from mother to newborn) increased slightly in 2006 (from 8.2 per 100,000 live births in 2005 to 8.5 in 2006). While it is too early to determine if the increase among newborns is a trend, increases in congenital syphilis have historically followed increases among women.

Health Consequences of Syphilis

Syphilis, a genital ulcerative disease, is highly infectious, but easily curable in its early (primary and secondary) stages. If untreated, it can lead to serious long-term complications, including brain, cardiovascular, and organ damage, and even death. Congenital syphilis can cause stillbirth, death soon after birth, and physical deformity and neurological complications in children who survive. Syphilis, like many other STDs, facilitates the spread of HIV by increasing the likelihood of transmission of the virus.[14]

Rising Rates Driven Largely by Cases among Men Who Have Sex with Men

The rate of P&S syphilis among men has risen 54% over the past five years (from 3.7 per 100,000 in 2002 to 5.7 per 100,000 in 2006), driving overall increases in syphilis rates for the nation. Several sources of data suggest that increased transmission of P&S syphilis among MSM may be largely responsible for these increases. Over time, the disparity between male and female case rates has grown considerably. The P&S syphilis rate among males is now nearly six times the rate among females, whereas the rates were almost equivalent a decade ago.

In 2005, CDC requested that case reports include the gender of sex partners for persons with syphilis. In 2006, the first full year for which data are available, 64% of all P&S syphilis cases were among MSM (based on data from 30 areas, 2006). More complete data on the gender of sex partners is expected in the coming years as a greater number of states report these findings.

Concerning Increases among Women

While P&S syphilis rates remained substantially lower among females than males, overall rates among females increased for the second year in a row, after a decade of declines, with an increase of 11.1% between 2005 and 2006 (from 0.9 to 1.0). This increase was largely driven by increased rates among African American females, which rose

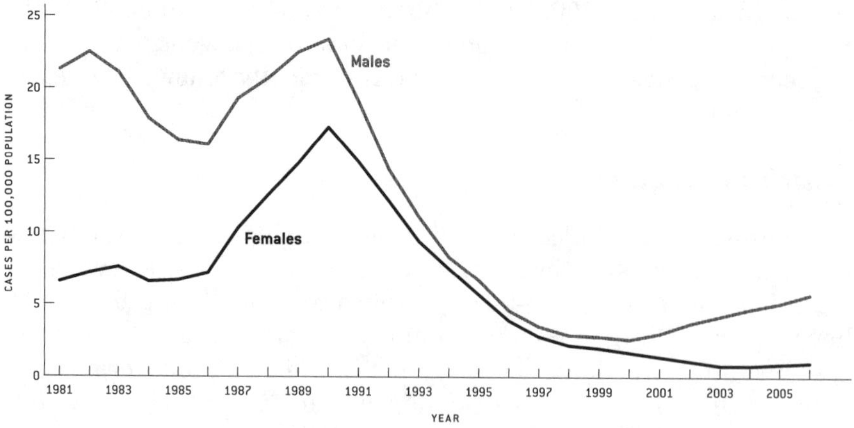

Figure 2.3. *P&S Syphilis Rates by Gender, 1981–2006*

11.4% (from 4.4 in 2005 to 4.9 in 2006). Rates among females in all other racial/ethnic groups declined or remained stable.

The reasons for these overall increases among females are not yet clear. However, CDC is currently analyzing this trend to better understand the factors driving this increase.

Eliminating syphilis as a health threat in the United States will require an ongoing commitment to syphilis education, testing, and treatment in all populations affected. In May 2006, CDC released its updated National Plan to Eliminate Syphilis, designed to sustain elimination efforts in populations traditionally at risk, including African Americans and women of all races and ethnicities, and to support innovative solutions to fight the resurgence of syphilis among MSM.[15]

Racial Disparities Persist across All Reportable STDs

Racial and ethnic minorities continue to be disproportionately affected by sexually transmitted diseases in the United States. These disparities may be, in part, because racial and ethnic minorities are more likely to seek care in public health clinics that report STDs more completely than private providers. However, this reporting bias does not fully explain these differences. Other contributing factors include limited access to quality health care, poverty, and higher prevalence of disease in these populations.

Data in CDC's 2006 STD Surveillance Report show higher rates of all STDs among minority racial and ethnic populations when compared to whites, with the exception of Asians/Pacific Islanders.

Chlamydia

In 2006, the rate of chlamydia among African Americans was more than eight times higher than the rate among whites (1,275.0 vs. 153.1 per 100,000 population), with approximately 46% of all chlamydia cases reported among African Americans. Additionally, the rates among American Indians/Alaska Natives (797.3 per 100,000) and Hispanics (477.0 per 100,000) were five times and three times higher than whites, respectively. In 2006, chlamydia rates increased for all racial/ethnic groups, except for Asians/Pacific Islanders.

Gonorrhea

Racial disparities in gonorrhea rates are even greater and racial gaps in diagnosis of gonorrhea are more pronounced than any other disease. The gonorrhea rate among African Americans was 18 times greater than that for whites in 2006 (658.4 per 100,000 vs. 36.5 per 100,000). From 2005 to 2006, the gonorrhea rate among African Americans increased by 6.3%—the first increase since 1998. In 2006, African Americans accounted for 69% of reported cases of gonorrhea.

In that same year, American Indians/Alaska Natives had the second-highest gonorrhea rate (138.3 per 100,000), followed by Hispanics (77.4), whites (36.5), and Asians/Pacific Islanders (21.1). In 2006, there were increases in gonorrhea rates among all racial and ethnic groups, except Asians/Pacific Islanders.

Syphilis

Although racial gaps in syphilis rates are narrowing, disparities remain, with rates in 2006 approximately six times higher among blacks than among whites. This represents a substantial decline from 1999, when the rate among blacks was 29 times greater than among whites. It is important to note that this narrowing reflects both declining disease rates among African Americans as well as significant increases among white males in recent years.

Despite some progress, African Americans continue to remain disproportionately affected by syphilis with a rate of 11.3 cases per 100,000 population in 2006. This is more than three times the rate for Hispanics, who have the second highest rate (3.6 cases per 100,000) as well as American Indians/Alaska Natives (3.3 cases per 100,000).

In 2006, the P&S syphilis rate among blacks increased for the third consecutive year, following more than a decade of declines. Between 2005 and 2006, the rate among blacks increased 16.5% (from 9.7 to 11.3), with the largest increase among black males (15.5 to 18.3, an increase of 18.1%).

In 2006, the rate of P&S syphilis in black females was 16 times higher than in white females. In that same year, 43.2% of all reported P&S syphilis cases occurred among African Americans, while whites accounted for 38.4%. Syphilis rates increased for all races and ethnicities in 2006.

CDC Efforts to Address Racial and Ethnic Disparities

CDC continues to work with partners from multiple sectors to increase awareness and identify and implement new solutions to reducing the impact of STDs in communities of color. In June 2007, CDC convened a consultation to address STD disparities in African American communities as part of its accelerated efforts to bring community leaders and other partners together to address racial and ethnic disparities in STD rates.

Continuing to highlight these disparities is one critical step in increasing awareness of the problem among health care providers and affected communities, which can lead to developing solutions to reduce the spread of STDs.

References

1. Weinstock H, et al. Sexually transmitted diseases among American youth: incidence and prevalence estimates, 2000. *Perspectives on Sexual and Reproductive Health* 2004;36(1): 6–10.

2. HW Chesson, JM Blandford, TL Gift, G Tao, KL Irwin. The estimated direct medical cost of STDs among American youth, 2000. 2004 National STD Prevention Conference. Philadelphia, PA. March 8–11, 2004. Abstract P075.

3. Hillis SD and Wasserheit JN. Screening for chlamydia—a key to the prevention of pelvic inflammatory disease. *New England Journal of Medicine* 1996;334(21):1399–1401.

4. CDC. Sexually transmitted diseases treatment guidelines, 2006. *Morbidity and Mortality Weekly Report* 2006;55(RR-11).

5. Scholes D, et al. Prevention of pelvic inflammatory disease by screening for cervical chlamydial infection. *New England Journal of Medicine* 1996334(21):1362–1366.

6. National Committee for Quality Assurance. The State of Health Care Quality 2006. Washington, DC, 2006:30, 57–67. Available at: http://www.ncqa.org/communications/SOHC2006/SOHC_2006.pdf.

7. Burstein G, et al. Chlamydia screening in a health plan before and after a national performance measure introduction. *Obstetrics & Gynecology* 2005;106(2):327–334.

8. Klinger E, et al. Burden of repeat chlamydia trachomatis infection in young women in New York City. 2006 National STD Prevention Conference. Jacksonville, FL. May 8–11, 2006. Abstract A1e.

9. Chow J, et al. Repeat chlamydia and gonorrhea infection using case-based surveillance reports and laboratory-based prevalence monitoring data, California, 2003–2004. 2006 National STD Prevention Conference. Jacksonville, FL. May 8–11, 2006. Abstract P32.

10. CDC. Increases in fluoroquinolone-resistant Neisseria gonorrhoeae among men who have sex with men—United States, 2003, and revised recommendations for gonorrhea treatment, 2004. *Morbidity and Mortality Weekly Report* 2004;53(16):335–338.

11. CDC. Gonococcal Isolate Surveillance Project. Available at: www.cdc.gov/std/gisp.

12. Fleming DT and Wasserheit JN. From epidemiological synergy to public health policy and practice: the contribution of other sexually transmitted diseases to sexual transmission of HIV infection. *Sexually Transmitted Infections* 1999;75:3–17.

13. CDC. Update to CDC's Sexually Transmitted Diseases Treatment Guidelines, 2006: Fluoroquinolones No Longer Recommended for Treatment of Gonococcal Infections. *Morbidity and Mortality Weekly Report* 2007;56(14):332–336. Available at: http://www.cdc.gov/mmwr/preview/mmwrhtml/mm5614a3.htm.

14. CDC. HIV prevention through early detection and treatment of other sexually transmitted diseases—United States recommendations of the Advisory Committee for HIV and STD Prevention. *Morbidity and Mortality Weekly Report* 1998;47(RR-12):1–24.

15. CDC. Together we can: the national plan to eliminate syphilis from the United States, May 2006. Available at: http://www.cdc.gov/stopsyphilis/SEEPlan2006.pdf.

Section 2.2

Estimates of New HIV Infections in the United States

"Estimates of New HIV Infections in the United States," Centers for Disease Control and Prevention (www.cdc.gov), August 2008.

Accurately tracking the HIV epidemic is essential to the nation's HIV prevention efforts. Yet monitoring trends in new HIV infections has historically posed a major challenge, in part because many HIV infections are not diagnosed until years after they occur.

Now, new technology developed by the Centers for Disease Control and Prevention can be used to distinguish recent from long-standing HIV infections. CDC has applied this advanced technology to develop the first national surveillance system of its kind that is based on direct measurement of new HIV infections. This new system represents a major advance in HIV surveillance and allows for more precise estimates of HIV incidence (the annual number of new infections) than ever before possible.

CDC's first estimates from this system reveal that the HIV epidemic is—and has been—worse than previously known. Results indicate that approximately 56,300 new HIV infections occurred in the United States in 2006 (95% confidence interval: 48,200–64,500). This figure is roughly 40% higher than CDC's former estimate of 40,000 infections per year, which was based on limited data and less precise methods.

It is important to note that the new estimate does not represent an actual increase in the annual number of new HIV infections. In fact, CDC's analysis suggests that the epidemic has been roughly stable since the late 1990s, though the number of new HIV infections remains unacceptably high. These findings underscore the ongoing challenges in confronting this disease and the urgent need to expand access to effective HIV-prevention programs.

Breakthrough Technology Allows Clearest Picture to Date

CDC's new HIV surveillance system is based on an approach known as STARHS (Serological Testing Algorithm for Recent HIV Seroconversion), which uses innovative testing technology to determine, at the population level, which positive HIV tests represent new HIV infections (those that occurred within approximately the past five months). Before the widespread availability of this technology, HIV diagnosis data provided the best indication of recent trends in key populations. However, diagnosis data only indicate when a person is diagnosed with HIV, not when an individual is actually infected, which can occur many years before a diagnosis.

By applying this technology to new HIV diagnoses in 22 states with name-based HIV-reporting systems, CDC was able—for the first time—to identify those diagnoses in a given year that represented new infections. Using a complex statistical model, these data were extrapolated to the general population to provide the first national estimate of HIV incidence based on direct measurement.

CDC researchers also used a separate method called "extended back-calculation" to confirm the official 2006 STARHS estimate and to examine historical trends in HIV infections in the United States from 1977 to 2006. The method uses a statistical model that considers all HIV and AIDS cases diagnosed in the U.S. through 2006 and reported to CDC, as well as HIV testing patterns. Extended back-calculation has become possible in the United States because of an expanded name-based HIV reporting system, which provides a population-based system for identifying new diagnoses. However, the method is an indirect measure of incidence and is most reliable for earlier years; data for the most recent years (2003–2006) must be interpreted with caution. Additionally, extended back-calculation does not generate single-year estimates, instead providing averages over multiple-year periods.

The statistical methods used to develop the 2006 incidence estimate, as well as the extended back-calculation historical trends, were developed in consultation with outside experts, and both the methods and their application underwent rigorous external scientific review.

Moving forward, the STARHS-based surveillance system will provide the most reliable way to monitor incidence trends. Over time, the picture will become even more clear as analyses for specific populations are completed (e.g., black women, young men who have sex with men). Now that this system is in place, CDC will be able to provide an updated estimate of HIV incidence in the United States on an annual basis. Over time, trend information from this system will allow for improved targeting and evaluation of prevention efforts for the populations at greatest risk.

The New Estimates

U.S. HIV Epidemic Worse Than Previously Known

Approximately 56,300 new HIV infections occurred in the U.S. in 2006, according to the new surveillance system. This number is approximately 40% higher than CDC's previous estimate of 40,000 new infections per year, which was based on less precise methods.

It is important to note that the new estimate does not reflect an increase in HIV incidence. In fact, CDC's separate analysis of historical trends, using the extended back-calculation model, indicates that the annual number of new HIV infections has been roughly stable since the late 1990s. CDC's trend analysis provides a clearer picture of how the nation's epidemic evolved to its current point. The analysis shows that new infections peaked in the mid-1980s at approximately

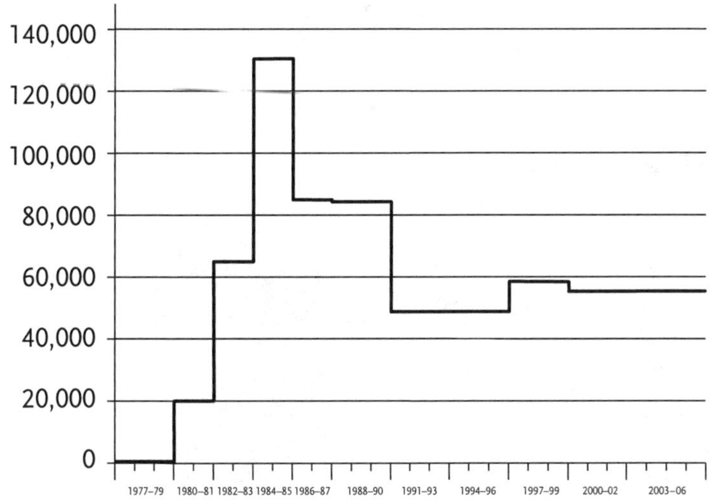

Note: Estimates are for 2-year intervals during 1980–1987, 3-year intervals during 1977–1979 and 1988–2002, and a 4-year interval for 2003–2006.

Figure 2.4. *Estimated New HIV Infections, Extended Back-Calculation Model, 1977–2006, Overall*

130,000 infections per year and reached a low of about 50,000 in the early 1990s. Incidence then appears to have increased in the late 1990s, but has stabilized since that time (with estimates ranging between 55,000 and 58,500 during the three most recent time periods analyzed).

Data Confirm Most Severe Impact Is among Gay and Bisexual Men of All Races and Black Men and Women

Gay and Bisexual Men of All Races Are Most Heavily Affected by HIV

Gay and bisexual men—referred to in CDC surveillance systems as men who have sex with men (MSM)—represented a significantly greater proportion of estimated new infections in 2006 than any other risk group. These findings underscore the need to expand access to HIV testing and other proven interventions, and to continue research to identify new interventions to address the evolving needs of diverse populations of gay and bisexual men in the U.S. Many factors likely contribute to high risk of HIV among MSM, including the challenge of maintaining consistently safe behaviors over time, inaccurate knowledge of HIV status, underestimating personal risk, stigma that may prevent access to needed services, substance abuse, and depression.

Analysis by Transmission Category

- **MSM:** MSM accounted for 53% (28,700) of estimated new HIV infections in 2006. CDC's historical trend analysis indicates that HIV incidence has been increasing steadily among gay and bisexual men since the early 1990s, confirming a trend suggested by other data showing increases in risk behavior, sexually transmitted diseases, and HIV diagnoses in this population.

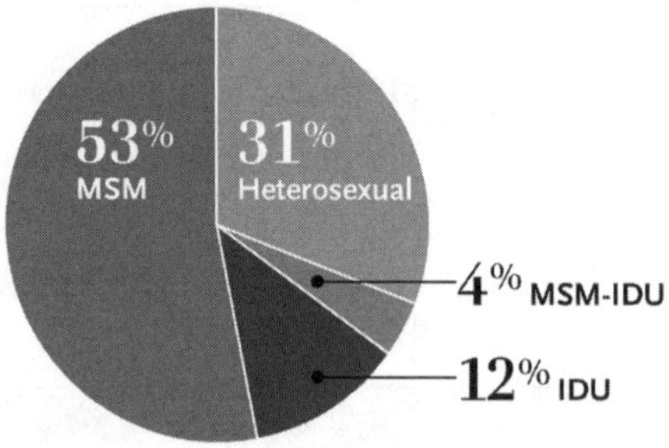

***Figure 2.5.** Estimated New HIV Infections, 2006, by Transmission Category*

- **Heterosexuals:** Heterosexuals accounted for 31% (16,800) of estimated new HIV infections in 2006. The historical analysis suggests that the number of new infections in this population fluctuated somewhat throughout the 1990s and has declined in recent years.
- **IDUs:** Injection drug users (IDUs) accounted for 12% (6,600) of estimated new HIV infections. CDC's historical trend analysis indicates that new infections have declined dramatically in this population over time; between 1988–1990 and 2003–2006, HIV infections among IDUs declined overall by 80%. These declines confirm the substantial evidence to date of success in reducing HIV infections among IDUs. The term men who have sex with men is used in CDC surveillance systems because it indicates the behaviors that transmit HIV infection, rather than how individuals self-identify in terms of their sexuality.

Impact of HIV Greater among Blacks Than Any Other Racial or Ethnic Group

CDC's new estimates confirm that blacks are more heavily and disproportionately affected by HIV than any other racial/ethnic group in the U.S. Trend analyses show that HIV incidence among blacks has been roughly stable at an unacceptably high level since the early 1990s (except for a brief fluctuation up and back down in the late 1990s). The continued severity of the epidemic among blacks underscores the need to sustain and accelerate prevention efforts in this population. While race itself is not a risk factor for HIV infection, a range of issues contribute to the disproportionate HIV risk for African Americans in the U.S., including poverty, stigma, higher rates of other STDs, and drug use.

Analysis by Race/Ethnicity

- **Blacks:** The rate of new infections among non-Hispanic blacks was seven times as high as that among whites in 2006 (83.7 versus 11.5 new infections per 100,000 population). Blacks also accounted for the largest share of new infections (45%, or 24,900). Historical trend data show that the number of new infections among blacks peaked in the late 1980s and has exceeded the number of infections in whites since that time.

- **Hispanics:** The rate of new HIV infections among Hispanics in 2006 was three times as high as that among whites (29.3 versus 11.5 per 100,000), and Hispanics accounted for 17% of new infections (9,700). Historically, the number of new infections among Hispanics has been lower than for whites and blacks. Incidence trends among Hispanics over time have mirrored those among blacks.
- **Whites:** Whites accounted for 35% (19,600) of estimated new HIV infections in 2006. After declining significantly in the late 1980s, the historical trend analysis suggests that new infections among whites increased slightly during the 1990s and have remained stable since 2000.
- **Asians/Pacific Islanders and American Indians/Alaska Natives:** Data suggest that Asians/Pacific Islanders accounted for roughly 2% of new infections and American Indians/Alaska Natives accounted for roughly 1% of new HIV infections in 2006. The relatively small number of infections in these populations makes it difficult to draw reliable conclusions about trends over time in these populations.

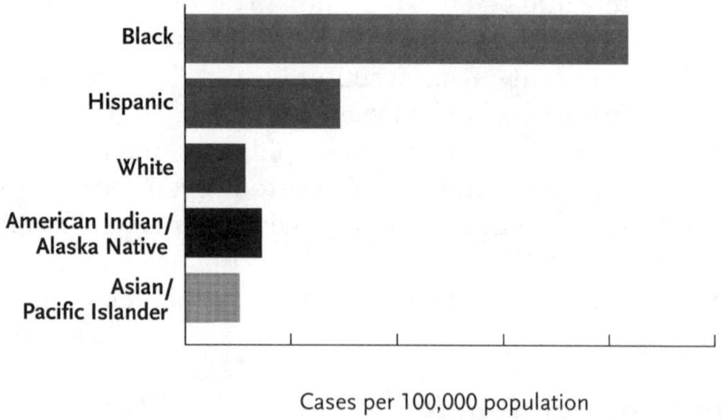

Figure 2.6. *Estimated Rates of New HIV Infections, 2006, by Race/Ethnicity*

Analysis by Gender and Age Group

Gender: Men accounted for the large majority of estimated new HIV infections in the U.S. in 2006 (73%, or 41,400). CDC's historical analysis indicates that the number of infections among men has mirrored the overall trend in HIV incidence, peaking at around 1984–1985 and reaching a low point in the early 1990s. Among women, incidence rose gradually until the late 1980s, declined towards the early 1990s, and has remained relatively stable since then.

Age: More infections occurred among young people under 30 (aged 13–29) than any other age group (34%, or 19,200), followed by individuals 30–39 (31%, or 17,400). These data confirm that HIV is an epidemic primarily of young people and underscores the critical need to reach each new generation of young people with HIV prevention services. Individuals over age 50 continue to represent a relatively small proportion of new infections.

Historical Challenges in Tracking HIV Incidence

Tracking HIV incidence has been a long-standing challenge in the U.S. and around the world. Historically, researchers relied on indirect methods to estimate the number of new infections. In the early 1990s, for example, data on U.S. AIDS diagnoses could be used to estimate the number of new HIV infections occurring over time, since the period from initial HIV infection to the development of AIDS was well-documented and understood (i.e., about 8–10 years). However, following the advent of highly active antiretroviral therapy (HAART) in the mid-1990s, the period between HIV infection and AIDS was no longer predictable, and AIDS cases could no longer be used as the primary basis for estimating HIV incidence.

Since that time, it has been necessary to rely on extrapolation from small studies of HIV infections among high-risk populations to estimate HIV incidence for the nation. Based on these limited data, CDC estimated that at least 40,000 Americans were infected annually since the early 1990s. However, because these data were so limited, they were not robust enough to give a precise picture of HIV incidence or to detect changes in incidence over time.

Implications of the New Estimates

While the new incidence estimates illustrate the challenges of fighting HIV, there is significant evidence that prevention can—and does—work when we apply what we know.

Stability in the number of new HIV infections since 2000 is an important sign of progress. With more people living with HIV than ever before, there are more opportunities for transmission. Yet HIV transmission has not increased, which indicates that people are taking steps to protect themselves and their partners. The relatively stable number of new infections suggests that significant efforts in recent years to reach people living with HIV/AIDS with effective prevention services are having a beneficial impact. In addition, the historical trends analysis shows encouraging signs of progress in reducing new infections among IDUs and heterosexuals over time.

Nonetheless, rates of HIV infection in the U.S. are unacceptably high, and far too many individuals at risk are not yet being reached. For example, a CDC study of gay and bisexual men in 15 cities found that 80% had not been reached by the intensive HIV prevention interventions that are known to be most effective. And the high rates of infection among young people highlight the urgent need to reach a new generation with prevention services.

In addition, CDC estimates that one-quarter of HIV-infected people are unaware of their HIV infection, and account for more than half of all new infections. To help ensure that everyone knows their status, CDC recommends that everyone in the U.S. between the ages of 13 and 64—regardless of perceived risk—get tested for HIV to help stop the spread of this disease. CDC also recommends that sexually active gay and bisexual men be tested for HIV at least annually.

Accelerating progress in HIV prevention will require a collective response that matches the severity of the epidemic. There is an urgent national need to reach all populations at risk with effective prevention programs.

To help prevent new HIV infections among MSM, CDC provides resources to state and local health departments and community-based organizations to help them reach MSM with effective testing and prevention services. Additionally, CDC is working to increase the use of successful prevention interventions for MSM across the country; adapting proven interventions for new populations of MSM, especially MSM of color; and continuing research to understand barriers and opportunities for more effectively reaching this population.

CDC is working to fight HIV among African Americans through the Heightened National Response, a partnership of CDC, public health partners, and black community leaders to intensify prevention efforts nationwide. The partnership is designed to build upon progress to date in four key areas: expanding prevention services, increasing testing, developing new interventions, and mobilizing broader community action.

Chapter 3

STDs in Men

Chapter Contents

Section 3.1

STDs among Heterosexual Men

This section begins with "Heterosexual Men and HIV/AIDS," © 2000 Canadian AIDS Society (www.cdnaids.ca), reprinted with permission. For more information on how to prevent HIV infection please contact the Canadian AIDS Society at 1-800-499-1986 or visit http://www.cdnaids.ca. Additional information from the Center for AIDS Prevention Studies, University of California – San Francisco is cited within the section. These documents were reviewed in January 2009 by Dr. David A. Cooke, M.D., Diplomate, American Board of Internal Medicine. The medical information contained in these documents is relevant; however, updated statistics regarding STDs can be found at the Centers for Disease Control and Prevention's STD Surveillance 2007 website at http://www.cdc.gov/std/stats07/.

Heterosexual Men and HIV/AIDS

Key Issues

- Men are encouraged to take risks that can jeopardize their health and increase the risk for contracting HIV and other sexually transmitted diseases.
- In Canada, a 1995 study showed that only 22% of men used condoms.
- The Canadian rate of condom use by males is one of the lowest in the industrialized world.

The different gender roles of men and women in our society are reflected in different attitudes and behavior. Social norms, upbringing, peers, and the media socialize men to meet standards of masculinity that set them apart from women. Men are generally expected to project the image of being strong, assertive, dominant, self-reliant, and willing to take risks.[1] When these patterns of thinking and acting are expressed as attitudes towards sex and in sexual behavior, they often increase men's chances of contracting and transmitting HIV.

The main patterns of behavior that place heterosexual men at greatest risk of contracting HIV/AIDS are having multiple sexual partners, injecting drugs, and the failure to practice safer sex.

Heterosexual men generally have more sexual partners than heterosexual women do.[2] In part this reflects a double standard: It is socially more acceptable for men to be sexually active than for women.[3] Men may even derive status (as "studs") from having multiple partners, while women who have multiple partners are often labeled negatively (as "sluts").

Married men are more likely than married women to have extramarital relationships. Studies estimate that between one-half and two-thirds of married men have at least one affair, compared to between one-third and one-half of married women.[4]

Having multiple partners increases the risk of contracting sexually transmitted diseases (STDs) including HIV. Although safer sex practices reduce this risk, many men do not practice safer sex.

Studies show consistent condom use is not widely practiced by men. For example, a 1992 U.S. study found that 46% of a sample of unmarried heterosexual men in San Francisco never used condoms. A 1998 study found that 33% of teenage heterosexual males did not use condoms.

In Canada, a 1995 study showed that only 22% of men used condoms as their primary form of contraception. Young men and unmarried men were more likely than older men and married (or formerly married) men to use condoms. The Canadian rate of condom use by males is one of the lowest in the industrialized world.[5]

The reasons for failure to use condoms range from embarrassment at buying them to a belief that they reduce sensitivity and pleasure.[6] Moreover, condoms are associated not only with the prevention of sexually transmitted disease but also with contraception, and many heterosexual men believe that condoms are unnecessary if their partner is using a contraceptive such as the pill. In addition to this, many men who do use condoms regularly, have sex without one on some occasions.

It may be that there is less chance of changing men's tendency to have multiple sexual relationships than persuading them to practice safer sex. But in order to encourage such a change, sex education campaigns must be maintained. It may be that condom use has declined as men have become used to the safer sex campaigns that were prominent when HIV/AIDS first became a major public health issue in the late 1980s.

Studies have shown that sexual health education can be effective in delaying first intercourse, increased use of condoms for first intercourse, and increased reporting of condom use for the most recent intercourse. Canadian research has also confirmed that the majority of parents support sexual health education in schools. Despite these findings, a Health Canada report indicates that the average number of hours spent on sexual health education is very low (between 2 and

2.5 hours) and that not all schools require that HIV prevention education be provided at any grade level. Parents and citizens need to raise concerns about the quality and quantity of sexual health education available in schools.[7]

These behavior patterns are made even more serious because men tend to be less concerned than women about health issues.[8] Men are less likely than women to visit a doctor regularly and many are reluctant to seek professional advice even when they suspect they may have a problem. This reflects men's sense of themselves as self-reliant and not in need of help. One result is that many men do not know that they have sexually transmitted diseases or HIV, because they have not been tested.

Men should be encouraged to understand and take responsibility for the consequences of their sexual actions—for themselves and their partners. Healthy peer support among men may allow men to become more comfortable discussing issues related to their sex lives and personal relationships.

There are precautions that can be taken to prevent HIV infection. They include, using a new condom with each sexual act, and if injecting drugs, using needles and other injection drug equipment that are sterile.

Society must also take some responsibility for permitting and encouraging men to behave in ways that are considered "male" or "masculine," but that are potentially unsafe to themselves and others. Instead, safer and more responsible behavior should be encouraged.

1. Men & AIDS—A Gendered Approach, 2000 World AIDS Campaign. UNAIDS, 2000. p. 6.
2. Ibid. p. 5.
3. Ibid. p. 8.
4. Lawson, A. *Adultery, An Analysis of Love and Betrayal*, New York: Basic Books, 1988.
5. General Social Survey, Statistics Canada, 1995.
6. Men & AIDS—A Gendered Approach, 2000 World AIDS Campaign. UNAIDS, 2000. p. 9.
7. Schools, Public Health, Sexuality and HIV: A Status Report. (1999). Council of Ministers of Education: Toronto.
8. Men & AIDS—A Gendered Approach, 2000 World AIDS Campaign. UNAIDS, 2000. p. 1.

What Are Heterosexual Men's HIV Prevention Needs?

"What Are Heterosexual Men's HIV Prevention Needs?" reprinted with permission from the Center for AIDS Prevention Studies, University of California – San Francisco. © 2001 University of California – San Francisco.

Are heterosexual men at risk?

Yes. In the U.S., new AIDS cases are increasing among people who were infected through injecting drug use (IDU) and heterosexual sexual contact.[1] The rise in IDU infections in heterosexual men has led to the rise in HIV infections in women, as more women become infected from men who are IDUs. For this reason, sexual behavior change among heterosexual men will be key to controlling the HIV epidemic for heterosexual men, women, and children.

Over one-fourth (28%) of all AIDS cases among men in the U.S. occurred through injection drug use and heterosexual sexual contact. Over three-fourths of those cases were among men of color, with African American men comprising more than half (55%).[2] AIDS and HIV cases are classified by drug use and sexual act, and not by self-identification. Heterosexually identified men that engage in sex with other men are classified as "men who have sex with men." However, they may not relate to programs targeting gay men.

Prevention programs in the U.S. have addressed the drug-using risks of heterosexual men. However, few have addressed their sexual behavior. Women have been the primary focus of sexual behavior change among heterosexuals. If heterosexually identified men are reached, often it is by default because the intervention was targeting another audience.

What puts men at risk?

Injection drug use poses the highest risk to heterosexual men.[2] Use of other non-injected substances such as methamphetamines, crack cocaine, and alcohol can increase sexual risk taking, which increases risk of HIV infection. A study of out-of-treatment IDUs in California found that heterosexual men who used methamphetamines reported more sex partners, more sexual activity—including anal intercourse with men and women—and less condom use than men who did not use methamphetamines. In addition, half of their regular female partners did not inject drugs.[3]

Men can get infected from having unprotected intercourse with an HIV+ woman, although the risk is much lower than the risk from sharing infected injection equipment or having sex with an HIV+ man. The risk increases when men or their female partners have STD infections.[4] The greatest sexual risk behavior for heterosexual men is unprotected anal sex with an HIV+ man. Because of homophobia and fear of rejection, men may be unlikely to report having sex with men, identifying sex with women as their only risk factor.[5]

Men in certain settings are at greater risk. In the U.S., 90% of prisoners are men. Among the incarcerated, rates of HIV are 8–10 times higher than in the general population.[6] Injection drug use, other illicit drug use, tattooing, and unprotected anal sex with other men are all risk behaviors for HIV in prison or jail. Clean needles are not available in jail and prisons in the U.S. and condoms are only available in a few.

What makes prevention difficult?

Men in this society are not trained or coached to develop a health plan for themselves. Between childhood vaccinations and post–middle age checks for prostate cancer, many heterosexual men typically do not visit a doctor's office.[7] Heterosexual men and African Americans in particular, are least likely to be tested for HIV, enter into treatment, and keep medical appointments.[8,9]

Many heterosexual men do not have enough knowledge about HIV and other STDs, and do not believe it concerns them. HIV is still seen as a "gay white man's" problem because of the lack of materials targeted to straight men and lack of heterosexual peer educators. Men may be reluctant to use HIV/AIDS services that are run by or targeted to gay men.

Men wear the (male) condom and ultimately have the power to use them or not. Men may be concerned about pregnancy, STD, and HIV prevention, but may have difficulty bringing up the subject of condoms with their partners. Some men wait for the female partner to begin that discussion—if she doesn't, they often do not mention condoms themselves.[10]

Young men of color often see themselves as an "endangered species."[11] For many inner-city youth, the dangers and concerns of daily survival far outweigh any future concerns such as HIV. The realities of poverty, violence, and addiction enforce Black men's belief that they will not live past the age of 25. For many inner-city youth, the likelihood of being shot or sent to prison is their greatest concern.[11]

How can heterosexual men be reached?

Peer educators can help address HIV prevention to heterosexual men, yet very few heterosexual men are involved in HIV prevention. Fear and misunderstanding about gay culture further inhibit involvement. Sensitivity training is necessary for all men to understand and respect sexual cultures and boundaries.

Recruiting heterosexual men can be a difficult task. For instance, approaching African American men individually may not be as effective as recruiting them through their employer, mentor, religious leader, or social group.[12] Heterosexual men also may need encouragement from girlfriends or wives to participate in HIV prevention programs.[12]

Campaigns that target heterosexual men should focus on general health issues, not sexual issues. Campaigns should encourage men to talk about and take responsibility for their health and well-being, instead of highlighting the negative side of sex (HIV kills, sex with a minor can land you in jail). Education should begin before adolescence to help young men protect themselves as they are confronted with the world of sexuality and substance use.

What's being done?

A video-based, skills-building HIV prevention program for African American heterosexual men in Atlanta, GA, helped increase rates of condom use and lower unprotected vaginal intercourse. The program showed videotaped HIV information, questions and answers about HIV, and condom use demonstrations. It also incorporated live facilitators. Because men were unlikely to participate in sexual role-playing with other men, the program used clips from popular movies and asked the men to suggest dialogue for safer sex.[13]

Le Penseur Youth Services reaches out to young people and families in Southeast Chicago, IL. One program targets young male gang members by using gang leaders as peer educators. Le Penseur trained gang leaders and members to deliver safer sex messages. A key component of the program is giving young men clear roles and opportunities for advancement and leadership. Using gang members drove home the point that HIV affects heterosexual men, and increased awareness of HIV in the community.[14]

In Baltimore, MD, the health department opened a free Men's Health Center to address the health care needs of uninsured men ages 19–64. The clinic provides primary and dental care, substance abuse counseling, job placement, and prevention education. The doctor, nurse, and physician's assistant are all men. When it opened, it was the only clinic targeting uninsured men in the U.S. The Center focuses on helping men stay healthy, which will help build healthier families.[15]

What should be done?

Heterosexual men are still in need of basic HIV/AIDS information. Programs are needed for heterosexual men that address their health and well-being and teach them how to advocate for their own health care. Programs also need to acknowledge that heterosexual men may engage in sex with men, and encourage safer sex in all sexual encounters. Finally, programs for heterosexual men need to be developed in conjunction with women, so that female partners' needs and concerns are incorporated.

Drug treatment and access to sterile syringes through needle exchange programs and pharmacy exchanges are crucial for heterosexual men. Incarcerated men need access to drug treatment, condoms, clean syringes, HIV prevention education, and transitional case management to help ease risks both while incarcerated and upon release.

Heterosexual men need to take more responsibility for trying to stop the spread of HIV. Because men have not traditionally been involved in health care and prevention issues, training and support for heterosexual men will be necessary to ensure and sustain their involvement in HIV prevention.

Says who?

1. CDC. HIV/AIDS Surveillance Report. 1995;7:10.

2. CDC. HIV/AIDS Surveillance Report. 2001;13:16.

3. Molitor F, Ruiz JD, Flynn N, et al. Methamphetamine use and sexual and injection risk behaviors among out-of-treatment injection drug users. *American Journal of Drug and Alcohol Abuse*. 1999;25:475–493.

4. Wasserheit JN. Epidemiological synergy. Interrelationships between human immunodeficiency virus infection and other sexually transmitted diseases. *Sexually Transmitted Diseases*. 1992;19:61–77.

5. Sternberg S. 'Secret' bisexuality among Black men contributes to rising number of AIDS cases in Black women. *USA Today*. March 15, 2001.

6. Hammett TM, Harmon P, Maruschak L. 1996–1997 Update: HIV/AIDS, STDs and TB in correctional facilities. Abt Associates, Inc.: Cambridge, MA; 1999.

7. Sandman D, Simantov E, An C. Out of Touch: American Men and the Health Care System. Published by The Commonwealth Fund. March 2000.

8. Fichtner RR, Wolitski RJ, Johnson WD, et al. Influence of perceived and assessed risk on STD clinic clients' acceptance of HIV testing, return for test results, and HIV serostatus. *Psychology, Health & Medicine*. 1996;1:83–98.

9. Israelski D, Gore-Felton G, Wood MJ, et al. Factors associated with keeping medical appointments in a public health AIDS clinic. Presented at the 8th International AIDS Conference, Durban, South Africa. Abst# WePeD4570.

10. Carter JA, McNair LD, Corbin WR. Gender differences related to heterosexual condom use: the influence of negotiation styles. *Journal of Sex & Marital Therapy*. 1999;25:217–225.

11. Parham TA, McDavis RJ. Black men, an endangered species: Who's really pulling the trigger? *Journal of Counseling & Development*. 1987;66:24–27.

12. Summerrise R, Wilson W. "The Black Print" model for recruitment of African-American males. Published by the Chicago, IL, Prevention Planning Group. 2000.

13. Kalichman SC, Cherry C, Brown-Sperling F. Effectiveness of a video-based motivational skills-building HIV risk-reduction intervention for inner-city African American men. *Journal of Consulting and Clinical Psychology*. 1999;67:959–966.

14. Summerrise R. Valuing the lives of men: HIV prevention for heterosexual men. Presented at the U.S. Conference on AIDS, Atlanta, GA. October, 2000.

15. Sugg DK. A first for men: clinic opens in Baltimore. *The Baltimore Sun*. May 11, 2000.

Section 3.2

Methamphetamine Use in Heterosexual Men Increases Risk of STDs

"Methamphetamine Use and HIV Risk Behaviors among Heterosexual Men—Preliminary Results from Five Northern California Counties, December 2001–November 2003," Centers for Disease Control and Prevention (www.cdc.gov), March 17, 2006.

Methamphetamine (meth) is a highly addictive stimulant that gained widespread popularity in California in the 1980s and has since spread to most regions of the United States, including rural areas.[1] Analyses of survey data among noninjection-drug users from California in the mid-1990s determined that, among heterosexual persons and among men who had sex with men (MSM), meth users reported more sex partners, were less likely to report condom use, and were more likely to report sex in exchange for money or drugs, sex with an injection-drug user, and history of a sexually transmitted disease (STD).[2] Subsequent studies among MSM have indicated an association between meth use and sexual risk behaviors, syphilis infection, and incidence of human immunodeficiency virus (HIV) infection.[3–5] Subsequent studies among heterosexual populations[6] have been less extensive than those among MSM and often have not used population-based samples nor adjusted for possible confounders. To further assess the association between meth use and high-risk sexual behaviors among heterosexual men, the California Department of Health Services, Office of AIDS, analyzed population-based data from five northern California counties in the HEY-Man (Health Evaluation in Young Men) Study. This report summarizes the results of that analysis, which determined that recent meth use was associated with high-risk sexual behaviors, including sex with a casual or anonymous female partner, anal intercourse, and sex with an injection-drug user. The results suggest the need for states to consider including referrals to meth prevention and treatment programs in their HIV prevention programs and for broader assessment of the relation between meth use and high-risk sexual behaviors.

HEY-Man is a population-based, cross-sectional evaluation of HIV infection, STDs, and associated risk behaviors among men aged 18–35 years residing in low-income neighborhoods of Alameda, Contra Costa, San Francisco, San Joaquin, and San Mateo counties in northern California. The study protocol was approved by the institutional review boards of the State of California Health and Welfare Agency and the University of California, San Francisco. Within the five counties, low-income neighborhoods were defined as census block groups with median household incomes below the 10th percentile on the basis of data from the 2000 U.S. Census. City blocks were randomly sampled, without replacement, from these census-defined block groups. Trained field staff enumerated dwelling places in each sampled city block, then went door-to-door to locate male residents and request their participation. Repeat visits, including visits during evening hours and weekends, were made as necessary to identify all eligible men and request their participation. During December 2001–November 2003, the period for which data were available, 2,132 men were contacted; 1,692 (79%) were determined eligible (i.e., aged 18–35 years and residing in the selected neighborhoods), and 1,068 (63%) of those agreed to participate and were enrolled. A total of 1,011 participants completed a staff-administered interview conducted in English or Spanish. The study is scheduled for completion in June 2006.

The HEY-Man questionnaire included a sexual-activity matrix in which field staff recorded the first name, nickname, initials, or alias of up to 10 persons with whom participants said they had vaginal or anal sex during the preceding six months. Questions were asked to determine the sex and category (i.e., main, casual, or anonymous) of each sex partner and whether acts included vaginal or anal intercourse with the partner. For this report, analyses were restricted to men who reported having female sex partners exclusively during the preceding six months; 43 men (4.1%) who reported having one or more male sex partners during the preceding six months were excluded, leaving 968 participants. Frequency of condom use was derived from the study's matrix as the sum of reported acts of vaginal and anal intercourse during which condoms were used, divided by the total number of acts of vaginal and anal intercourse. Meth use was divided into two categories: recent use (any use during the preceding six months) and historical use (use but not during the preceding six months). Participants also were asked if they had ever been tested for HIV or chlamydial infection and if they had ever given or received money or drugs for sex or been forced into sex by another male or female.

Chi-square tests were conducted to compare the characteristics of participants (i.e., recent versus no reported meth use, historical versus no reported meth use, and recent versus historical meth use). Separate regression models were used to examine associations between meth use (independent variable) and dichotomously categorized sexual risk and protective behaviors. Regression models were adjusted for demographic characteristics that were significantly associated with recent or historical meth use and use of any other illicit drugs. Prevalence ratios and 95% confidence intervals were calculated using regression procedures for binomially distributed variables.[7]

Among the 968 participants, a larger percentage were non-white (Hispanic [51.1%] or non-Hispanic black [19.0%]), born in the United States (48.0%) or in Mexico (36.8%), single/never married (73.0%), and employed full- (47.8%) or part-time (34.4%). Meth use was reported among 151 (15.6%) participants, including 93 (9.6%) who reported historical use and 58 (6.0%) who reported recent use. The prevalence of recent meth use was higher among participants who were non-Hispanic white (11.9%), born in the United States (8.6%), single/never married (6.6%), and employed part-time (7.2%) or unemployed (8.3%).

A greater percentage of recent meth users (93.1%) than men who reported never using meth (72.2%) had been sexually active with a female partner during the preceding six months ($p<0.001$). A greater percentage of meth users reported having anal sex with a female during this period than never users (recent users [29.6%; $p<0.001$] and historical users [24.3%; $p<0.01$] versus never users [11.9%]). Statistically significant differences with respect to other high-risk sexual behaviors were observed between recent meth users and never users. These differences included having a casual or anonymous female sex partner (recent users [64.8%] versus never users [44.4%]; $p<0.01$), having multiple partners (56.9% versus 26.3%; $p<0.001$), having a partner who injected drugs (11.1% versus 1.7%; $p<0.01$) during the preceding six months, and ever having received drugs or money for sex with a male or female partner (15.5% versus 3.5%; $p<0.001$).

Regression analyses determined that recent meth users were more likely than men who had never used meth to be sexually active with a female partner, have multiple female partners, have a casual or anonymous female partner, have anal intercourse with a casual or anonymous female partner, have a female partner who injected drugs, or have ever received money or drugs for sex from a male or female partner. Recent meth use was not associated with reported condom use during the preceding six months, but this might reflect overall infrequent condom use among the 968 men in the study population, who had a median of 48 reported acts of vaginal intercourse and a median of five uses of condoms during vaginal intercourse. Recent meth users were no more likely to have been tested for HIV or chlamydial infection than were men who had never used meth. Among historical meth users, sexual activity with higher HIV-transmission risk (i.e., anal sex) was identified primarily among those with main female sex partners only. Both recent and historical meth users were more likely to report they had ever been forced into sex by a male or female than men who had never used meth. After adjustment for demographic characteristics, recent and historical meth use was associated with recent use of one or more other illicit drugs,* use of club drugs,† and specific use of marijuana, ecstasy, hallucinogens (e.g., LSD), crack cocaine, and cocaine.

Editorial Note [in original]

The population-based estimates of meth use among low-income men aged 18–35 years presented in this section support previous cross-sectional surveys linking meth use to sexual risk behaviors among heterosexual populations.[2] Recent research on meth use has focused on MSM populations because of the greater prevalence of HIV in this population. Meth use was associated with increased HIV infections among MSM in San Francisco who were tested for HIV during 2001–2002.[3] Results from the study described in this section and additional data suggest that further attention should be given to the association between meth use and STD and HIV infection among heterosexuals. In southern California, 9.5% of primary and secondary syphilis cases in heterosexuals during 2004 were among persons with a history of meth use, continuing a trend of increases from 3.1% in 2001, 6.4% in 2002, and 7.3% in 2003.§ A gonorrhea outbreak in six central California counties in 2004 noted substantial meth use among heterosexual patients (men [38%], women [28%]), particularly when compared with MSM patients (8%).

Similar observations regarding STD incidence among MSM subpopulations (e.g., young minorities) often have indicated future trends of HIV incidence among MSM. Such projections typically have not been made for heterosexuals because of the lesser prevalence of HIV in that population. However, HIV/AIDS surveillance data from CDC and southern California indicate a growing burden of HIV among heterosexuals, particularly among females, non-Hispanic blacks, and Hispanics.[8,9] Data from California HIV counseling and testing facilities also suggest the potential for meth use to connect populations with higher HIV prevalence to those with lower HIV prevalence; among bisexual males tested in California, meth users were 5.5 times more likely (99% CI = 1.4–22.3) to test HIV-positive compared with users of other stimulant drugs (CS Krawczyk, PhD, C Dahlgren, MA, unpublished data, 2002–2003). Increased HIV burden among heterosexuals, coupled with the increased use of meth nationwide and the findings of this section, suggest the potential for meth to influence heterosexual transmission of HIV. Users might initially use meth for either nonsexual (e.g., mental "escape" or weight loss) or sexual (e.g., increased sex drive, performance, and pleasure) effects; regardless of reason for use, the effects of the drug might lead to risk behaviors for transmission of STDs and HIV. In one study, 74% of male meth users reported that their sexual thoughts, feelings, and behaviors became associated with meth, 77% indicated that meth made them obsessed with having sex, and 53% said they had participated in riskier sexual acts (i.e., anal sex) while under the influence of meth.[10]

The findings in this section are subject to at least three limitations. First, because of the cross-sectional design of the study, no temporal or causal relations between meth use and sexual risk behaviors can be evaluated. Second, multiple data comparisons were used, increasing the potential for identifying associations by chance. Finally, because these analyses were conducted before completion of data collection, the current results might differ from the results that will be obtained by analyzing data from the entire targeted study population.

The public health implications of a potential association between meth use and high-risk sexual behaviors among heterosexuals suggests the need for a broader approach in addressing meth use and risk for infection with HIV and STDs. States should consider enhancing HIV and STD prevention and treatment programs to include assessment for meth use, with referrals to meth treatment, primary meth prevention activities, and substance use treatment programs incorporating STD/HIV screening, testing, and sexual health promotion. In addition, policy initiatives should be considered to support further collaborations between professionals focusing on substance use and HIV/STDs, integrated prevention and treatment services, and research and demonstration projects evaluating the impact of treatment for meth use on sexual risk behavior reduction.

References

1. Kraman P. Drug abuse in America—rural meth. TrendsAlert: critical information for state decision-makers. Lexington, KY:

The Council of State Governments; 2004. Available at http://www.csg.org/csg/products/trends+alerts/default.htm.

2. Molitor F, Truax SR, Ruiz JD, Sun RK. Association of methamphetamine use during sex with risky sexual behaviors and HIV infection among non-injection drug users. *West J Med* 1998;168:93–7.

3. Buchacz K, McFarland W, Kellogg TA, et al. Amphetamine use is associated with increased HIV incidence among men who have sex with men in San Francisco. *AIDS* 2005;19:1423–4.

4. Wong W, Chaw JK, Kent CK, Klausner JD. Risk factors for early syphilis among gay and bisexual men seen in an STD clinic: San Francisco, 2002–2003. *Sex Transm Dis* 2005;32:458–63.

5. Purcell DW, Moss S, Remien RH, Woods WJ, Parsons JT. Illicit substance use, sexual risk, and HIV-positive gay and bisexual men: differences by serostatus of casual partners. *AIDS* 2005;19(Suppl 1):S37–47.

6. Semple SJ, Patterson TL, Grant I. The context of sexual risk behavior among heterosexual methamphetamine users. *Addict Behav* 2004;29:807–10.

7. Spiegelman D, Hertzmark E. Easy SAS calculations for risk and prevalence ratios and differences. *Am J Epidem* 2005;162:199–200.

8. County of San Diego Health and Human Services Agency. HIV/AIDS epidemiology report, 2004. San Diego, CA: County of San Diego Health and Human Services Agency; 2004. Available at http://www2.sdcounty.ca.gov/hhsa/documents/2004hiv_aidsrpt.pdf.

9. CDC. HIV/AIDS surveillance report, 2004. Vol. 16. Atlanta, GA: U.S. Department of Health and Human Services, CDC; 2005.

10. Rawson RA, Washton A, Domier CP, Reiber C. Drugs and sexual effects: role of drug type and gender. *J Subst Abuse Treat* 2002;22:103–8.

* Marijuana, barbiturates, cocaine, crack cocaine, heroin, or phencyclidine (PCP).

† Viagra®, ecstasy, nitrites, lysergic acid diethylamide (LSD), or gamma hydroxybutyrate (GHB).

§ Syphilis Elimination Surveillance Data, available at http://www.dhs.ca.gov/ps/dcdc/std/mqreports.htm.

Section 3.3

STDs among Men Who Have Sex with Men (MSM)

"Surveillance 2006: Special Focus Profiles: Men Who Have Sex with Men," Centers for Disease Control and Prevention (www.cdc.gov), November 13, 2007.

Public Health Impact

Data from several U.S. cities and projects, including syphilis outbreak investigations and the GISP, suggest that an increasing number of MSM are acquiring STDs.[1–7] Data also suggest that an increasing number of MSM engage in sexual behaviors that place them at risk for STDs and HIV infection.[8] Several factors may be contributing to this change, including the availability of highly active antiretroviral therapy (HAART) for HIV infection.[9] Because STDs and the behaviors associated with acquiring them increase the likelihood of acquiring and transmitting HIV infection,[10] the rise in STDs among MSM may be associated with an increase in HIV diagnoses among MSM.[11]

Observations

Most nationally notifiable STD surveillance data reported to CDC do not include information regarding sexual behaviors; therefore, national trends in STDs among MSM in the United States are not currently available. Data from enhanced surveillance projects are presented in this section to provide information regarding STDs in MSM.

Monitoring Trends in Prevalence of STDs, HIV, and Risk Behaviors among Men Who Have Sex with Men (MSM Prevalence Monitoring Project), STD Clinics, 1999–2006

From 1999 through 2006, eight U.S. cities participating in the MSM Prevalence Monitoring Project submitted syphilis, gonorrhea, chlamydia, and HIV test data to CDC from 120,164 MSM visits to STD clinics; data from 98,866 MSM visits were submitted from five public STD clinics (Denver, New York City, Philadelphia, San Francisco, and Seattle) and data from 21,298 MSM visits were submitted from three STD clinics in community-based, gay men's health clinics (Chicago, the District of Columbia, and Houston).

Changes in testing technology for gonorrhea and chlamydia have occurred in recent years with the advent of nucleic acid amplification tests (NAATs), which achieve greater sensitivity than traditional culture methods.[12,13] The MSM Prevalence Monitoring Project includes data from culture and non-culture tests collected during routine care and reflects testing practices at participating clinics. Tests for gonorrhea included culture, NAATs, or nucleic acid hybridization tests (DNA probes). Tests for chlamydia included culture, NAATs, DNA probes, or direct fluorescent antibody tests (DFAs). Nontreponemal syphilis tests included the Rapid Plasma Reagin (RPR) test and the Venereal Disease Research Laboratory (VDRL).

All statistics were based on data collected from clinic visits and may reflect multiple visits by a patient rather than individual patients. City-specific medians and ranges were calculated for the proportion of tests done and for STD and HIV test positivity.

Gonorrhea

Between 1999 and 2006 the number of gonorrhea tests for all anatomic sites combined increased in all eight cities. The trend in the number of positive gonorrhea tests for all anatomic sites varied by city. For all cities, the number of symptomatic positive gonorrhea tests accounts for the majority of the overall positive tests.

In 2006, 75% (range: 56–94%) of MSM were tested for urethral gonorrhea, 40% (range: 3–61%) were tested for rectal gonorrhea, and 53% (range: 6–87%) were tested for pharyngeal gonorrhea.

In 2006, median clinic urethral gonorrhea positivity in MSM was 10% (range: 8–13%), median rectal gonorrhea positivity was 7% (range: 2–13%), and median pharyngeal gonorrhea positivity was 7% (range: 1–15%).

Chlamydia

In 2006, a median of 75% (range: 58–93%) of MSM visiting participating STD clinics were tested for urethral chlamydia, compared to 65% (range: 58–68%) in 1999. In 2006, the median urethral chlamydia positivity was 6% (range: 5–8%).

Syphilis

In 2006, 83% (range: 61–94%) of MSM visiting participating STD clinics had a nontreponemal serologic test for syphilis (RPR or VDRL) performed, compared with 69% (range: 54–93%) in 1999.

Overall, median seroreactivity among MSM tested for syphilis increased from 4% (range: 4–13%) in 1999 to 10% (range: 6–18%) in 2006.

Syphilis seroreactivity is used to estimate syphilis prevalence and is correlated with prevalence of P&S syphilis in this population.[14]

HIV Infection

Trends: Overall, the percent of MSM tested for HIV in STD clinics increased between 1999 and 2006. In 2006, a median of 73% (range: 28–85%) of MSM visiting STD clinics that were not previously known to be HIV-positive were tested for HIV, while 44% (range: 21–55%) were tested in 1999. In 2006, median HIV positivity in MSM was 4% (range: 2–7%).

In 2006, median HIV prevalence among MSM, including persons previously known to be HIV-positive and persons testing HIV-positive at their current visit, was 12% (range: 10–16%).

HIV/STDs by Race/Ethnicity

HIV positivity varied by race/ethnicity, but was highest in African American MSM. HIV positivity was 3% (range: 1–4%) in whites, 10% (range: 3–13%) in African Americans, and 4% (range: 2–6%) in Hispanics.

HIV prevalence was 11% (range: 7–16%) in whites, 21% (range: 15–25%) in African Americans, and 14% (range: 8–19%) in Hispanics.

In 2006, urethral gonorrhea positivity was 9% (range: 6–12%) in whites, 14% (range: 9–19) in African Americans, and 7% (range: 4–21%) in Hispanics. Rectal gonorrhea positivity was 8% (range: 3–11%) in whites, 10% (range: 2–12%) in African Americans, and 9% (range: 2–11%) in Hispanics.

Pharyngeal gonorrhea positivity was 8% (range: 1–15%) in whites, 6% (range: 1–12%) in African Americans, and 7% (range: 1–28%) in Hispanics.

Urethral chlamydia was 5% (range: 3–8%) in whites, 7% (range: 5–13%) in African Americans, and 6% (range: 4–8%) in Hispanics.

Median syphilis seroreactivity was 7% (range: 6–11%) in whites, 15% (range: 8–26%) in African Americans, and 14% (range: 7–26%) in Hispanics.

STDs by HIV Status, STD Clinics, 2006

In 2006, urethral gonorrhea positivity was 14% (range: 12–31%) in HIV-positive MSM and 8% (range: 7–12%) in MSM who were HIV-negative or of unknown HIV status; rectal gonorrhea positivity was 11% (range: 3–18%) in HIV-positive MSM and 6% (range: 2–14%) in MSM who were HIV-negative or of unknown HIV status; pharyngeal gonorrhea positivity was 6% (range: 1–19%) in HIV-positive MSM and 7% (range: 1–14%) in MSM who were HIV-negative or of unknown HIV status.

Median urethral chlamydia positivity was 7% (range: 5–9%) in HIV-positive MSM and 6% (range: 4–8%) in MSM who were HIV-negative or of unknown HIV status.

Median syphilis seroreactivity was 30% (range: 17–44%) in HIV-positive MSM and 7% (range: 5–13%) in MSM who were HIV-negative or of unknown HIV status.

Nationally Notifiable Syphilis Surveillance Data

P&S syphilis increased in the United States between 2002 and 2006, with a 54.1% increase in the number of P&S syphilis cases among men and a 9.1% decrease in the number of cases among women. In 2006, the rate of reported P&S syphilis among men (5.7 cases per 100,000 males) was 5.7 times greater than the rate among women (1.0 cases per 100,000 females). Trends in the syphilis male-to-female rate ratio, which are assumed to reflect, in part, syphilis trends among MSM,[7] have been increasing in the United States during recent years. The overall male-to-female syphilis rate ratio has risen steadily from 3.4 in 2002 to 5.7 in 2006. The increase in the male-to-female rate ratio occurred among all racial and ethnic groups between 2002 and 2006.

In recent years, MSM have accounted for an increasing number of estimated syphilis cases in the United States[15] and in 2006 accounted for 64% of P&S syphilis cases in the United States based on information reported from 29 states and Washington, D.C.[16]

Gonococcal Isolate Surveillance Project (GISP)

The GISP, a collaborative project among selected STD clinics, was established in 1986 to monitor trends in antimicrobial susceptibilities of strains of *Neisseria gonorrhoeae* in the United States.[17,18]

GISP also reports the percentage of *N. gonorrhoeae* isolates obtained from MSM. Overall, the proportion of isolates from MSM in GISP clinics increased steadily from 4% in 1988 to 21.5% in 2006.

The proportion of isolates coming from MSM varies geographically with the largest percentage from the West Coast.

References

1. Centers for Disease Control and Prevention. Gonorrhea among men who have sex with men—selected sexually transmitted disease clinics, 1993–1996. *MMWR* 1997;46:889–92.

2. Centers for Disease Control and Prevention. Resurgent bacterial sexually transmitted disease among men who have sex with men—King County, Washington, 1997–1999. *MMWR* 1999;48:773–7.

3. Centers for Disease Control and Prevention. Outbreak of syphilis among men who have sex with men—Southern California, 2000. *MMWR* 2001;50:117–20.

4. Fox KK, del Rio C, Holmes K, et. al. Gonorrhea in the HIV era: A reversal in trends among men who have sex with men. *Am J Public Health* 2001;91:959–964.

5. Centers for Disease Control and Prevention. Primary and secondary syphilis among men who have sex with men—New York City, 2001. *MMWR* 2002;51:853–6.

6. Centers for Disease Control and Prevention. Primary and secondary syphilis—United States, 2003–2004. *MMWR* 2006;55:269–73.

7. Beltrami JF, Shouse RL, Blake PA. Trends in infectious diseases and the male to female ratio: possible clues to changes in behavior among men who have sex with men. *AIDS Educ Prev* 2005;17:S49–S59.

8. Stall R, Hays R, Waldo C, Ekstrand M, McFarland W. The gay '90s: a review of research in the 1990s on sexual behavior and HIV risk among men who have sex with men. *AIDS* 2000;14:S1–S14.

9. Scheer S, Chu PL, Klausner JD, Katz MH, Schwarcz SK. Effect of highly active antiretroviral therapy on diagnoses of sexually transmitted diseases in people with AIDS. *Lancet* 2001;357:432–5.

10. Fleming DT, Wasserheit JN. From epidemiologic synergy to public health policy and practice: the contribution of other sexually transmitted diseases to sexual transmission of HIV infection. *Sex Transm Infect* 1999;75:3–17.

11. Centers for Disease Control and Prevention. HIV/AIDS Surveillance Report, 2003, (Vol. 15). Atlanta: U.S. Department of Health and Human Services, Centers for Disease Control and Prevention; 2004.

12. Renault CA, Hall C, Kent CK, Klausner JD. Use of NAATs for STD diagnosis of GC and CT in non-FDA-cleared anatomic specimens. *MLO Med Lab Obs* 2006; 38(7):10, 12–6, 21–2.

13. Jespersen DJ, Flatten KS, Jones MF, Smith TF. Prospective comparison of cell cultures and nucleic acid amplification tests for laboratory diagnosis of *Chlamydia trachomatis* Infections. *J Clin Microbiol* 2005; 43(10):5324–6.

14. Helms DJ, Weinstock HS, et. al. Increases in syphilis among men who have sex with men attending STD clinics, 2000–2005. In: program and abstracts of the 17 Biennial meeting of the ISSTDR, Seattle, WA, July 29–August 1, 2007 [abstract P-608].

15. Heffelfinger JD, Swint EB, Berman SM, Weinstock HS. Trends in primary and secondary syphilis among men who have sex with men in the United States. *Am J Public Health* 2007;97:1076–1083.

16. Beltrami JF, Weinstock HS. Primary and secondary syphilis among men who have sex with men in the United States, 2005. In: program and abstracts of the 17 Biennial meeting of the ISSTDR, Seattle, WA, July 29–August 1, 2007 [abstract O-069].

17. Schwarcz S, Zenilman J, Schnell D, et. al. National Surveillance of Antimicrobial Resistance in *Neisseria gonorrhoeae*. *JAMA* 1990; 264(11): 1413–1417.

18. Centers for Disease Control and Prevention. Sexually Transmitted Disease Surveillance 2006 Supplement: Gonococcal Isolate Surveillance Project (GISP) Annual Report 2006. Atlanta, GA: U.S. Department of Health and Human Services (available first quarter 2008).

Section 3.4

Racial/Ethnic and Age Disparities in Human Immunodeficiency Virus (HIV) among MSM

"Research Summary: Racial/Ethnic and Age Disparities in HIV Prevalence and Disease Progression among Men Who Have Sex with Men in the United States," Centers for Disease Control and Prevention (www.cdc.gov), May 25, 2007.

CDC researchers published a new study in the *American Journal of Public Health* that highlights racial, ethnic, and age differences within the HIV/AIDS epidemic among men who have sex with men.

What does the study show?

The study shows the following statistics for the years 2001–2004*:

- Black and Hispanic MSM had higher rates of HIV/AIDS diagnoses across all age groups compared to white MSM.
- The percentage of men who progressed to AIDS within three years of their HIV diagnoses was higher among black and Hispanic MSM than among white MSM.
- Three-year survival among black MSM was lower than that for Hispanic or white MSM.

- Overall, HIV/AIDS diagnoses rates remained stable during this time period, but the rates for younger MSM showed large increases.

* This study uses data from the 33 states with confidential, long-term, name-based HIV reporting.

Why is the study important?

This study is further evidence of the racial and ethnic disparities within the HIV/AIDS epidemic as well as the urgency of educating young MSM about HIV/AIDS.

What is CDC doing about the problem?

On a national level, CDC funds special initiatives, interventions, and research addressing these disparities. CDC provides funding to state and local health departments and community-based organizations to better address the needs and gaps of the epidemic locally.

Research Summary

During the years 2001–2004, black and Hispanic men who have sex with men had higher rates of HIV/AIDS diagnoses across all age groups than did white MSM, according to a new CDC study to be published in the June 2007 issue of the *American Journal of Public Health*. Additionally, even though overall HIV/AIDS diagnoses rates remained stable for MSM during this time period, the rates for younger MSM (between the ages of 13 and 24) showed large increases.

The study, led by H. Irene Hall, PhD of CDC's Division of HIV/AIDS Prevention, also showed that the percentage of men who progressed to AIDS within three years of their HIV diagnosis was higher among black and Hispanic MSM than among white MSM. Three-year survival after an AIDS diagnosis was lower for black than for white or Hispanic MSM.

The study's authors said the poorer outcomes for minority men may be tied to later diagnosis or lack of adequate access to treatment.

This study was performed using data from the national HIV/AIDS surveillance system that consists of 33 states that have conducted HIV surveillance for at least five years. The study sought to determine the interaction between race/ethnicity and age as well as to examine differences in late HIV diagnosis and progression to AIDS or progression from AIDS to death among racial/ethnic groups of MSM diagnosed with HIV.

It found that among all age groups, HIV/AIDS diagnosis rates were higher for black and Hispanic MSM than for white MSM. In 2004, the rate of HIV/AIDS diagnosis per 100,000 was 70.8 for black MSM, 39.0 for Hispanic MSM, and 14.6 for white MSM.

The rates also varied by age. In 2004, the HIV/AIDS diagnosis rate for MSM aged 13 through 19 was 23.5 for black MSM, 6.1 for Hispanic MSM, and 1.2 for white MSM. From 2001 to 2004, there were no differences by race/ethnicity in trends within age groups. By age group alone, for MSM aged 13 to 19 years, HIV/AIDS diagnosis rates increased about 14% per year; for those aged 20 to 24 years, they increased about 13% per year.

Of the 43,994 MSM with a reported HIV diagnosis during 1996 through 2002, 15,174 (34.5%) had a diagnosis of AIDS by 2004. HIV was significantly more likely to progress to AIDS within three years of HIV diagnosis among black and Hispanic MSM than among white MSM. AIDS did not develop within three years for 66.8% of black MSM and 68.1% of Hispanic MSM compared with 74.7% of white MSM.

Of the 62,045 MSM with a diagnosis of AIDS during 1996 through 2002, 13,962 (22.5%) had died by the end of 2004. Black MSM were significantly less likely to be alive three years after AIDS diagnosis (80.6%) than were Hispanic (85.2%) or white (84.5%) MSM.

The 1990s saw a reduction in new HIV diagnoses, most likely due to better treatments coupled with prevention behaviors. However, since 1999, the downward trend in new HIV and AIDS diagnoses has leveled off, primarily because of increases in the number of HIV diagnoses among MSM. Other reports have noted that increasing rates of primary and secondary syphilis among MSM may be attributable to increases in risky sexual behaviors among members of this community and may explain the resurgence of new HIV diagnoses among MSM. Increased rates of HIV testing may also play a role in increased HIV/AIDS diagnoses in certain populations.

This report highlights the need for increased prevention efforts to reach young gay and bisexual men. These prevention efforts need to be tailored to individual populations and behaviors and will require a combination of strategies to reduce new HIV infections among MSM.

CDC is Addressing the Disparities of HIV/AIDS

CDC is addressing the disparities in HIV/AIDS diagnoses through a number of mechanisms.

Increasing HIV testing: In September 2006, CDC released Revised Recommendations for HIV Testing of Adults, Adolescents, and Pregnant Women in Health-Care Settings, which encourage routine HIV screening of adults, adolescents, and pregnant women in health care settings in the United States. CDC also recommends that MSM get tested at least annually.

Increased testing will enable those who are infected with HIV to get into treatment that can improve their health and extend their lives and reduce further transmission of the virus. HIV testing is especially important for MSM of racial or ethnic minorities, as research has shown that black and Hispanic MSM who are infected with HIV enter treatment at a later stage than their white counterparts.

CDC is also supporting research to assess the effectiveness of different strategies to identify undiagnosed HIV infection among African American MSM. CDC has shown social networks to hold much promise in reaching MSM.

Community mobilization: CDC provides resources to state and local health departments and community-based organizations to reach MSM of all races and ethnicities. CDC has worked to mobilize African American leaders across the country to implement a heightened national response to the AIDS epidemic among African Americans. CDC is also working internally and with external partners to examine and further improve HIV prevention efforts for Hispanic populations.

Supporting research-based interventions: CDC creates and supports interventions to help people reduce the risk of getting HIV and to help those infected with HIV to live healthy lives and reduce the transmission to others. A catalogue of those interventions can be found at http://www.effectiveinterventions.org. An example of an intervention is Many Men, Many Voices, which is an HIV/STD prevention program for African American MSM that has been proven to reduce risk behaviors. CDC is encouraging its nationwide implementation. Together Learning Choices is an example of an intervention specifically for young people.

Adapting proven interventions: Interventions, such as Popular Opinion Leader, which trains opinion leaders to encourage safer sexual norms and behaviors within their social networks, is being adapted for African American MSM and has been successfully adapted for Latino MSM. Other interventions have also been translated for use with Hispanic populations.

Researching new interventions: CDC is studying new behavioral interventions for MSM and evaluating strategies for increasing testing rates and decreasing risky behaviors. For example, Brothers Y Hermanos is a study of African American and Hispanic MSM conducted in Los Angeles, New York, and Philadelphia. The first phase of the study consisted of epidemiologic research to identify and understand risk-promoting and risk-reducing sexual behaviors. The second phase, which is taking place in six U.S. cities, will create interventions.

CDC is also conducting research evaluating community-level interventions of Mpowerment for African American MSM and research to look at risk behaviors among non-gay identified MSM of all races and ethnicities. CDC's ARTAS II study is evaluating the effects of linkage case management on those newly diagnosed with HIV.

Chapter 4

STDs in Women and Children

Chapter Contents

Section 4.1

Pregnancy, Infertility, and STDs

This section includes "STDs and Pregnancy—CDC Fact Sheet", January 4, 2008; and "Infertility and STDs," Centers for Disease Control and Prevention (www.cdc.gov), April 8, 2008.

Can pregnant women become infected with STDs?

Yes, women who are pregnant can become infected with the same sexually transmitted diseases (STDs) as women who are not pregnant. Pregnancy does not provide women or their babies any protection against STDs. The consequences of an STD can be significantly more serious, even life threatening, for a woman and her baby if the woman becomes infected with an STD while pregnant. It is important that women be aware of the harmful effects of STDs and know how to protect themselves and their children against infection.

How common are STDs in pregnant women in the United States?

Some STDs, such as genital herpes and bacterial vaginosis, are quite common in pregnant women in the United States. Other STDs,

Table 4.1. Estimated number of pregnant women with specific STDs

STDs	Estimated Number of Pregnant Women
Bacterial vaginosis	1,080,000
Herpes simplex virus 2	880,000
Chlamydia	100,000
Trichomoniasis	124,000
Gonorrhea	13,200
Hepatitis B	16,000
HIV	6,400
Syphilis	<1,000

notably HIV and syphilis, are much less common in pregnant women. Table 4.1 shows the estimated number of pregnant women in the United States who are infected with specific STDs each year.

How do STDs affect a pregnant woman and her baby?

STDs can have many of the same consequences for pregnant women as women who are not pregnant. STDs can cause cervical and other cancers, chronic hepatitis, pelvic inflammatory disease, infertility, and other complications. Many STDs in women are silent; that is, without signs or symptoms.

STDs can be passed from a pregnant woman to the baby before, during, or after the baby's birth. Some STDs (like syphilis) cross the placenta and infect the baby while it is in the uterus (womb). Other STDs (like gonorrhea, chlamydia, hepatitis B, and genital herpes) can be transmitted from the mother to the baby during delivery as the baby passes through the birth canal. HIV can cross the placenta during pregnancy, infect the baby during the birth process, and unlike most other STDs, can infect the baby through breastfeeding.

A pregnant woman with an STD may also have early onset of labor, premature rupture of the membranes surrounding the baby in the uterus, and uterine infection after delivery.

The harmful effects of STDs in babies may include stillbirth (a baby that is born dead), low birth weight (less than five pounds), conjunctivitis (eye infection), pneumonia, neonatal sepsis (infection in the baby's blood stream), neurologic damage, blindness, deafness, acute hepatitis, meningitis, chronic liver disease, and cirrhosis. Most of these problems can be prevented if the mother receives routine prenatal care, which includes screening tests for STDs starting early in pregnancy and repeated close to delivery, if necessary. Other problems can be treated if the infection is found at birth.

Should pregnant women be tested for STDs?

Yes, STDs affect women of every socioeconomic and educational level, age, race, ethnicity, and religion. The CDC 2006 Guidelines for Treatment of Sexually Transmitted Diseases recommend that pregnant women be screened on their first prenatal visit for STDs that may include chlamydia, gonorrhea, hepatitis B, HIV, and syphilis.

In addition, some experts recommend that women who have had a premature delivery in the past be screened and treated for bacterial vaginosis at the first prenatal visit.

Pregnant women should ask their doctors about getting tested for these STDs, since some doctors do not routinely perform these tests. New and increasingly accurate tests continue to become available. Even if a woman has been tested in the past, she should be tested again when she becomes pregnant.

Can STDs be treated during pregnancy?

Chlamydia, gonorrhea, syphilis, trichomoniasis, and bacterial vaginosis (BV) can be treated and cured with antibiotics during pregnancy. There is no cure for viral STDs, such as genital herpes and HIV, but antiviral medication may be appropriate for pregnant women with herpes and definitely is for those with HIV. For women who have active genital herpes lesions at the time of delivery, a cesarean delivery (C-section) may be performed to protect the newborn against infection. C-section is also an option for some HIV-infected women. Women who test negative for hepatitis B may receive the hepatitis B vaccine during pregnancy.

How can pregnant women protect themselves against infection?

The surest way to avoid transmission of sexually transmitted diseases is to abstain from sexual contact, or to be in a long-term mutually monogamous relationship with a partner who has been tested and is known to be uninfected.

Latex condoms, when used consistently and correctly, are highly effective in preventing transmission of HIV, the virus that causes AIDS. Latex condoms, when used consistently and correctly, can reduce the risk of transmission of gonorrhea, chlamydia, and trichomoniasis. Correct and consistent use of latex condoms can reduce the risk of genital herpes, syphilis, and chancroid only when the infected area or site of potential exposure is protected by the condom. Correct and consistent use of latex condoms may reduce the risk for genital human papillomavirus (HPV) and associated diseases (e.g., warts and cervical cancer).

Sources

Centers for Disease Control and Prevention (CDC). Sexually Transmitted Diseases Treatment Guidelines 2006. *MMWR* 2006;55(no. RR-11).

Goldenberg RL, Andrews WW, Yuan AC, MacKay HT, St. Louis ME. Sexually transmitted diseases and adverse outcomes of pregnancy. *Clinics in Perinatology* 1997; 24(1): 23–41.

Institute of Medicine. *The Hidden Epidemic: Confronting Sexually Transmitted Diseases.* Eng TR, Butler WT, eds. Washington: National Academy Press. 1997.

CDC Recommends Screening of All Sexually Active Women 25 and Under

Chlamydia and gonorrhea are the most important preventable causes of infertility. Untreated, up to 40% of women with chlamydia or gonorrhea will develop pelvic inflammatory disease (PID). PID can lead to infertility and potentially fatal tubal (ectopic) pregnancy.

- An estimated 2.8 million cases of chlamydia and 718,000 cases of gonorrhea occur annually in the United States.
- Most women infected with chlamydia or gonorrhea have no symptoms.

CDC recommends annual chlamydia screening for all sexually active females 25 and under and for women older than 25 with risk factors such as a new sex partner or multiple partners.

Section 4.2

Long-Term Consequences for Women and Infants with STDs and AIDS

This section begins with "Surveillance 2006 Special Focus Profiles: Women and Infants," Centers for Disease Control and Prevention (www.cdc.gov), November 13, 2007. Additional information from the Center for AIDS Prevention Studies, University of California – San Francisco is cited separately within the section.

Women and Infants: Public Health Impact

Women and infants disproportionately bear the long-term consequences of STDs. Women infected with *Neisseria gonorrhoeae* or *Chlamydia trachomatis* can develop PID, which, in turn, may lead to reproductive system morbidity such as ectopic pregnancy and tubal factor infertility. If not adequately treated, 20% to 40% of women infected with chlamydia[1] and 10% to 40% of women infected with gonorrhea[2] may develop PID. Among women with PID, tubal scarring can cause involuntary infertility in 20%, ectopic pregnancy in 9%, and chronic pelvic pain in 18%.[3] Approximately 70% of chlamydial infections and 50% of gonococcal infections in women are asymptomatic.[4-6] These infections are detected primarily through screening programs. The vague symptoms associated with chlamydial and gonococcal PID cause 85% of women to delay seeking medical care, thereby increasing the risk of infertility and ectopic pregnancy.[7] Data from a randomized controlled trial of chlamydia screening in a managed care setting suggest that such screening programs can reduce the incidence of PID by as much as 60%.[8]

Human papillomavirus (HPV) infections are highly prevalent, especially among young sexually active women. While the great majority of HPV infections in women resolve within one year, they are a major concern because persistent infection with specific types are causally related to cervical cancer; these types also cause Pap smear abnormalities. Other types cause genital warts, low-grade Pap smear abnormalities and, rarely, recurrent respiratory papillomatosis in infants born to infected mothers.[9]

Direct Impact on Pregnancy

Gonorrhea and chlamydia can result in adverse outcomes of pregnancy, including neonatal ophthalmia and, in the case of chlamydia, neonatal pneumonia. Although topical prophylaxis of infants at delivery is effective for prevention of gonococcal ophthalmia neonatorum, prevention of neonatal pneumonia requires prenatal detection and treatment.

Genital infections with herpes simplex virus are extremely common, may cause painful outbreaks, and may have serious consequences for pregnant women including potentially fatal neonatal infections.[10]

When a woman has a syphilis infection during pregnancy, she may transmit the infection to the fetus in utero. This may result in fetal death or an infant born with physical and mental developmental disabilities. Most cases of congenital syphilis are easily preventable if women are screened for syphilis and treated early during prenatal care.[11]

Observations

Chlamydia: United States

Between 2005 and 2006, the rate of chlamydial infections in women increased from 492.2 to 515.8 per 100,000 females. Chlamydia rates exceed gonorrhea rates among women in all states.

Chlamydia: Infertility Prevention Program

Prenatal clinics: In 2006, the median state-specific chlamydia test positivity among 15- to 24-year-old women screened in selected prenatal clinics in 23 states, Puerto Rico, and the Virgin Islands was 8.1% (range 3.5% to 16.7%).

Family planning clinics: In 2006, the median state-specific chlamydia test positivity among 15- to 24-year-old women who were screened during visits to selected family planning clinics in all states and outlying areas was 6.7% (range 2.8% to 16.9%).

Gonorrhea: United States

Gonorrhea rates among women were higher than the overall HP 2010 target of 19.0 cases per 100,000 population[12] in 46 states, Washington, D.C., and two outlying areas in 2006.

Like chlamydia, gonorrhea is often asymptomatic in women. Gonorrhea screening, therefore, is an important strategy for the identification of gonorrhea among women. Large-scale screening programs for gonorrhea in women began in the 1970s. After an initial increase in cases detected through screening, gonorrhea rates for both women and men declined steadily throughout the 1980s and early 1990s, and then reached a plateau. The gonorrhea rate for women (124.3 per 100,000 females) increased slightly in 2006 for the second consecutive year.

Although the gonorrhea rate in men has historically been higher than the rate in women, the gonorrhea rate among women has been higher than the rate among men for six consecutive years.

Gonorrhea: Infertility Prevention Program

Prenatal clinics: In 2006, the median state-specific gonorrhea test positivity among 15- to 24-year-old women screened in selected prenatal clinics in 20 states, Puerto Rico, and the Virgin Islands was 1.0% (range 0.0% to 3.2%). Median gonorrhea positivity in prenatal clinics has shown minimal change in recent years.

Family planning clinics: In 2006, the median state-specific gonorrhea test positivity among 15- to 24-year-old women screened in selected family planning clinics in 43 states, Puerto Rico, the District of Columbia, and the Virgin Islands was 1.1% (range 0.0%–4.8%). Median gonorrhea positivity in family planning clinics has shown minimal change in recent years.

Primary and Secondary Syphilis by State

The HP 2010 target for primary and secondary (P&S) syphilis is 0.2 cases per 100,000 population. In 2006, 32 states, the District of Columbia, and two outlying areas had rates of P&S syphilis for women that were greater than 0.2 case per 100,000 population.

Congenital Syphilis

The HP 2010 target for congenital syphilis is 1.0 case per 100,000 live births. In 2006, 26 states, the District of Columbia, and Puerto Rico had rates higher than this target.

Trends in congenital syphilis usually follow trends in P&S syphilis among women, with a lag of one to two years. The congenital syphilis rate peaked in 1991 at 107.3 cases per 100,000 live births, and declined by 92.4% to 8.2 cases per 100,000 live births in 2005. The rate of P&S syphilis among women declined 94.8% (from 17.3 to 0.9 cases per 100,000 females) during 1990–2005.

After 14 years of decline in the United States, the rate of congenital syphilis increased 3.7% between 2005 and 2006 (from 8.2 to 8.5 cases per 100,000 live births).

The 2006 rate of congenital syphilis for the United States is currently 8.5 times higher than the HP 2010 target of 1.0 case per 100,000 live births.

While most cases of congenital syphilis occur among infants whose mothers have had some prenatal care, late or limited prenatal care has been associated with congenital syphilis. Failure of health care providers to adhere to maternal syphilis screening recommendations also contributes to the occurrence of congenital syphilis.[13]

Pelvic Inflammatory Disease

Accurate estimates of pelvic inflammatory disease and tubal factor infertility resulting from gonococcal and chlamydial infections are difficult to obtain. Definitive diagnoses of these conditions can be complex. Hospitalizations for PID have declined steadily throughout the 1980s and early 1990s, but have remained relatively constant between 1995 and 2005. Accurate estimates of PID and tubal factor infertility resulting from gonococcal and chlamydial infections are difficult to obtain. Definitive diagnoses of these conditions can be complex. Hospitalizations for PID have declined steadily throughout the 1980s and early 1990s[14,15] but have remained relatively constant between 1995 and 2005.[14]

The estimated number of initial visits to physicians' offices for PID from the National Disease and Therapeutic Index (NDTI) has generally declined from 1993 through 2006.

In 2004, an estimated 170,076 cases of PID were diagnosed in emergency departments among women 15 to 44 years of age. In 2005 this estimate decreased to 147,642 (National Hospital Ambulatory Medical Care Survey, NCHS). As of the date of publication of this report, 2006 data are not available.

Racial disparities in diagnosed PID have been observed in both ambulatory and hospitalized settings. Black women had rates of disease that were two to three times those in white women. Because of the subjective methods by which PID is diagnosed, racial disparity data should be interpreted with caution.[15]

Ectopic Pregnancy

Evidence suggests that health care practices associated with clinical management of ectopic pregnancy changed in the late 1980s and early 1990s. Before that time, treatment of ectopic pregnancy usually required admission to a hospital. Hospitalization statistics were therefore useful for monitoring trends in ectopic pregnancy. From 1996 to 2005, hospitalizations for ectopic pregnancy have remained generally stable. As of the date of publication of this report, 2006 data are not available. Data suggest that nearly half of all ectopic pregnancies are treated on an outpatient basis.[16]

References

1. Stamm WE, Guinan ME, Johnson C. Effect of treatment regimens for Neisseria gonorrhoeae on simultaneous infections with *Chlamydia trachomatis*. *N Engl J Med* 1984;310:545–9.
2. Platt R, Rice PA, McCormack WM. Risk of acquiring gonorrhea and prevalence of abnormal adnexal findings among women recently exposed to gonorrhea. *JAMA* 1983;250:3205–9.
3. Westrom L, Joesoef R, Reynolds G, et al. Pelvic inflammatory disease and fertility: a cohort study of 1,844 women with laparoscopically verified disease and 657 control women with normal laparoscopy. *Sexually Transmitted Diseases* 1992;9:185–92.
4. Hook EW III, Handsfield HH. Gonococcal infections in the adult. In: Holmes KK, Mardh PA, Sparling PF, et al, eds. *Sexually Transmitted Diseases*, 2nd edition. New York City: McGraw-Hill, Inc, 1990:149–65.
5. Stamm WE, Holmes KK. *Chlamydia trachomatis* infections in the adult. In: Holmes KK, Mardh PA, Sparling PF, et al, eds. *Sexually Transmitted Diseases*, 2nd edition. New York City: McGraw-Hill, Inc, 1990:181–93.
6. Zimmerman HL, Potterat JJ, Dukes RL, et al. Epidemiologic differences between chlamydia and gonorrhea. *Am J Public Health* 1990;80:1338–42.
7. Hillis SD, Joesoef R, Marchbanks PA, et al. Delayed care of pelvic inflammatory disease as a risk factor for impaired fertility. *Am J Obstet Gynecol* 1993;168:1503–9.

8. Scholes D, Stergachis A, Heidrich FE, Andrilla H, Holmes KK, Stamm WE. Prevention of pelvic inflammatory disease by screening for cervical chlamydial infection. *N Engl J Med* 1996;34(21):1362–6.

9. Division of STD Prevention. *Prevention of Genital HPV Infection and Sequelae: Report of an External Consultants' Meeting.* National Center for HIV, STD, and TB Prevention, Centers for Disease Control and Prevention, Atlanta, December 1999.

10. Handsfield HH, Stone KM, Wasserheit JN. Prevention agenda for genital herpes. *Sexually Transmitted Diseases* 1999;26:228–231.

11. Centers for Disease Control. Guidelines for prevention and control of congenital syphilis. *MMWR* 1988;37(No.S-1).

12. U.S. Department of Health and Human Services. *Healthy People 2010*. 2nd ed. With Understanding and Improving Health and Objectives for Improving Health. 2 vols. Washington, DC: U.S. Government Printing Office, November 2000.

13. Centers for Disease Control and Prevention. Congenital syphilis—United States, 2002. *MMWR* 2004;53:716–9.

14. Rolfs RT, Galaid EI, Zaidi AA. Pelvic inflammatory disease: trends in hospitalization and office visits, 1979 through 1988. *Am J Obstet Gynecol* 1992;166:983–90.

15. Sutton MY, Sternberg M, Zaidi A, St. Louis ME, Markowitz LE. Trends in pelvic inflammatory disease hospital discharges and ambulatory visits, United States, 1985–2001. *Sexually Transmitted Diseases* 2005;32(12)778–784.

16. Centers for Disease Control and Prevention. Ectopic pregnancy in the United States, 1990–1992. *MMWR* 1995;44:46–8.

What Are U.S. Women's HIV Prevention Needs?

"What Are U.S. Women's HIV Prevention Needs?" reprinted with permission from the Center for AIDS Prevention Studies, University of California – San Francisco. © 2008 University of California – San Francisco.

Are women at risk?

Yes. HIV is taking an increasing toll on women and girls in the U.S. In 1985, women comprised 8% of all AIDS cases in the U.S., while by 2005, women made up 27% of all AIDS cases.[1]

In 2005, women accounted for 30% of all new HIV infections. Of these, 60% occurred among African Americans, 19% among Whites, 19% among Hispanics, and 1% each among Asian/Pacific Islanders and American Indian/Alaska Natives.[2]

Who are women most affected by HIV?

African American and Hispanic women in particular are disproportionately affected by HIV/AIDS. Although African American and Hispanic women comprise only 23% of the total female population in the U.S., in 2005 they accounted for 79% of all new HIV infections (African American women: 60%, Hispanic women: 19%).[2,3] Accordingly, in 2004 HIV infection was the leading cause of death for Black women (including African American women) aged 25–34 years.[3]

Younger women are also affected by HIV/AIDS. In recent years, the largest number of HIV/AIDS diagnoses among women occurred in women 15–39 years old.[3] In 2005, young women represented 28% of AIDS cases among young men and women aged 20–24.[1]

What places women at risk?

Most women are infected with HIV through heterosexual contact, especially women with injection drug using partners. In 2005, 80% of all new infections in women were from heterosexual contact.[3] Women are more likely than men to acquire HIV via sexual intercourse, due to greater exposed surface area in the female genital tract.[4]

Injection and non-injection drug use places women at an increased risk for HIV and is strongly linked to unsafe sexual practices. Approximately 20% of new HIV cases in women are related to injection drug use.[3] Women who use crack cocaine may also be at high risk of sexual transmission of HIV, particularly if they sell or trade sex for drugs.[5]

Sexually transmitted infections (STIs) other than HIV can increase the likelihood of getting or transmitting HIV.[6] In the U.S., chlamydia and gonorrhea (both asymptomatic) are the most commonly reported STIs, with highest rates in women of color and young women and adolescents.[7]

Sexual abuse (both childhood and adult) and domestic violence play a substantial role in placing women at risk for HIV infection. In the U.S., annually 2.1 million women are raped and 4 million become victims of domestic violence; of these women, more than 10,000 rape victims and 79,000 violence victims require hospitalization.[8] Women who report early and chronic sexual abuse are seven times more likely to engage in HIV-related risk behaviors compared to women without trauma history.[9]

Women disproportionately suffer from poverty, in particular women of color who are affected by HIV. Because of this, women are less likely than men to have health insurance and access to quality healthcare or prevention services. Approximately two-thirds of women with HIV in the U.S. have an annual income of less than $10,000.[10] Poverty can increase HIV risks such as exchanging sex for money, shelter, or drugs. In a survey of young and low-income women in California, women who reported sex work were more likely to have syphilis, herpes, hepatitis C, and a history of sexual abuse.[11]

Abuse, violence, and poverty can all lessen a woman's power to negotiate condom use or choose safer partners. They also can lead to psychological distress, such as depression, anxiety, and post-traumatic stress disorder (PTSD).[9]

Having relationships that overlap in time (concurrent partners) can increase women's risk of HIV transmission. Concurrency is more likely to occur among women who are not married, are young adults, and are poor.[12]

What can help?

Involving male partners: For women to protect themselves from HIV, they must not only rely on their own skills, attitudes, and behaviors regarding condom use, but also on those of their male partner. Often, men and women in relationships may find intimacy to be more important than protection against HIV. Involving women's partners in HIV prevention programs can help strengthen intimacy and trust and improve sexual communication and negotiation, including asking about past and current partners.

Support from other women: Many prevention programs for women offer groups to reduce women's isolation and allow women to support each other and normalize safer behaviors. Greater social support can increase self esteem and allow women to make healthier choices. A program in Washington, DC, helped build support and empowerment for HIV+ African American women by holding educational groups during shared meals and providing small gifts (along with condoms) as incentives or thank-yous.[13]

Help with non-HIV factors: Women at risk for HIV face many behavioral and structural challenges beyond HIV: poverty and economic strain, unemployment, violence and unhealthy gender relations, migration, STIs, drug use, and caring for children and family members.[14] HIV prevention programs for women should provide transportation, child care, nutritious food, and compensation such as money, phone or store cards, or gift packs. Programs should provide up-to-date referrals for employment, housing, medical care and mental health services, trauma, abuse, and depression.

What is being done?

Currently 17 women-specific interventions exist that have been approved by the CDC as best evidence or promising evidence or are part of the Diffusion of Effective Behavioral Interventions (DEBI) project: CHOICES, Communal Effectance-AIDS Prevention, Female and Culturally Specific Negotiation, Project FIO, Project SAFE, RAPP, SiHLE, SISTA, Sisters Saving Sisters, Sister to Sister, WHP, WiLLOW, Women's Co-op, Condom Promotion, Insights, Safer Sex, and SEPA.[15]

The Women's Leadership and Community Planning project in San Francisco offered a two-day training for women with HIV in California who want to take greater leadership roles in state Planning Councils. At the training, women network with each other, as well as learn skills in public speaking, decision-making, and conflict management. Women stay in touch through monthly conference calls. After the first training, 6 of 13 women moved into leadership positions on their local or state Councils.[16]

Respeto/Proteger: Respecting and Protecting our Relationships is an HIV prevention program for Latino teen mothers and fathers in Los Angeles, CA. Developed and tested with a community agency and academic researchers, the program recognizes risks young women face, including poverty, drug and alcohol use, history of STIs, and physical or sexual abuse. The six-session intervention focuses on healing the wounded spirit and builds on feelings of maternal and paternal protectiveness using cultural and traditional teachings.[17]

What needs to be done?

Because women are more likely to get HIV from their male partners, programs that target men (especially injection drug users) will have a beneficial impact on women. Needle exchange and drug treatment strategies are critical. Public health agencies need to raise awareness about sexual abuse and domestic violence to not only help men and women develop the skills to prevent it, but also to curb its effect on the HIV epidemic. HIV testing campaigns that target women and women-friendly testing sites are also needed.

Behavioral and structural HIV prevention interventions for women continue to be necessary, given the lack of evidence from biomedical interventions (microbicides, vaccines).[18] However, research needs to continue on how women can protect themselves with an accessible, affordable, comfortable, and discrete tool for safer sex.

Although research has highlighted the subpopulations of women most affected by HIV/AIDS, it is even more important to translate and materialize study findings into tangible public health programs and effective policies. Interventions that address sexuality, family, culture, empowerment, self-esteem, and negotiating skills, as well as interventions located in varying community settings, are especially valuable.

Says who?

1. Kaiser Family Foundation. Women and HIV/AIDS in the United States. Policy Fact Sheet. July 2007.

2. Centers for Disease Control and Prevention. Cases of HIV infection and AIDS in the United States and Dependent Areas, 2005. HIV/AIDS Surveillance Report. 2007;17.

3. Centers for Disease Control and Prevention. HIV/AIDS fact sheet: HIV/AIDS among women. June 2007.

4. National Institute of Allergy and Infectious Diseases at National Institutes of Health. Research on HIV infection in women. 2006.

5. Theall KP, Sterk CE, Elifson KW, et al. Factors associated with positive HIV serostatus among women who use drugs: continued evidence for expanding factors of influence. Public Health Reports. 2003;118:415–424.

6. Sangani P, Rutherford G, Wilkinson D. Population-based interventions for reducing sexually transmitted infections, including HIV infection. Cochrane Database of Systematic Reviews. 2004; 2:CD001220.

7. Weinstock H, Berman S, Cates W. Sexually transmitted diseases among American youth: incidence and prevalence estimates, 2000. *Perspectives in Sexual and Reproductive Health*. 2004;36:6–10.

8. Koenig LJ, Moore J. Women, violence, and HIV: A critical evaluation with implications for HIV services. *Maternal and Child Health Journal*. 2000;4:103–109.

9. Wyatt GE, Myers HF, Loeb TB. Women, trauma, and HIV: an overview. *AIDS and Behavior*. 2004;8:401–403.

10. Bozzette SA, Berry SH, Duan N, et al. The care of HIV-infected adults in the United States. HIV Cost and Services Utilization Study Consortium. *New England Journal of Medicine*. 1998;339:1897–1904.

11. Cohan DL, Kim A, Ruiz J, et al. Health indicators among low income women who report a history of sex work: the population based Northern California Young Women's Survey. *Sexually Transmitted Infections*. 2005;81:428–433.

12. Adimora AA, Schoenbach VJ, Bonas DM, et al. Concurrent sexual partnerships among women in the United States. *Epidemiology*. 2002;13:320–327.

13. Prosper! The Women's Collective, Washington DC.

14. Dworkin SL, Ehrhardt AA. Going beyond "ABC" to include "GEM": critical reflections on progress in the HIV/AIDS epidemic. *American Journal of Public Health*. 2007;97:13–18.

15. Centers for Disease Control and Prevention. Updated Compendium of Evidence-Based Interventions, 2007.

16. Women's Leadership and Community Planning project, CompassPoint, San Francisco, CA.

17. Lesser J, Koniak-Griffin D, Gonzalez-Figueroa E, et al. Childhood abuse history and risk behaviors among teen parents in a culturally rooted, couple-focused HIV prevention program. *Journal of the Association of Nurses in AIDS Care*. 2007;18:18–27.

18. Landovitz RJ. Recent efforts in biomedical prevention of HIV. *Topics in HIV Medicine*. 2007;15:99–103.

Section 4.3

STDs in Children and Child Sexual Abuse

"Sexually Transmitted Diseases and Child Sexual Abuse: Key Facts," U.S. Department of Justice (www.ncjrs.gov), December 2002. Reviewed in January 2009 by Dr. David A. Cooke, M.D., Diplomate, American Board of Internal Medicine.

When presented with a child with an STD, law enforcement officials must attempt to determine absolutely if the infection was associated with sexual contact and, for the purposes of prosecution, whether appropriate diagnostic methods were used. The following facts should be kept in mind:

- STDs may be transmitted during sexual assault.
- Multiple episodes of abuse increase the risk of STD infection, probably by increasing the number of contacts with an infected individual, and rates of infection also vary by the type of assault. For example, vaginal or rectal penetration is more likely to lead to detectable STD infection than fondling.
- Sexual assault is a violent crime that affects children of all ages, including infants.
- The majority of children who are sexually abused will have no physical complaints related either to trauma or STD infection. Most sexually abused children do not indicate that they have genital pain or problems.
- In children the isolation of a sexually transmitted organism may be the first indication that abuse has occurred.
- In most cases, the site of infection is consistent with a child's history of assault.
- Although the presence of a sexually transmissible agent in a child over the age of one month is suggestive of sexual abuse, exceptions do exist. Rectal and genital chlamydia infections in young children may be due to a persistent perinatally acquired infection, which may last for up to three years.

- The incidence and prevalence of sexual abuse in children are difficult to estimate.
- Most sexual abuse in childhood escapes detection.
- Patterns of childhood sexual abuse appear to depend on the sex and age of the victim.
- Between 80 and 90% of sexually abused children are female (average age: seven to eight years).
- Between 75 and 85% of sexually abused children were abused by a male assailant, an adult or minor known to the child. This individual is most likely a family member such as the father, stepfather, mother's boyfriend, or an uncle or other male relative.
- Victims of unknown assailants tend to be older than children who are sexually abused by someone they know and are usually only subjected to a single episode of abuse.
- Sexual abuse by family members or acquaintances usually involves multiple episodes over periods ranging from one week to years.
- Most victims describe a single type of sexual activity, but over 20% have experienced more than one type of forced sexual act. Vaginal penetration has been reported to occur in approximately one-half and anal penetration in one-third of female victims of sexual abuse.
- Over 50% of male victims of sexual abuse have experienced anal penetration.
- Other types of sexual activity, including oral-genital contact and fondling, occur in 20 to 50% of victims of sexual abuse.
- Children who are sexually abused by known assailants usually experience less physical trauma, including genital trauma, than victims of assaults by strangers because such trauma might arouse suspicion that abuse is occurring.

Section 4.4

Child Sexual Abuse and Long-Term HIV Prevention

"How Does Childhood Sexual Abuse Affect HIV Prevention?" reprinted with permission from the Center for AIDS Prevention Studies, University of California – San Francisco. © 2003 University of California – San Francisco. Reviewed in January 2009 by Dr. David A. Cooke, M.D., Diplomate, American Board of Internal Medicine.

What is childhood sexual abuse?

Childhood sexual abuse (CSA) may be defined in many ways, but this section refers to unwanted sexual body contact prior to age 18, the age of consent to engage in sex. CSA is a painful experience on many levels that can have a profound and devastating effect on later physiological, psychosocial, and emotional development.

CSA experiences can vary with respect to duration (multiple experiences with the same perpetrator), degree of force/coercion or degree of physical intrusion (from fondling to digital penetration to attempted or completed oral, anal, or vaginal sex). The identity of the perpetrator—ranging from a stranger to a trusted figure or family member—may also impact the long-term consequences for individuals. To distinguish CSA from exploratory sexual experimentation, the contact should be unwanted/coerced or there should be a clear power difference between the victim and perpetrator, often defined as the perpetrator being at least five years older than the victim.

Many more children are sexually abused than are reported to authorities.[1] Estimates of the prevalence of CSA in the U.S. are about 33% for females under the age of 18 and 10% in males under 18 years of age.[2] Men are significantly less likely than women to report CSA when it occurs.[3]

CSA is more likely to occur in families under duress. Children are at risk for CSA in families that experience stress, poverty, violence, and substance abuse and whose parents and relatives have histories of CSA.

Does CSA affect HIV risk?

Yes. Because childhood and early adolescence are critical times in a person's sexual, social, and personal development, CSA can distort survivors' physical, mental, and sexual images of themselves. These distortions, combined with coping mechanisms adopted to offset the trauma of CSA, can lead CSA survivors into high-risk sexual and drug-using behaviors that increase the likelihood of HIV infection.[4]

Persons who experience CSA may feel powerless over their sexuality and sexual communication and decision-making as adults because they were not given the opportunity to make their own decisions about their sexuality as children or adolescents. As a result, they may engage in more high-risk sexual behavior, be unable to refuse sexually aggressive partners, and have less sexual satisfaction in relationships.

CSA survivors may have difficulties forming attachments and long term relationships and may dissociate from their feelings, resulting in having multiple sexual partners, "one night stands," and short-term sexual relationships. Adults who perceive positive aspects of their own CSA (such as gaining attention) may also use sex as a soothing or comforting strategy, which can lead to promiscuity and compulsive sexual patterns.[5]

The effects of CSA may be different for adult men and women. Female survivors of CSA may have lower condom self-efficacy with partners, use condoms less frequently, exhibit more sexual passivity, and attract or be attracted to overly controlling partners.[6] Male survivors of CSA may experience higher levels of eroticism, exhibit aggressive, hostile behavior, and victimize others.[7]

Adults with CSA histories may use dissociation and other coping efforts to avoid negative thoughts, emotions, and memories associated with the abuse. One of the most common dissociation methods is alcohol and drug abuse. A study of men and women with a history of substance abuse found that 34% had experienced CSA. CSA survivors with substance abuse problems were more likely than substance abusers who had not experienced CSA to exchange sex for money or drugs, have an HIV+ or high-risk partner, and not use condoms.[8]

Sexual revictimization can also influence high-risk sexual behavior. One study of African American and white women found that CSA survivors who experience revictimization as adults had more unintended pregnancies, abortions, STDs, and high-risk sexual behaviors than those who experienced only CSA.[9]

What's being done?

There are many resources for CSA survivors, but few programs exist to reduce HIV-related sexual and drug-using risk behaviors and increase psychological well being. Most of these programs focus on women; there are even fewer programs for male CSA survivors.

Good-Touch/Bad-Touch is a comprehensive child abuse prevention intervention designed for pre-school and kindergarten through sixth grade students. The program uses a variety of materials to teach children prevention skills including personal body safety rules, what abuse is, and what action to take if threatened.[10]

The Children's Medical Center in Dallas, TX, provides HIV/STD prevention for young female sexual abuse victims at a child abuse clinic. Adolescent females between 12 and 16 years old receive one-on-one evaluation and personalized education from an adolescent-focused HIV/STD counselor. Providing sensitive counseling close to the time of recognition of abuse can be a good method for prevention education.[11]

At Stanford University, CA, a trauma-focused group therapy intervention seeks to reduce HIV risk behavior and revictimization among adult women survivors of CSA. The groups focus on survivors' memories of CSA to see if this helps increase safer behaviors and reduce stress. The women also receive case management.[12]

The Visiting Nurse Service of New York offers comprehensive in-home services to HIV-infected families. The children in these families are at high risk for repeating the histories and behaviors of their parents, including HIV infection, substance abuse, sexual abuse, and mental illness. The program provides home-based interventions that include play therapy, health and safe sex education, family and individual counseling, relapse prevention for the parent, and drug awareness and prevention for the children. Helping the child deal with anger and resentment towards the parent lessens the likelihood that their anger will be displaced on themselves, thus repeating the behavior of the parent. Supporting each family member is key to breaking the cycle of HIV and abuse in these families.[13]

At the University of California, Los Angeles, and King-Drew University, CA, a psychoeducational intervention aims to increase healthy behavior and decrease HIV risk behaviors in HIV+ women with histories of CSA. Women are taught communication and problem-solving tools and link CSA experiences to past and current areas of risk.[14]

What needs to be done?

Although dealing with CSA may seem like a daunting task for many HIV prevention programs, there are a variety of usable approaches to address CSA in adults. Programs can include questions on abuse during routine client screening, reassess clients over time, provide basic education on the effects of CSA, and offer referrals for substance abuse and mental health services. Program staff need basic training and support to help cope with the effects of CSA counseling and the relative high prevalence in certain populations.[15]

Persons who are likely to interact with CSA survivors such as medical and other health professionals, religious and peer counselors, including alcohol, substance abuse and rape counselors, and probation officers need to be educated on the effects of CSA on sexual and drug risk behaviors. They also need training on how to recognize symptoms of CSA and how to address these issues or provide appropriate referrals for treatment.

Professionals should look beyond CSA symptoms and inquire about other childhood experiences that may have been problematic. CSA survivors often are forced to contend with other types of abuse and a dysfunctional family environment. A poor family environment may set the tone for abuse to occur and leave the survivor with little support to cope with the experience.

Says who?

1. Green AH. Overview of child sexual abuse. In SJ Kaplan (ed.), Family violence: A clinical and legal guide. Washington, DC: American Psychiatric Press. 1996;73–104.

2. Finkelhor D. The international epidemiology of child sexual abuse. *Child Abuse & Neglect*. 1994;18:409–417.

3. Roesler TA, McKenzie N. Effects of childhood trauma on psychological functioning in adults sexually abused as children. *Journal of Nervous and Mental Disease*. 1994;182:145–150.

4. Prillo KM, Freeman RC, Collier C, et al. Association between early sexual abuse and adult HIV-risky behaviors among community-recruited women. *Child Abuse & Neglect*. 2001; 25:335–346.

5. Paul J. Understanding childhood sexual abuse as a predictor of sexual risk-taking among men who have sex with men: The

Urban Men's Health Study. *Child Abuse & Neglect.* 2001;125:557–584.

6. Watkins B, Bentovim A. The sexual abuse of male children and adolescents: a review of current research. *Journal of Child Psychology & Psychiatry & Allied Disciplines*. 1992;33: 197–248.

7. Wyatt GE, Guthrie D, Notgrass CM. Differential effects of women's child sexual abuse and subsequent revictimization. *Journal of Consulting and Clinical Psychology*. 1992;60:167–173.

8. Morrill AC, Kasten L, Urato M, et al. Abuse, addiction and depression as pathways to sexual risk in women and men with a history of substance use. *Journal of Substance Abuse*. 2001;13: 169–184.

9. Wyatt GE, Myers HF, Williams JK, et al. Does a history of trauma contribute to HIV risk for women of color? Implications for prevention and policy. *American Journal of Public Health*. 2002;92:1–7.

10. Harvey P, Forehand R, Brown C, et al. The prevention of sexual abuse: Examination of the effectiveness of a program with kindergarten-age children. *Behavior Therapy*. 1988;19:429–435.

11. Squires J, Persaud DI, Graper JK. HIV and STD prevention counseling for adolescent girls seen in a child abuse clinic. Presented at the 14th International AIDS Conference, Barcelona, Spain. 2002. Abst # TuPeF5249.

12. Group Interventions to Prevent HIV in High Risk Women. www.med.stanford.edu/school/ Psychiatry/PSTreatLab/ TraumaStudy.php

13. Mills R, Samuels KD, Bob-Semple N, et al. Breaking the cycle: multigenerational dysfunction in families affected with HIV/ AIDS. Presented at the 14th International AIDS Conference, Barcelona, Spain. 2002. Abst #. ThPeE7828.

14. Wyatt GE, Myers H, Longshore D, et al. Examining the effects of trauma on HIV risk reduction: the women's health intervention. Presented at the International Conference on AIDS, Barcelona, Spain. 2002. Abst# WePeF6853.

15. Paul JP. Coerced childhood sexual episodes and adult HIV prevention. *FOCUS*. 2003;18:1–4.

Chapter 5

STDs in Teens

Chapter Contents

Section 5.1

Information for Teens about STDs

Sexually transmitted diseases (also known as STDs and once called venereal diseases or VD) are infectious diseases that spread from person to person through intimate contact. STDs can affect guys and girls of all ages and backgrounds who are having sex—it doesn't matter if they're rich or poor.

Unfortunately, STDs have become common among teens. Because teens are more at risk for getting some STDs, it's important to learn what you can do to protect yourself.

STDs are more than just an embarrassment. They're a serious health problem. If untreated, some STDs can cause permanent damage, such as infertility (the inability to have a baby) and even death (in the case of HIV/AIDS).

How STDs Spread

One reason STDs spread is because people think they need to have sexual intercourse to become infected. That's wrong. A person can get some STDs, like herpes or genital warts, through skin-to-skin contact with an infected area or sore. Another myth about STDs is that you can't get them if you have oral or anal sex. That's also wrong because the viruses or bacteria that cause STDs can enter the body through tiny cuts or tears in the mouth and anus, as well as the genitals.

STDs also spread easily because you can't tell whether someone has an infection. In fact, some people with STDs don't even know that they have them. These people are in danger of passing an infection on to their sex partners without even realizing it.

Some of the things that increase a person's chances of getting an STD are:

- Sexual activity at a young age. The younger a person starts having sex, the greater his or her chances of becoming infected with an STD.
- Lots of sex partners. People who have sexual contact—not just intercourse, but any form of intimate activity—with many different partners are more at risk than those who stay with the same partner.
- Unprotected sex. Latex condoms are the only form of birth control that reduce your risk of getting an STD. Spermicides, diaphragms, and other birth control methods may help prevent pregnancy, but they don't protect a person against STDs.

Preventing and Treating STDs

As with many other diseases, prevention is key. It's much easier to prevent STDs than to treat them. The only way to completely prevent STDs is to abstain from all types of sexual contact. If someone is going to have sex, the best way to reduce the chance of getting an STD is by using a condom.

People who are considering having sex should get regular gynecological or male genital examinations. There are two reasons for this. First, these exams give doctors a chance to teach people about STDs and protecting themselves. And second, regular exams give doctors more opportunities to check for STDs while they're still in their earliest, most treatable stage.

In order for these exams and visits to the doctor to be helpful, people need to tell their doctors if they are thinking about having sex or if they have already started having sex. This is true for all types of sex—oral, vaginal, and anal.

Don't let embarrassment at the thought of having an STD keep you from seeking medical attention. Waiting to see a doctor may allow a disease to progress and cause more damage. If you think you may have an STD, or if you have had a partner who may have an STD, you should see a doctor right away.

If you don't have a doctor or prefer not to see your family doctor, you may be able to find a local clinic in your area where you can get an exam confidentially. Some national and local organizations operate STD hotlines staffed by trained specialists who can answer your questions and provide referrals. Calls to these hotlines are confidential. One hotline you can call for information is the National STD Hotline at 800-227-8922.

Not all infections in the genitals are caused by STDs. Sometimes people can get symptoms that seem very like those of STDs, even though they've never had sex. For girls, a yeast infection can easily be confused with an STD. Guys may worry about bumps on the penis that turn out to be pimples or irritated hair follicles. That's why it's important to see a doctor if you ever have questions about your sexual health.

Section 5.2

Statistics on STDs in Youth

This section begins with "Sexual Health of Adolescents and Young Adults in the United States," September 2008. This information was reprinted with permission from the Henry J. Kaiser Family Foundation. The Kaiser Family Foundation is a non-profit private operating foundation, based in Menlo Park, California, dedicated to producing and communicating the best possible information, research, and analysis on health issues. "Nationally Representative CDC Study Finds One in Four Teenage Girls Has a Sexually Transmitted Disease," is reprinted from Centers for Disease Control and Prevention (www.cdc.gov), April 7, 2008.

Sexual Health of Adolescents and Young Adults in the United States

Following a decade of decline, the share of adolescents engaging in sexual activity has leveled off in recent years. Recent data indicate that sexually transmitted infection rates are very high for young adults and that teen birth rates may be trending upwards after years of steady decline. This section provides key data on teen and young adult sexual activity rates, pregnancy and birth rates, contraceptive use, and prevalence of sexually transmitted infections. It also discusses some of the central policies that affect access to reproductive health care services for youth.

Sexual Activity

- Nearly half (48%) of all high school students in 2007 reported ever having had sexual intercourse, a decline from 54% in 1991. Males (50%) are slightly more likely than females (46%) to report having had sex.[1] The median age at first intercourse is 16.9 years for boys and 17.4 years for girls.[2]
- There are racial/ethnic differences in sexual activity rates. African American high school students are more likely to have had intercourse (67%) compared to White (44%) and Hispanic students (52%). 16% of African American high school students and 8% of Latino students initiated sex before age 13 compared to 4% of White students.[1]
- Many young adults consider oral sex to be less risky in terms of health, social, and emotional consequences than vaginal sex.[3] Over half of males (55%) and females (54%) ages 15 to 19 report having had oral sex with someone of the opposite sex. About 24% of males and 22% of females ages 15–19 had oral sex but not vaginal intercourse.[4]
- Approximately one in 10 males and females ages 15 to 19 have engaged in anal sex with someone of the opposite sex;[4] and about 5% of males ages 15 to 19 have had oral or anal sex with a male.[5]
- The percentage of high school students who report having had four or more sexual partners declined from 18% in 1995 to 15% in 2007. Males (18%) are more likely than females (12%) to report having had four or more sexual partners.[1]
- Among those ages 20 to 24, males have a higher average number of partners (3.8) than females (2.8). Men in this age group are also more likely (30%) than women (21%) to report having had seven or more sexual partners.[5]
- Almost one quarter (23%) of currently sexually active high school students reported using alcohol or drugs during their most recent sexual encounter, with males having a higher percentage (28%) compared to females (18%).[1]
- One in 10 high school students reported having experienced dating violence. Nine percent of students have been physically forced to have sexual intercourse, with females (11%) more likely than males (5%) to report this experience.[1]

- The average age of first marriage continues to rise, reaching 25.6 for women and 27.5 for men in 2007.[6]

Pregnancy

- Despite the decline in teen pregnancy rates over the past decade, the U.S. continues to have one of the highest teen pregnancy, birth, and abortion rates in the developed world.[7]
- The teen pregnancy rate fell from 77 pregnancies per 1,000 girls ages 15 to 17 in 1990 to 42 in 2004. The rate also dropped for girls ages 18 to 19 from 168 pregnancies per 1,000 girls in 1990 to 119 in 2004.[8]
- However, the teen birth rate increased 3% between 2005 and 2006 to 42 births per 1,000 girls (15–19 years old), the first increase following a long-term decline.[9]
- By age 20, 32% of Latinas, 24% of African American women, and 21% of Native Americans have had a birth, compared to 11% of White and 7% of Asian American women.[10]
- Of the approximately 729,000 pregnancies of girls 15 to 19 years old in 2004, 57% ended in live births, 27% in induced abortions, and 16% in fetal losses.[8]
- The teen abortion rate has been falling.[11] The abortion rate for teens ages 15 to 19 and young adults ages 20 to 24 years old was 19.8 and 39.9 per 1,000 women, respectively, in 2004. About 17% of women having abortions in the U.S. are teens and 33% are between the ages of 20 and 24.[12]
- Thirty-five states require parental involvement in a minor's decision to have an abortion, up from 18 states in 1991. Twenty-two of these states require parental consent, 11 require parental notification, and 2 require both.[13]
- In contrast, 35 states and DC allow a minor to obtain confidential prenatal care that includes regular medical visits and routine services for labor and delivery without parental consent or notification.[14] In 12 of these states, however, physicians can inform parents that their minor daughters are seeking or receiving prenatal care, if deemed in the best interest of the minor.

Contraceptive Use and Services

- In 2007, among the 35% of currently sexually active high school students, 62% reported using a condom the last time they had sexual intercourse, up from 57% in 1997.[1] African American students (67%) were more likely to report using condoms compared to White (60%) and Hispanic (61%) students. Males (69%) were more like to report condom use than females (55%).[1]

- Oral contraceptive use was much lower, with 16% of currently sexually active high school students reporting they or their partner had used birth control pills. White students (21%) were more likely to use birth control pills compared to African American (9%) and Hispanic (9%) students.[1]

- Using a dual method of a condom and hormonal contraceptive is becoming more prevalent for teenage females. The percentage of currently sexually active never-married females 15–19 years of age reporting use of dual methods rose from 8% in 1995 to 20% in 2002.[15]

- About one quarter of teen females and 18% of teen males used no method of contraception at first intercourse.[15] Research has shown that those who reported condom use at their sexual debut were more likely than those who did not use condoms to engage in subsequent protective behaviors.[16]

- Emergency contraception can prevent pregnancy when taken shortly after unprotected intercourse. This drug, sold as Plan B, remains a prescription-only drug for minors, but is available as an over-the-counter medication for those aged 18 and older.

- Health insurance coverage and the ability to pay directly for services influence teen access to contraceptive services. Older adolescents and young adults have the highest uninsured rate of any age group.[17] Approximately 29% of young adults 18–24 years old were uninsured and 13% were covered by Medicaid in 2006. One-third (32%) of young adults lived below the poverty level and an additional 23% were near-poor (100–199% federal poverty level).[18]

- The Federal Title X program funds confidential contraceptive services and STD screening and treatment for low-income teens and young adults by providing funding to approximately 4,600 clinics, public health departments, and hospitals.

- Currently, Medicaid provides over 6 in 10 public dollars for family planning services in the U.S.[19] Twenty-six states operate special Medicaid family-planning waiver programs that offer contraceptive services to individuals (mostly women) who otherwise would not qualify for Medicaid. Of those, 20 states provide these benefits to individuals based on income, with most states setting the income eligibility ceiling at or near 200% of poverty. Seventeen states extend their services to all teens.[20]

- Confidentiality is important for youth access to health care services. Twenty-one states and DC have enacted policies that explicitly allow all minors to consent to contraceptive services.[21]

- Currently, there are 1,700 school-based health centers in the country that provide on-site services including pregnancy testing, STD diagnosis and treatment, and HIV testing and counseling. Contraception is often provided only by referral.[22]

Sexually Transmitted Infections (STIs)

- Compared to older adults, sexually active adolescents and young adults are at higher risk for acquiring STIs, which is attributable to a combination of behavioral, biological, and cultural factors.[23]

- An estimated 9.1 million adolescents and young adults ages 15–24 were newly infected with a STI in 2000 (the most recent year for which data is available), which represented almost one-half of all new STI cases. The human papillomavirus (HPV) was the most common STI (51% of new infections), followed by trichomoniasis (21%) and chlamydia (16%).[24]

- An unpublished 2008 CDC study finds that among female adolescents ages 14 to 19, one in four (26%) either has HPV, chlamydia, HSV-2 infection, or trichomoniasis, with HPV accounting for the vast majority of infections. African American girls had a higher STI prevalence (48%) than Whites (20%) and Latinas (20%).[25]

- Despite the higher risk for acquiring STIs among youth, only one-third (31%) of sexually active teens ages 15 to 17 and half (53%) of sexually active young adults ages 18 to 24 say they have been tested for STDs.[26]

- In 2006, the Food and Drug Administration approved a new vaccine that protects against infection for certain strains of HPV associated with cervical cancer and genital warts. A CDC advisory committee has recommended that all girls be vaccinated at age 11 or 12, and that girls and women ages 13 to 26 be given a "catch-up" vaccination.[27] A recent CDC survey found that only 10% of women ages 18 to 26 had received the HPV vaccine as of summer 2007.[28]

HIV/AIDS

- The CDC estimates that almost 46,000 young people, ages 13 to 24, were living with HIV in the U.S. (in the 45 states and 5 dependent areas with confidential name-based HIV reporting) in 2006.[29] Women comprised 28% of these HIV/AIDS cases among 13- to 24-year-olds.[30]
- African American young adults are disproportionately affected by HIV infection, accounting for 60% of HIV/AIDS diagnoses in 13- to 24-year-olds in 2006.[30]
- More HIV infections occurred among adolescents and young adults 13–29 years old (34%) of new HIV infections than any

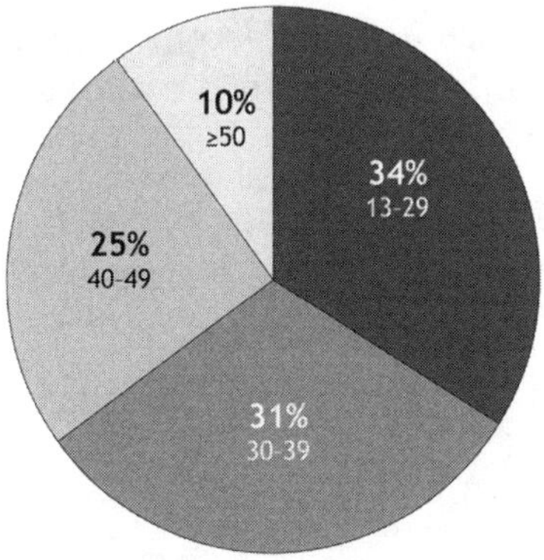

Total = 56,300 new HIV infections

Source: CDC. Estimates of new HIV infections in the United States. *CDC HIV/AIDS Facts*. 2008.

Figure 5.1. *Estimated New HIV Infections in the U.S., by Age, 2006*

other age group. Most young people with HIV/AIDS were infected by sexual transmission.[31]

- In 2006, 16% of young adults ages 18 to 24 reported that they had been tested for HIV in the past 12 months.[32]

References

1. CDC. Youth Risk Behavior Surveillance System—United States, 2007. *MMWR*, 57(SS-4). 2008.

2. Guttmacher Institute. *In Their Own Right: Addressing the Sexual and Reproductive Health Needs of American Men*. 2002.

3. Halpern-Felsher BL, Cornell JL, Kropp RY & Tschann JM. Oral versus vaginal sex among adolescents: Perceptions, attitudes, and behavior. *Pediatrics*, 115(4). 2005.

4. Lindberg LD, Jones R & Santelli JS. Non-coital sexual activities among adolescents. *Journal of Adolescent Health*, 43(3). 2008.

5. Mosher WD, Chandra A & Jones J. Sexual behavior and selected health measures: Men and women 15–44 years of age, United States, 2002. CDC Advance Data, No. 362. 2005.

6. U.S. Census Bureau. Estimated Median Age at First Marriage, by Sex: 1890 to the Present. 2007.

7. Singh S & Darroch JE. Adolescent pregnancy and childbearing: Levels and trends in developed countries. *Family Planning Perspectives*, 32(1). 1999.

8. Ventura SJ, Abma JC, Mosher WD & Henshaw SK. Estimated pregnancy rates by outcome for the United States, 1990–2004. CDC National Vital Statistics Reports, 56(15). 2008.

9. Hamilton BE, Martin JA & Ventura SJ. Births: Preliminary data for 2006. CDC National Vital Statistics Reports, 56(7). 2007.

10. National Campaign to Prevent Teen and Unplanned Pregnancy analysis of Martin JA, Hamilton BE et al. Births: Final data for 2005. CDC National Vital Statistics Reports, 56(6). 2007.

11. Jones RK, Darroch JE & Henshaw SK. Patterns in the socioeconomic characteristics of women obtaining abortions in

2000–2001. *Perspectives on Sexual and Reproductive Health*, 34(5). 2002.

12. Guttmacher Institute. Henshaw SK adjustments to Strauss LT et al. Abortion surveillance—United States, 2004. *MMWR*, 56(SS-9). 2007.

13. Guttmacher Institute. Parental involvement in minors' abortions. State Policies in Brief. 2008.

14. Guttmacher Institute. Minors' access to prenatal care. State Policies in Brief. 2008.

15. Abma JC, Martinez GM, Mosher WD, & Dawson BS. Teenagers in the United States: Sexual activity, contraceptive use, and childbearing, 2002. *Vital Health Statistics,* 23(24). 2004.

16. Shafii T, Stovel K & Holmes K. Association between condom use at sexual debut and subsequent sexual trajectories: A longitudinal study using biomarkers. *American Journal of Public Health,* 97(6). 2007.

17. Kaiser Commission on Medicaid and the Uninsured. Uninsured Young Adults: A Profile and Overview of Coverage Options. 2008.

18. Kaiser Family Foundation. Unpublished analysis of Urban Institute tabulations of 2007 ASEC Supplement to the CPS. 2008.

19. Gold RB. Stronger together: Medicaid, Title X bring different strengths to family planning effort. *Guttmacher Policy Review,* 10(2). 2007.

20. Guttmacher Institute. State Medicaid family planning eligibility expansions. State Policies in Brief. 2008.

21. Guttmacher Institute. Minors' access to contraceptive services. State Policies in Brief. 2008.

22. Santelli JS, Nystrom RJ, Brindis C et al. Reproductive health in school-based health centers: Findings from the 1998–99 census of school-based health centers. *Journal of Adolescent Health,* 32(6). 2003.

23. CDC. Sexually Transmitted Disease Surveillance. 2006.

24. Weinstock H, Berman S & Cates W. Sexually transmitted diseases among American youth: Incidence and prevalence

estimates, 2000. *Perspectives on Sexual and Reproductive Health,* 36(1). 2004.

25. CDC Press Release. Prevalence of sexually transmitted infections and bacterial vaginosis among female adolescents in the United States: data from the National Health and Nutritional Examination Survey (NHANES) 2003–2004. 2008.
26. Kaiser Family Foundation. National Survey of Adolescents and Young Adults. 2003.
27. CDC. Advisory Committee on Immunization Practices Provisional Recommendations for the Use of Quadrivalent HPV Vaccine. 2006.
28. CDC & National Foundation for Infectious Diseases. Adult Immunization News Conference. 2008.
29. CDC. HIV/AIDS Surveillance Report, 2006, 18. 2008.
30. Calculation based on CDC's HIV/AIDS Surveillance in Adolescents and Young Adults (Through 2006) Slide Series.
31. CDC. HIV/AIDS Surveillance in Adolescents and Young Adults (Through 2006) Slide Series.
32. CDC. Persons tested for HIV—United States, 2006. *MMWR.* 2008.

Nationally Representative CDC Study Finds One in Four Teenage Girls Has a Sexually Transmitted Disease

3.2 Million Female Adolescents Estimated to Have at Least One of the Most Common STDs

A CDC study released today estimates that one in four (26%) young women between the ages of 14 and 19 in the United States—or 3.2 million teenage girls—is infected with at least one of the most common sexually transmitted diseases (human papillomavirus (HPV), chlamydia, herpes simplex virus, and trichomoniasis). The study, presented at the 2008 National STD Prevention Conference, is the first to examine the combined national prevalence of common STDs among adolescent women in the United States, and provides the clearest picture to date of the overall STD burden in adolescent women.

Led by CDC's Sara Forhan, MD, MPH, the study also finds that African American teenage girls were most severely affected. Nearly half of the young African American women (48%) were infected with an STD, compared to 20% of young white women.

The two most common STDs overall were human papillomavirus, or HPV (18%), and chlamydia (4%). Data were based on an analysis of the 2003–2004 National Health and Nutrition Examination Survey.

"Today's data demonstrate the significant health risk STDs pose to millions of young women in this country every year," said Kevin Fenton, MD, director of CDC's National Center for HIV/AIDS, Viral Hepatitis, STD and TB Prevention. "Given that the health effects of STDs for women—from infertility to cervical cancer—are particularly severe, STD screening, vaccination, and other prevention strategies for sexually active women are among our highest public health priorities."

"High STD infection rates among young women, particularly young African American women, are clear signs that we must continue developing ways to reach those most at risk," said John M. Douglas, Jr., MD, director of CDC's Division of STD Prevention. "STD screening and early treatment can prevent some of the most devastating effects of untreated STDs."

CDC recommends annual chlamydia screening for sexually active women under the age of 25. CDC also recommends that girls and women between the ages of 11 and 26 who have not been vaccinated or who have not completed the full series of shots be fully vaccinated against HPV.

The study of STDs among teenage girls is one of several presented at the 2008 National STD Prevention Conference that highlights the significant burden of STDs among girls and women, and identifies creative prevention strategies for reducing the toll of STDs in the United States.

Contraceptive Services Represent Missed Opportunities for STD Screening, Prevention

Two other studies featured at the conference point to missed opportunities for STD testing, and underscore that it is critical for STD screening to be included in comprehensive reproductive health services for young women.

A study by CDC's Sherry L. Farr and colleagues found that while the majority of sexually active 15- to 24-year-old young women (82%) receive contraceptive or STD/HIV services, few receive both (39%). In addition, only 38% of a subset of young women who reported receiving contraceptive services associated with unprotected sex (e.g., pregnancy testing) also received STD/HIV counseling, testing, or treatment, which indicates that many women at high risk are not receiving necessary prevention services.

A separate study, by CDC's Shoshanna Handel and the New York City Department of Health and Mental Hygiene, examined STD screening rates among young women seeking emergency contraception, which would suggest recent unprotected sex. The study found that just 27% were screened for chlamydia or gonorrhea. A significant proportion of those women (12%) had a positive test result, highlighting the need for routine chlamydia and gonorrhea screening at emergency contraception visits.

Innovative Programs Provide Models for Effective STD Prevention

Other research from the conference highlighted creative programs that are effectively screening and treating people with STDs, and identifying those most at risk.

A CDC-funded confidential chlamydia screening program in high school–based health clinics in California resulted in high rates of screening among those seeking contraceptive or STD services (range: 85–94%). It also revealed significantly higher infection rates among African American women than white women (9.6% versus 1.7%).

A study by New York City health officials assessed the effectiveness of an express visit option, allowing patients at city clinics to be tested for STDs without a doctor's exam. Comparing data before and after express visits were routinely offered, researchers found that the express visit option made it possible for an additional 4,588 tests to be performed, and increased STD diagnoses by 17% (2,617 versus 2,231).

Section 5.3

Attitudes of Teens toward STDs and Sex

"National Survey of Adolescents and Young Adults: Sexual Health Knowledge, Attitudes, and Experiences," May 2003. This information was reprinted with permission from the Henry J. Kaiser Family Foundation. The Kaiser Family Foundation is a non-profit private operating foundation, based in Menlo Park, California, dedicated to producing and communicating the best possible information, research, and analysis on health issues.

Introduction

The past decade has produced an increased use of condoms among sexually active young people and a small but significant decline in teen birth rates. This good news is offset by the fact that 10% of girls between 15 and 19 become pregnant, nearly two-thirds of high school seniors have had sex, and an alarming percentage of sexually active adolescents and young adults engage in unsafe sexual behaviors. Nearly one in four sexually active young people contract a sexually transmitted disease every year, and one-half of all new HIV infections in this country occur among people under the age of 25.

These facts indicate that there is much more yet to be known about the sexual behavior of today's young people, their knowledge about sex and sexual health risks, and the social pressures and influences they experience around sexual issues. The Henry J. Kaiser Family Foundation's National Survey of Adolescents and Young Adults: Sexual Health Knowledge, Attitudes, and Experiences takes a new approach to studying the problems and choices that today's young people face by moving beyond standard questions about sexual behavior (e.g., "Are you sexually active? Do you practice safe sex?") and tapping directly into the minds of America's young people with detailed questions about their knowledge and attitudes toward sex and sexual health (e.g., "Do you feel pressure to have sex? Do you think condoms are effective in preventing STDs and HIV/AIDS?").

The survey builds on a nationally representative sample of more than 1,800 young people in three key age groups—young adolescents (ages 13–14), adolescents (ages 15–17), and young adults (ages 18–24)—and representative oversamples of racial and ethnic subgroups. Parents, educators, health professionals, policymakers, the media, and the public can use this survey as a comprehensive national index of what young people know about sex and decisions they are making about important sexual health issues so that we can effectively address the needs and concerns of a generation at risk. To keep the nation attuned to changing patterns in sexual knowledge, attitudes, and behavior among the nation's young people, this survey will be updated periodically.

The report's key findings reveal that young people are more concerned about sex and sexual health than any other health issues in their lives. Young people also feel great pressure to have sex, with a majority saying that while putting off sex may be a "nice idea, nobody really does."

Moreover, many young people are misinformed about the health risks associated with unprotected sexual activity. While three-fourths of sexually active adolescents engage in oral sex, one-fifth of adolescents are unaware that STDs can be transmitted through this activity. Many young people have misperceptions about the health risks associated with STDs and HIV/AIDS and have incomplete information on safer sex practices, the relative effectiveness of condoms versus other forms of birth control in preventing disease, and the frequency and availability of testing for STDs and HIV.

While America's teen birth rate has declined, a significant percentage of young people are still having unprotected sex and engaging in other dangerous risk behaviors. Three in five sexually active young people report that they or a partner have had a pregnancy scare, one in six say that sex without a condom once in a while is not a "big deal," and one in five say that they have had unprotected sex after drinking or taking drugs.

The survey reveals that young people want to know more about how to use condoms, how to recognize the signs of STD and HIV infection, what STD and HIV testing involves, and where they can go to get tested. Young people also want more instruction on communicating effectively with partners about sensitive sexual concerns and relationship issues.

Due to the sensitive nature of some questions—specifically those that ask participants to discuss their own sexual experiences—young adolescents did not participate in certain parts of the survey. The analysis reported here thus focuses on young people between the ages of 15 and 24, an age range that corresponds with higher rates of sexual activity. There is also a special section focusing on the knowledge and attitudes of young adolescents.

Summary of Key Findings

Sexual Issues Dominate the Concerns of Young People

More young people say that sexual health issues—namely STDs, HIV/AIDS, and unintended pregnancy—are "big concerns" for people their age than any other issue. And perhaps more importantly, four in five adolescents and young adults—including 79% of those who are not sexually active—say they are personally concerned about how sexual health issues may affect them.

Young People Report Considerable Pressure to Have Sex

Across the age spectrum, young people report considerable pressure to have sex. For both adolescents and young adults pressure to have sex is exceeded only by pressure to drink, and nearly a third of adolescents say that they have experienced pressure to have sex. These pressures are even greater among those who are sexually active, and adolescent males report experiencing more pressure to have sex than their female peers.

The pressures that young people feel in regard to sex may be reflected in the attitudes they hold toward sexual activity, what they report about their own sexual behavior, and the health risks they take. Three in five adolescents and young adults state that while delaying sex may be a "nice idea, nobody really does," and 9% of sexually active adolescents say that they were 13 or younger when they first had sexual intercourse.

A Third of Adolescents Have Engaged in Oral Sex, but One in Five Are Unaware That Oral Sex Can Transmit STDs

The survey also indicates that oral sex plays an important role in the sexual lives of America's young people and suggests that many adolescents and young adults are unaware of the serious health risks associated with this type of sexual contact. While a third of adolescents (including three-fourths of sexually active adolescents) say they have engaged in oral sex, one in five does not know that STD transmission can occur through oral sex and two in five considers oral sex to be "safer sex." About a quarter of sexually active adolescents also report engaging in oral sex as a strategy to avoid sexual intercourse. And more than two in five do not consider it to be as big of a deal as sexual intercourse.

Pregnancy Remains a Serious Concern for Young People and Many Have Faced Pregnancy Scares or Been Pregnant Themselves

Despite recent declines in teen birth rates, the report shows that pregnancy and pregnancy scares remain a big concern for adolescents and young adults. The survey data show that 7 in 10 sexually active young adults and 4 in 10 sexually active adolescents have had a pregnancy test or have had a partner who took a pregnancy test, and nearly two in five young adults and 8% of adolescents report that they or a partner have been pregnant. Furthermore, females were twice as likely as males in both age groups to report that they had faced a pregnancy.

Many Young People Remain Reluctant to Discuss Sexual Health Issues with Partners, Family, and Health Providers

The divergence in pregnancy reporting between females and males underscores the fact that many adolescents and young adults feel extremely uncomfortable talking about essential issues related to sex and their sexual health even though open discussions with partners, parents, and health care providers could yield great benefits for their personal health and emotional well-being. While a majority of adolescents and young adults report having discussions with their partners about contraception and their comfort level with specific types of sexual activity, fewer have engaged in dialogue about STDs and HIV/AIDS. Females are much more likely to take the lead in initiating dialogue with their male partners about a broad range of sexual issues, but it is important to note that a third of respondents say they have been in relationships where sexual activity has moved forward faster than they wanted.

Young People Report Alcohol and Drugs Often Play a Dangerous Role in Their Sex Lives

Another significant challenge to communication and decision making in regard to sex is the strong role that alcohol and drugs play in sexual activity. This report shows that four out of five adolescents believe that people their age usually drink or use drugs before having sex. It also reveals that almost third of young adults have "done more" sexually under the influence of alcohol and drugs than they planned while sober and more than one in five sexually active young people report having engaged in unprotected sex while intoxicated.

Many Young People Have Serious Misperceptions about STDs and HIV/AIDS

While three-quarters of adolescents and young adults say they know at least "something" about STDs and HIV/AIDS and one-quarter say they know "a lot," half of those surveyed did not know that 25% of sexually active young people contract an STD, and one-third were unaware that people their age account for 50% of all new HIV infections. And while most adolescents and young adults are aware that STDs can cause serious health problems, between one-fifth and three-fifths of those surveyed do not know the specific complications of certain diseases. There are also dangerous gaps in young people's knowledge of STD transmission; one-fifth of young people believe they would simply "know" if someone else had an STD even if they were not tested, and one-sixth believe that STD transmission can only occur when obvious symptoms are present.

A Surprisingly High Number of Young People Are Misinformed about Safer Sex

While 9 out of 10 adolescents and young adults regard sex with a condom as "safer sex," 71% consider sex with other forms of birth control safer sex despite the fact that many other contraceptive measures do not offer protection from STDs. Also, more than one-third regard oral sex as safer sex even though STDs can be transmitted through this activity. One-fifth consider "pulling out" prior to ejaculation or sex during a woman's menstrual cycle safer sex despite the fact that these methods do not provide adequate protection against either pregnancy or STD transmission.

Many Young People Mistakenly Believe That Testing for STDs and HIV Is a Standard Part of Routine Medical Exams and May Not Know They Are Infected

While half of sexually active young people say they have been tested for STDs and HIV, the virus that causes AIDS, 3 in 10 mistakenly believe these tests are a standard feature of routine medical exams. One in 10 young adults and 2% of adolescents disclosed that they had contracted an STD. These figures are significantly lower than national estimates for STD incidence among young people. While the gap in reporting may reflect discomfort with revealing personal information, it may also indicate that a significant number of young people are unaware that they have contracted an STD.

Many Young People Are Misinformed about the Relative Protection That Condoms and Other Birth-Control Measures Provide

Nine out of 10 sexually active adolescents report using birth control or protection at least most of the time and 70% say they use birth control or protective measures every time. However, a significant percentage of young people—one-fifth of adolescents and only slightly fewer young adults—believe that condoms are "not effective" in preventing the transmission of STDs and HIV/AIDS. Many young people are also seriously misinformed about the type of protection they receive from birth control pills. One in five young people believe that birth control pills offer protection from STDs and HIV/AIDS.

While Most Young People Agree That Sex without a Condom Is Risky, Many Young People See Sex without Condoms Occasionally as "Not a Big Deal"

Adolescents and young adults have some mixed feelings about the importance of using condoms. While more than three-quarters of those surveyed say that sex without a condom is not worth the risk, one-sixth believe that sex without out a condom once in a while is "not that big of a deal" and 1 in 10 say that "unless you have a lot of sexual partners you do not need to use condoms." Males are twice as likely as females to say that unprotected sex occasionally is no "big deal."

Most Young People Say That Using a Condom Is a Sign of Respect and Caring, but about Half Say That Suggesting Condom Use Can Raise Mistrust and Suspicion

While 9 out of 10 adolescents say that using condoms is a sign of respect, caring, and responsibility, about half of those surveyed also say that bringing up the subject of condoms can raise suspicions about one's own sexual history or suggest that one is suspicious of a partner's sexual history. The discomfort associated with talking about and buying condoms may also pose hurdles. More than a third of adolescents and young adults say that buying condoms is embarrassing and a similar number say that it is hard to "bring up" the subject of condoms.

When It Comes to Sex and Relationships Young People Say They Get Their Information from a Variety of Places Including Their Parents, Sex Education, Friends, and the Media

Among adolescents, the top three sources of information are sex education in school, friends, and parents. These sources are followed closely by media sources like television, the movies, magazines, and the Internet. For young adults, sex education plays a much less prominent role—possibly because many last had sex education sometime during their high school career. Young adults also stress the importance of friends, the media, and boyfriends and girlfriends as their most important sources of information.

Young People Express a Strong Desire for More Information about Sex and Sexual Health

More than three-quarters of adolescents and young adults express a need for more information about sexual health topics. They are especially concerned with how to recognize STDs and HIV/AIDS infection, what STD and HIV testing involves, and where they can go to get tested. Two in five young people also want more information on how to communicate more effectively with partners about sensitive sexual concerns and issues. And one-quarter of those surveyed say they need more information on how to use condoms.

While Young Adolescents (13- to 14-Year-Olds) Are Less Sexually Active, They Are Deeply Concerned about Relationships and Sexual Health Issues

The survey found that even among 13- and 14-year-olds—the majority of whom are not yet sexually active—there is strong concern about sex and relationships. Four in five say they are personally concerned about sexual health issues, and three-quarters say they have concerns about sexual violence or other physical violence in relationships.

Chapter 6

STDs in Minorities

Chapter Contents

Section 6.1

Rates of STDs among Minorities

This section includes "HIV/AIDS Policy Fact Sheet: Black Americans and HIV/AIDS," and "HIV/AIDS Policy Fact Sheet: Latinos and HIV/AIDS," October 2008. This information was reprinted with permission from the Henry J. Kaiser Family Foundation. The Kaiser Family Foundation is a non-profit private operating foundation, based in Menlo Park, California, dedicated to producing and communicating the best possible information, research, and analysis on health issues.

Black Americans and HIV/AIDS

Black Americans have been disproportionately affected by HIV/AIDS since the epidemic's beginning, and that disparity has deepened over time.[1,2] Blacks account for more new HIV infections, AIDS cases, people estimated to be living with HIV disease, and HIV-related deaths than any other racial/ethnic group in the U.S.[1,3,4,5,6] The epidemic has also had a disproportionate impact on Black women, youth,

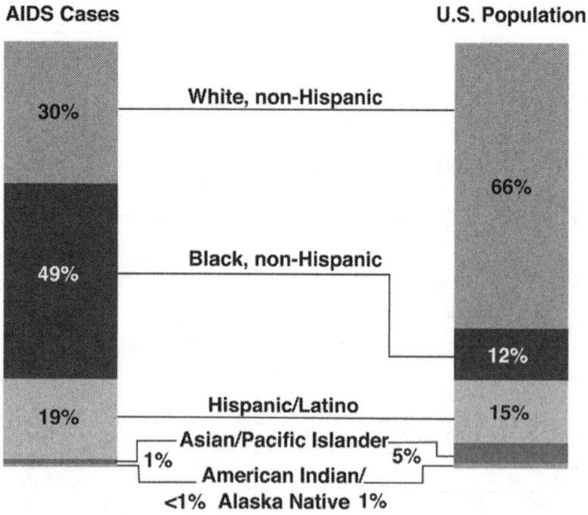

Figure 6.1. *AIDS Diagnoses & U.S. Population, by Race/Ethnicity, 2006[1,11,12]*

and men who have sex with men, and its impact varies across the country. Moreover, Blacks with HIV/AIDS may face greater barriers to accessing care than their white counterparts.[7,8,9] Today, there are approximately 1.1 million people living with HIV/AIDS in the U.S., including more than 500,000 who are Black.[5] Analysis of national household survey data found that 2% of Blacks in the U.S. were HIV positive, higher than any other group.[10]

Snapshot of the Epidemic

- Although Black Americans represent only 12% of the U.S. population,[12] they account for half of AIDS cases diagnosed in 2006.[1,11] Blacks also account for 45% of new HIV infections (24,900 of 56,300 total new infections) and 46% of people living with HIV disease in 2006.[3,4,5]

- The AIDS case rate per 100,000 among Black adults/adolescents was more than nine times that of whites in 2006.[1,13] The AIDS case rate for Black men (82.9) was the highest of any group, followed by Black women (40.4). By comparison, the rate among white men was 11.2.[1,13] The rate of new infections is also highest among Blacks and was seven times greater than the rate among whites in 2006.[3,4]

- HIV-related deaths and HIV death rates are highest among Blacks. Blacks accounted for 56% of deaths due to HIV in 2004[6] and their survival time after an AIDS diagnosis is lower on average than it is for most other racial/ethnic groups.[1] In 2004, Black men had the highest HIV death rate per 100,000 men aged 25–44 at 39.9; it was 5.5 for white men. The HIV death rate among Black women aged 25–44 was 23.1 compared to 1.3 for white women.[14]

- HIV was the fourth leading cause of death for Black men and third for Black women, aged 25–44, in 2005, ranking higher than for their respective counterparts in any other racial/ethnic group.[15]

Key Trends and Current Cases

- The number of new HIV infections per year among Blacks is down from its peak in the late 1980s, but has exceeded the number of infections among whites since that time; new infections have remained stable in recent years.[4]

- The share of AIDS diagnoses accounted for by Blacks has risen over time, rising from 25% of cases diagnosed in 1985 to 49% in 2006; in recent years, this share has remained relatively stable.[1,2]
- A recent analysis of 1999–2006 data from a national household survey found that 2% of Blacks in the U.S. (among those aged 18–49) were HIV positive, significantly higher than whites (0.23%). Also, the prevalence of HIV was higher among Black men (2.64%) than Black women (1.49%).[10]
- The number of Black Americans living with AIDS increased by 27% between 2002 and 2006, compared to a 19% increase among whites.[1]
- The number of deaths among both Blacks and whites with AIDS declined between 2002 and 2006, by 18% and 26%, respectively. Deaths among Hispanics remained stable.[1]

Women and Young People

- Black women account for the largest share of new HIV infections among women (61% in 2006) and the incidence rate among Black women is nearly 15 times the rate among white women.[16]

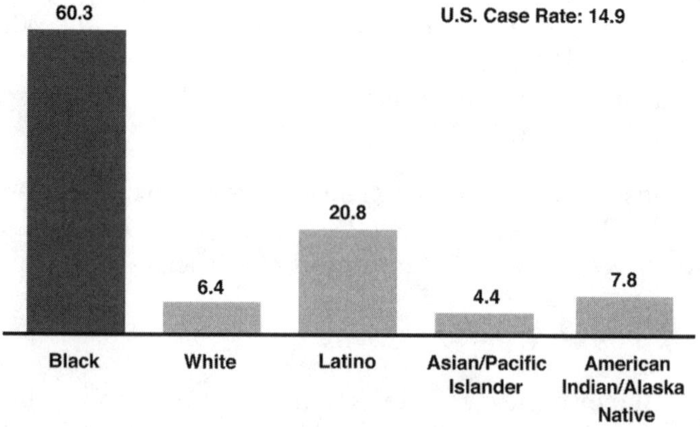

Figure 6.2. *AIDS Case Rate per 100,000 Population, by Race/Ethnicity, for Adults/Adolescents, 2006*[1,13]

- Black women account for the majority of new AIDS cases among women (66% in 2006); white and Latina women account for 17% and 16% of new AIDS cases, respectively.[1,11,13]
- Black women represent more than a third (36%) of AIDS cases diagnosed among Blacks (Black men and women combined) in 2006; by comparison, white women represent 15% of AIDS cases diagnosed among whites in 2006.[1,13]
- Although Black teens (aged 13–19) represent only 16% of U.S. teenagers, they account for 69% of new AIDS cases reported among teens in 2006.[17] A similar impact can be seen among Black children.[1]

Transmission

- HIV transmission patterns among Black men vary from those of white men. Although both groups are most likely to have been infected through sex with other men, white men are more likely to have been infected this way. Heterosexual transmission and injection drug use account for a greater share of infections among Black men than white men.[1,16,18]
- Black women are most likely to have been infected through heterosexual transmission, the most common transmission route for women overall. White women are somewhat more likely to have been infected through injection drug use than Black women.[1,16,18]
- Among men who have sex with men (MSM), Black MSM have been disproportionately affected. A recent study in five major U.S. cities found that 46% of Black MSM in the study were infected with HIV, compared to 21% of white MSM and 17% of Latino MSM. Knowledge of HIV status among those already infected was also very low, particularly among Black MSM.[19,20] In addition, newly infected Black MSM are younger than their white counterparts with those aged 13–29 accounting for 52% of new infections among Black MSM compared to 25% among whites.[16]

Geography

Although AIDS cases among Blacks have been reported throughout the country, the impact of the epidemic is not uniformly distributed:

- AIDS case rates per 100,000 among Blacks are highest in the eastern part of the U.S. The District of Columbia has the highest case rate for Blacks (277.5) in the country.[13,21]
- Over half (52%) of Blacks estimated to be living with AIDS and 58% of newly reported AIDS cases among Blacks in 2006 occurred in the South; by comparison, Blacks represent approximately 19% of the South's population.[21,22,23]
- Estimated AIDS prevalence among Blacks is clustered in a handful of states, with 10 states accounting for 71% of Blacks estimated to be living with AIDS in 2006. New York, Florida, and Georgia top the list.[21,22,23] Ten states also account for a majority of newly reported AIDS cases among Blacks (70% in 2006).[21,22]

Access to and Use of the Health Care System

- The HIV Cost and Services Utilization Study (HCSUS), the only nationally representative study of people with HIV/AIDS receiving regular or ongoing medical care for HIV infection, found that Blacks fared more poorly on several important measures of access and quality than whites; these differences diminished over time but were not completely eliminated.[7] HCSUS also found that Blacks were more likely to report postponing medical care because they lacked transportation, were too sick to go to the doctor, or had other competing needs.[8]
- A recent analysis of data from 2000–2002 in 11 HIV primary and specialty care sites in the U.S. found higher rates of hospitalization among Blacks with HIV/AIDS, but differences in outpatient utilization were not significant.[9]

Health Insurance

Having health insurance, either public or private, improves access to care. Insurance coverage of those with HIV/AIDS varies by race/ethnicity, as it does for the U.S. population overall.

- According to HCSUS, Blacks with HIV/AIDS were more likely to be publicly insured or uninsured than their white counterparts, with over half (59%) relying on Medicaid compared to 32% of whites. One fifth of Blacks with HIV/AIDS (22%) were uninsured compared to 17% of whites. Blacks were also much less likely to be privately insured than whites (14% compared to 44%).[24]

- Insurance status also varies at the time of HIV diagnosis. Analysis of data from 25 states between 1994 and 2000 found that Blacks were less likely than whites to have private coverage and more likely to be covered by Medicaid, or uninsured, at the time of their HIV diagnoses.[25]

HIV Testing

- Among the U.S. population overall, Blacks are more likely than whites to report ever having been tested for HIV (67% compared to 45%).[26]

- Among those who are HIV positive, CDC data indicate that 38% of Blacks were tested for HIV late in their illness—that is, diagnosed with AIDS within one year of testing positive for HIV (in those states/areas with HIV name reporting); by comparison, 35% of whites and 42% of Latinos.[1]

Concern about HIV/AIDS

- A recent survey found that Black Americans express concern about HIV/AIDS, and are the only racial/ethnic group to name it as the number one health problem in the U.S. However, half (49%) say the U.S. is "losing ground" on the domestic AIDS epidemic; half also say that HIV/AIDS is a more urgent problem in their community than it was a few years ago.[26]

- Personal concern about becoming infected with HIV is highest among Blacks, as is concern among Black parents about their children becoming infected. However, the proportion of Blacks saying they are personally concerned about becoming infected has declined since the mid-1990s.[26]

References

1. CDC, *HIV/AIDS Surveillance Report*, Vol. 18; 2008.
2. CDC, Special Data Request; 2006.
3. Hall HI et al., "Estimation of HIV Incidence in the United States." *JAMA*, Vol. 300, No. 5; August 2008.

4. CDC, Fact Sheet: Estimates of New HIV Infections in the United States; August 2008.
5. CDC, *MMWR*, Vol. 57, No. 39; 2008.
6. NCHS, "Deaths: Final Data for 2004." *NVSR*, Vol. 55, No. 19; 2007.
7. Shapiro MF et al., "Variations in the Care of HIV-Infected Adults in the United States." *JAMA*, Vol. 281, No. 24; 1999.
8. Cunningham WE et al., "The Impact of Competing Subsistence Needs and Barriers to Access to Medical Care for Persons with Human Immunodeficiency Virus Receiving Care in the United States." *Medical Care*, Vol. 37, No. 12; 1999.
9. Fleishman JA et al., "Hospital and Outpatient Health Services Utilization among HIV-Infected Adults in Care 2000-2002." *Medical Care*, Vol. 43, No. 9, Supplement; September 2005.
10. McQuillan GM et al., *NHCS Data Brief*, No. 4; January 2008.
11. Calculations based only on cases for which race/ethnicity data were provided.
12. U.S. Census Bureau, 2006 Population Estimates.
13. Includes estimated cases among those 13 years of age and older. Estimates do not include U.S. dependencies, possessions, and associated nations, and cases of unknown residence.
14. NCHS, Health, United States; 2007.
15. CDC, Slide Set: HIV Mortality (through 2005).
16. CDC, *MMWR*, Vol. 57, No. 36; 2008.
17. CDC, Slide Set: HIV/AIDS Surveillance in Adolescents and Young Adults (through 2006).
18. CDC, Slide Set: HIV/AIDS Surveillance by Race/Ethnicity (through 2006).
19. CDC, Fact Sheet: HIV/AIDS Among Men Who Have Sex with Men; June 2007.
20. CDC, *MMWR*, Vol. 54, No. 24; 2005.
21. The Kaiser Family Foundation, www.statehealthfacts.org. Data Source: Centers for Disease Control and Prevention, Division

of HIV/AIDS Prevention-Surveillance and Epidemiology, Special Data Request; March 2008.

22. Estimates include U.S. dependencies, possessions, and associated nations, and cases of unknown residence.
23. US Census Bureau, The Black Population: 2000; August 2001.
24. Fleishman JA. Personal Communication, Analysis of HCSUS Data; January 2002.
25. Kaiser Family Foundation analysis of CDC data.
26. Kaiser Family Foundation, *Survey of Americans on HIV/AIDS*; 2006.

Latinos and HIV/AIDS

Latinos in the United States continue to be disproportionately affected by the HIV/AIDS epidemic, accounting for higher rates of new HIV infections, AIDS cases, and people living with HIV/AIDS than their white counterparts.[1,2,3,4] The epidemic has also had a disproportionate impact on Latinas and on Latino youths, and the impact varies across the country and by place of birth.[1,5] Moreover, studies have shown that Latinos with HIV/AIDS may face additional barriers to accessing care than their white counterparts.[6,7,8] Today, there are approximately 1.1 million people living with HIV/AIDS in the U.S., including nearly 200,000 Latinos.[4] As the largest and fastest growing ethnic minority group in the U.S., addressing the impact of HIV/AIDS in the Latino community takes on increased importance in efforts to improve the nation's health.

Snapshot of the Epidemic

- Although Latinos represent approximately 15% of the U.S. population,[10] they account for 19% of the AIDS cases diagnosed in 2006.[1,9] Latinos also account for 17% of new HIV infections (9,700 of 56,300 total new infections) and nearly 18% of people living with HIV disease in 2006.[2,3,4]

- The AIDS case rate per 100,000 among Latino adults/adolescents was the second highest of any racial/ethnic group in the U.S. in 2006—about three times that of whites, but one-third that of Blacks.[1,11] The HIV incidence rate for Latinos follows a similar pattern.[3]

- HIV was the sixth leading cause of death for Latino men and fifth for Latinas, aged 25–44, in 2005.[12] HIV death rates per 100,000 among those aged 25–44 were higher among Latinos (9.3 for men and 3.1 for Latinas) than whites, although they were highest for Blacks in 2004.[13]

Key Trends and Current Cases

- The number of new infections among Latinos peaked in the late 1980s and has declined since then, and been fluctuating around 10,000 per year for most of the decade. Throughout the epidemic, the number of new HIV infections among Latinos has been lower than for whites and Blacks.[3]
- Latinos account for a growing share of AIDS diagnoses over the course of the epidemic, rising from 15% in 1985 to 19% in 2006; in recent years, this share has remained relatively stable.[1,14]
- The number of Latinos living with AIDS has also increased over time, in part due to treatment advances but also to the epidemic's continued impact on Latinos. Estimated AIDS prevalence among Latinos increased by 27% between 2002 and 2006, compared to a 19% increase among whites.[1]
- The number of deaths among Latinos with AIDS remained stable between 2002 and 2006 while both Blacks and whites experienced significant decreases.[1]

Women and Young People

- Among women, Latinas account for 16% of new HIV infections and their HIV incidence rate is nearly four times the rate for white women, but about a quarter of the rate for Black women.[15]
- In looking at new AIDS cases in 2006 among women, Latinas similarly account for 16% of new cases; Black women account for 66% and white women account for 17%.[1,9,11]
- Latinas represent 22% of AIDS cases diagnosed among all Latinos (men and women combined) in 2006; by comparison, white women represent 15% of cases among whites, and Black women represent 36% of cases diagnosed among Blacks.[1,11]
- The AIDS case rate per 100,000 among Latinas (9.5) is five times higher than the case rate for white women (1.9).[1,11]

- Latino teens, aged 13–19, account for 19% of AIDS cases among teens, slightly greater than their share of the U.S. teen population in 2006 (17%).[5] Latinos aged 20–24 account for 23% of new AIDS cases reported among young adults, but represent 18% of U.S. young adults, in 2006.[5]

Transmission

- HIV transmission patterns among Latino men vary from those of white men. Although both groups are most likely to be infected through sex with other men, white men are more likely to have been infected this way. Heterosexual transmission and injection drug use account for a greater share of infections among Latino men than white men.[1,15,16]
- Latinas are somewhat more likely to have been infected through heterosexual transmission than white women, although this is the most common transmission route for both groups and for women overall. White women are somewhat more likely to have been infected through injection drug use than Latinas.[1,15,16]
- Studies have found high HIV/AIDS prevalence among Latino men who have sex with men (MSM).[17] A study in five major U.S. cities found that 17% of Latino MSM in the study were infected with HIV. Prevalence among white MSM was 21% and among Black MSM, 46%, the highest of any group.[18] Knowledge of HIV status among those already infected is also very low.[17] In addition, newly infected Latino MSM are younger than their white counterparts, with those aged 13–29 accounting for 43% of new infections among Latino MSM compared to 25% among whites.[15]

Geography

Although AIDS cases among Latinos have been reported throughout the country, the impact of the epidemic is not uniformly distributed:

- AIDS case rates per 100,000 among Latinos are highest in the eastern part of the U.S., particularly in the Northeast.[19] The Northeast also has the greatest proportion of Latinos estimated to be living with AIDS (36% in 2006) and new AIDS cases among Latinos (31%).[19,20]
- AIDS prevalence among Latinos is clustered in a handful of states, with 10 states accounting for 88% of Latinos estimated

to be living with AIDS in 2006. New York, California, and Puerto Rico top the list. Ten states also account for the majority of newly reported AIDS cases among Latinos (84% in 2006).[19,20]

- AIDS cases among Latinos vary by place of birth. Latinos born in the U.S. account for 34% of estimated AIDS cases among Latinos in 2006, followed by Latinos born in Puerto Rico (17%) and Mexico (17%).[1,21] HIV transmission patterns among Latinos also vary by place of birth.[1]

Access to and Use of the Health Care System

The HIV Cost and Services Utilization Study (HCSUS), the only nationally representative study of people with HIV/AIDS receiving regular or ongoing medical care for HIV infection, found that Latinos fared more poorly on several important measures of access and quality, differences that diminished over time but were not completely eliminated.[6] In addition, HCSUS found that Latinos were more likely to report postponing medical care due to factors such as lack of transportation.[7] Latinos were also more likely than whites to delay care after HIV diagnosis.[8]

Health Insurance

Having health insurance, either public or private, improves access to care. Insurance coverage of those with HIV/AIDS varies by race/ethnicity, as it does for the U.S. population overall.

- The HCSUS study found that Latinos with HIV/AIDS were more likely to be publicly insured or uninsured than their white counterparts, with half relying on Medicaid compared to 32% of whites. Approximately one quarter of Latinos with HIV/AIDS (24%) were uninsured compared to 17% of whites. Latinos were also about half as likely to be privately insured than whites (23% compared to 44%).[22]

- Insurance status also varies at the time of HIV diagnosis. Analysis of data from 25 states between 1994 and 2000 found that Latinos were less likely than whites to have private coverage and more likely to be covered by Medicaid at the time of their HIV diagnosis. A third of Latinos were uninsured at the time of their diagnosis, higher than other groups.[23]

HIV Testing

- Among the U.S. population overall, Latinos are more likely than whites to report ever having been tested for HIV (54% compared to 45%).[24]
- Among those who are HIV positive, CDC data indicate that more than 4 in 10 Latinos (42%) were tested for HIV late in their illness—that is, diagnosed with AIDS within one year of testing positive (in those states/areas with HIV name reporting); by comparison, 38% of Blacks and 35% of whites were tested late.[1]

Concern about HIV/AIDS

- A recent survey found that Latinos express concern about HIV/AIDS. Nearly a quarter of Latinos named it as the most urgent health problem facing the nation, ranked second after cancer. More Latinos believe the U.S. is making progress on the domestic epidemic (39%) than losing ground (30%), as do whites; by contrast, Black Americans are more likely to say the U.S. is losing ground.[24]
- Almost half (46%) of Latinos say they think AIDS is a more urgent problem in their community than it was a few years ago compared to 15% of whites. Although 31% of Latinos say they are personally very concerned about becoming infected with HIV, this proportion has declined since the mid-1990s.[24]

References

1. CDC, *HIV/AIDS Surveillance Report*, Vol. 18; 2008.
2. Hall HI et al., "Estimation of HIV Incidence in the United States." *JAMA*, Vol. 300, No. 5; August 2008.
3. CDC, Fact Sheet: Estimates of New HIV Infections in the United States; August 2008.
4. CDC, *MMWR*, Vol. 57, No. 39; 2008.
5. CDC, Slide Set: HIV/AIDS Surveillance in Adolescents and Young Adults (through 2006).
6. Shapiro MF et al., "Variations in the Care of HIV-Infected Adults in the United States." *JAMA*, Vol. 281, No. 24; 1999.

7. Cunningham WE et al., "The Impact of Competing Subsistence Needs and Barriers to Access to Medical Care for Persons with Human Immunodeficiency Virus Receiving Care in the United States." *Medical Care*, Vol. 37, No. 12; 1999.

8. Turner BJ et al., "Delayed Medical Care After Diagnosis in a U.S. Probability Sample of Persons Infected with the Human Immunodeficiency Virus." *Archives of Internal Medicine*, Vol. 160; 2000.

9. Calculations based only on cases for which race/ethnicity data were provided.

10. U.S. Census Bureau, 2006 Population Estimates.

11. Includes reported cases among those 13 years of age and older. Estimates do not include cases from the U.S. dependencies, possessions, and associated nations, and cases of unknown residence.

12. CDC, Slide Set: HIV Mortality (through 2005).

13. NCHS, *Health, United States*, 2007.

14. CDC, Special Data Request; 2006.

15. CDC, *MMWR*, Vol. 57, No. 36; 2008.

16. CDC, Slide Set: HIV/AIDS Surveillance by Race/Ethnicity (through 2006).

17. CDC, Fact Sheet: HIV/AIDS Among Men Who Have Sex with Men; June 2007.

18. CDC, *MMWR*, Vol. 54, No. 24; 2005.

19. Kaiser Family Foundation, www.statehealthfacts.org. Data Source: Centers for Disease Control and Prevention, Division of HIV/AIDS Prevention-Surveillance and Epidemiology, Special Data Request; March 2008.

20. Estimates include U.S. dependencies, possessions, and associated nations, and cases of unknown residence.

21. Calculations based only on cases for which data by place of birth were provided.

22. Fleishman JA, Personal Communication, Analysis of HCSUS Data; January 2002.

23. Kaiser Family Foundation analysis of CDC data.

24. Kaiser Family Foundation, *Survey of Americans on HIV/AIDS*; 2006.

Section 6.2

Overcoming Racial Disparities in STDs

"Overcoming the Epidemics: Racial Disparities in HIV and STDs," September 2006, by Deana McRae, Health Policy Associate, National Black Caucus of State Legislators.

When compared to the U.S. population, African Americans and other minorities are contracting HIV and other sexually transmitted diseases (STDs) at a disproportionate rate despite the efforts of federal, state, and local agencies. While African Americans represent approximately 13% of the nation's population, they are the population group most disproportionately affected by HIV and STDs each year. This fact illustrates the ever-increasing need for education and prevention within the African American community.

The Centers for Disease Control and Prevention (CDC) estimates that in 2003, more than one million persons[1] in the United States were living with an HIV infection and about 40,000 new HIV infections occur each year.[2] According to CDC's 2004 HIV/AIDS Surveillance Report, African Americans accounted for 50% of all HIV/AIDS cases diagnosed in 2004. By the end of 2004, an estimated 415,000 individuals were living with AIDS in the United States and 43% of them were African Americans.

In addition to HIV, other STDs continue to be a major U.S. public health challenge. CDC estimates that 19 million new sexually transmitted infections occur each year.[3] Data in CDC's *2004 STD Surveillance Report* showed higher rates of all STDs among minority racial and ethnic populations when compared to whites. Additionally, the U.S. Department of Health and Human Services' *Healthy People 2010* chapter on Sexually Transmitted Diseases notes that race and ethnicity can be recognized as risk markers for prevalence of STDs in association with other important factors, such as poverty, access to quality health care, and living in urban settings in the United States.[4]

STD Epidemic Affecting African Americans

The three major nationally reportable STDs are chlamydia, gonorrhea, and syphilis. The most frequently reported bacterial STD in the U.S. is chlamydia; CDC estimates that there are approximately 2.8 million new cases of chlamydia each year in the U.S.[5] Chlamydia is easily cured, but is usually asymptomatic and often undiagnosed. If left untreated, it can cause severe health consequences for women, including pelvic inflammatory disease (PID) which can lead to ectopic pregnancy, chronic pelvic pain, and infertility. In addition, women infected with chlamydia are up to five times more likely to become infected with HIV, if exposed. African American women have the highest rate of reported chlamydial infection. In 2004, CDC reported that the rate of chlamydia among African American females was more than seven times higher than the rate among white females.[6]

With gonorrhea, the second most frequently reported bacterial STD, racial disparities are even more pronounced, and African Americans are the most heavily affected. While gonorrhea rates have continued to decline since 1975, and the rate among African Americans fell 3% between 2003 and 2004, the reported rate for African Americans remains 19 times greater than for whites. In 2004, African Americans accounted for 70% of the reported cases of gonorrhea. African American females ages 15 to 24 had the highest gonorrhea rate of any age and race/ethnic group in 2004, followed closely by African American females ages 20 to 24. Gonorrhea, like chlamydia, is easily curable, but is often untreated because it is asymptomatic. It can lead to severe health consequences in women; up to 40% of untreated cases of gonorrhea lead to PID.[1]

The third major reportable STD is syphilis. Syphilis is a highly infectious disease, but easily curable in its early (primary and secondary) stages. If left untreated, it can lead to serious long-term complications, including nerve and organ damage and even death. Congenital syphilis (the transmission from mother to child) can cause stillbirth, physical deformity, and neurological complications in children who survive. Syphilis also facilitates the spread of HIV, increasing transmission at least two- to five-fold.

During the 1990s, the rate of primary and secondary (P&S) syphilis reported in the U.S. decreased, and in 2000, the rate was the lowest since national reporting began in 1941. These historically low rates and the concentration of syphilis in a small number of geographical areas, led CDC to develop its *National Plan to Eliminate Syphilis.* Since its implementation in 1999, significant progress has been made in reducing racial disparities in syphilis.

In 2004:

- There was an 80% decrease in the disparity in P&S syphilis rates between African Americans and whites since 1999;
- African Americans still accounted for 41% of the reported cases of P&S syphilis;
- The P&S syphilis rate for African Americans was 5.6 times greater than the rate for whites;
- The disparity in congenital syphilis decreased 47% since 1999; and
- The congenital syphilis rate for African Americans was 16 times the rate for whites, compared with 30 times the rate in 1999.

While there has been progress, syphilis remains a problem among African Americans living in poverty and in the southern region of the United States.

Economic Burden

In addition to the physical and emotional toll associated with HIV/AIDS and STDs, these epidemics are an economic burden as well. The economic impact includes such things as the price of doctor's visits and medicines, as well as lost wages due to illness and lower on-the-job productivity.[7] In Fiscal Year (FY) 2006, the U.S. government has budgeted $12.6 billion for programs for people living with HIV/AIDS.[8] The majority of funding from the government goes to Medicaid and Medicare, the Ryan White CARE Act, and the AIDS Drug Assistance Program. About one in five people living with HIV receive Medicare coverage and most of those also receive Medicaid benefits. At least 15 million new cases of STDs are reported annually; while an estimated $8 billion is spent each year to diagnose and treat STDs and STD-related complications, not including HIV.[9] An estimated 18 million new cases of non-HIV STDs occur each year at an estimated annual cost of $11.4 billion in year 2000 dollars.[10]

National Programs Addressing These Epidemics

As health disparities persist, federal agencies have been working toward improving public health conditions within minority communities. The FY 2006 U.S. Federal Government budget invests more than $17 billion for domestic AIDS treatment, prevention and research, including $2.1 billion for the Ryan White program. The budget provides continued support in the AIDS Drug Assistance Program, which provides life-saving anti-retroviral drug treatments for individuals that cannot afford them. In addition, the U.S. Department of Health and Human Services (HHS) launched programs and initiatives targeting racial and ethnic minority communities in the fight against specific diseases, such as HIV/AIDS and STDs.

Within HHS, CDC's National Center for HIV/AIDS, Viral Hepatitis, STD, and TB Prevention (NCHHSTP—proposed) is responsible for public health surveillance, research, and programs to prevent and control HIV/AIDS, viral hepatitis, other STDs, and tuberculosis (TB). Additionally, in 1986, the Office of Minority Health (OMH) was created within HHS with the mission to improve and protect the health of racial and ethnic minority populations through the development of policies and programs that will eliminate health disparities. OMH coordinates programs to assist HHS in the implementation of initiatives addressing minority health disparities, such as the HHS HIV/AIDS Initiative for communities of color. One component of the initiative was the use of supplemental funding under the Ryan White CARE Act to establish AIDS Education and Training Centers at Historically Black Colleges and Universities (HBCUs) to provide ongoing AIDS education.[11] The Minority HIV/AIDS Initiative,[12] another OMH program, is part of HHS' larger initiative Eliminate Racial and Ethnical Disparities. The initiative provides funding to various areas, including community-based organizations (CBOs), state and local health departments, and correctional institutions to help address the HIV/AIDS epidemic within the minority populations.

CDC has established various initiatives and programs to address health disparities among minority communities.

- In 1999, CDC launched the Racial and Ethnic Approaches to Community Health (REACH 2010) Program, designed to eliminate health disparities in six areas, including HIV/AIDS, through community collaborations in designing, implementing, and evaluating community-driven and culturally appropriate strategies.

- In April 2003, CDC announced an initiative, "Advancing HIV Prevention (AHP): New Strategies for a Changing Epidemic," aimed at reducing the number of new HIV infections that occur each year in the United States. The AHP initiative expands on current HIV prevention strategies and includes four major strategies:
  - Make HIV testing a routine part of medical care;
  - Implement new models for diagnosing HIV infections outside medical settings;
  - Prevent new infections by working with persons diagnosed with HIV and other partners; and
  - Further decrease perinatal HIV transmission.

  Seven demonstration projects were funded to test the feasibility of the four AHP strategies. One project was Using Social Network Strategies for Reaching Persons at High Risk for HIV Infection in Communities of Color.

- Historically low rates and the concentration of syphilis cases in a small number of geographic areas in the U.S. led to the development of CDC's *National Plan to Eliminate Syphilis*, announced by Surgeon General David Satcher in 1999. The program gives priority funding to areas with high prevalence and morbidity in order to reduce P&S syphilis and increase the number of syphilis-free counties. It focuses on the improvement of a community's health by removing syphilis and reducing the risk of HIV transmission and other health threats associated with syphilis.

- In recent years, CDC funded various new projects to improve the health of minorities disproportionately affected by HIV and sexually transmitted diseases, including:
  - The HIV Prevention Survey for HBCUs which assesses the availability of HIV prevention and testing services and the willingness to offer routine HIV testing on each campus;
  - CDC's Prevention Response to the North Carolina HIV Infection Outbreak, which provides funding to support training for peer volunteers to adopt community level HIV prevention interventions;
  - In Robeson, N.C., the high rate of infectious syphilis was largely in African American and Native American communities and the county was recently ranked highest in infectious

syphilis among U.S. counties. Despite challenges associated with providing STD prevention and control services in a rural setting, Robeson County collaborated with the North Carolina State Health Department to conduct extensive outreach screening and STD health education activities, including both syphilis and HIV testing, as well as condom distribution and public information campaigns; and

- In addition to maintaining syphilis prevention and control efforts in predominantly poor and underserved minority communities, in 2002 CDC provided funding for projects in eight cities with the greatest number of syphilis cases among men who have sex with men (MSM). These projects worked with community organizations and local health departments to increase syphilis screening, symptom recognition, and outreach efforts among MSM. Results of the projects were published in a special issue of the journal *Sexually Transmitted Diseases* in October 2005.

How Can Legislators Address the Epidemics?

At a time when health disparities are overwhelming minority communities, states and local agencies cannot progress without a unified effort to integrate more prevention efforts into an already fragile health care system. African American state legislators should acknowledge that HIV and STD rates among African Americans have remained disproportionately high and demand increased efforts from federal, state, and local agencies. Data consistently show the effects of HIV and STD health disparities on African American communities. State officials should acknowledge these disparities in order to react and empower these communities to address the burden. An intergovernmental approach is necessary to combat the spread of HIV/AIDS and sexually transmitted diseases in the African American community.

To reduce the spread of HIV and STDs, state policymakers can take the following steps: 1) Implement a Call to Action, in which state officials are urged to put minority health as a priority on their agenda, and 2) Create a task force to work in partnership with federal agencies to improve health services and prevention programs within their states. Other strategies include:

- Increasing state resources to address specific minority health issues, such as HIV and STD infections;

- Reviewing state public health surveillance reports and plans to understand existing conditions and support resolutions as recommended by the National Association of County and City Health Officials (NACCHO);
- Reallocating state funding toward programs that improve access to care and address emerging health-related issues impacting minority communities;
- Establishing or utilizing programs to offer health services to low-income and minority populations, including: a safe HIV and STD testing environment, educating individuals on HIV and STDs, access to treatment and care, and prevention methods;
- Pushing for insurance plan coverage for women age 25 and younger to be routinely screened for STDs during annual gynecological visits; and
- Supporting collaboration among health departments, community organizations, and state and local agencies to launch education programs and prevention initiatives.

HIV and sexually transmitted diseases can be combated in African American communities, however it is urgent that state legislators, officials, and public health departments work together and take coordinated action.

1. Centers for Disease Control and Prevention, Division of HIV/AIDS Prevention, Basic Fact Sheet. Available at: http://www.cdc.gov/hiv/stats.htm#hivest. Accessed January 19, 2006.
2. Centers for Disease Control and Prevention. HIV/AIDS Surveillance Report, 2004. Vol. 16. U.S. Department of Health and Human Services, Centers for Disease Control and Prevention; 2005[6]. Also available at: http://www.cdc.gov/hiv/stats/hasrlink.htm.
3. Weinstock H, Berman S, Cates W. Sexually transmitted diseases among American youth; incidence and prevalence estimates, 2000. *Perspectives on Sexual and Reproductive Health* 2004;36(1):6-10.
4. Healthy People 2010: 25 Sexually Transmitted Diseases. The U.S. Department of Health and Human Services. Available at: www.healthypeople.gov/Document/word/Volume2/25STDs.doc.

5. Weinstock H, Berman S, Cates W. Sexually transmitted diseases among American youth; incidence and prevalence estimates, 2000. *Perspectives on Sexual and Reproductive Health* 2004; 36(1): 6-10.

6. Centers for Disease Control and Prevention. *Sexually Transmitted Diseases Surveillance, 2004.* Atlanta, GA: U.S. Department of Health and Human Services, September 2005. Available at: http://www.cdc.gov/std/stats/default.htm.

7. Centers for Disease Control and Prevention. *Tracking the Hidden Epidemics 2000: Trends in STDs in the United States.* Available at: http://www.cdc.gov/nchstp/od/news/RevBrochure1pdf faq.htm. Accessed March 23, 2006.

8. Fact Sheet: U.S. Federal Funding for HIV/AIDS, The FY 2006 Budget. The Kaiser Family Foundation. February 2005. http://www.kff.org/hivaids/.

9. Institute of Medicine. (1997). *The hidden epidemic–Confronting sexually transmitted disease* (edited by Thomas R. Eng and William T. Butler). Washington, DC: National Academy Press.

10. Chesson H, Blandford J, Gift T, Tao G, Irwin K. The estimated direct medical cost of STDs among American youth, 2000. *Perspectives on Sexual and Reproductive Health* 2004;36(1):11-19.

11. The United States Department of Health & Human Services. HHS Reshaping the Health of Minority Communities and Underserved Populations. January 18, 2001. Available at: http://www.hhs.gov/news/press/2001pres/01fsminhlth.html.

12. The United States Department of Health & Human Services: The Office of Minority Health. *About the Minority HIV/AIDS Initiative.* Modified: October 17, 2005. Available at: http://www.omhrc.gov/templates/content.aspx?ID=584.

Chapter 7

STDs in Older Patients

Chapter Contents

Section 7.1

Sexual Health and Aging

"Even in the Golden Years, STDs Remain a Concern," by Paul Beckman.

Three years ago, Mary Jones, not her real name, visited her doctor after experiencing vaginal pain. A professional woman in her 60s, Jones thought it was just "an infection people sometimes get." She was shocked to learn she'd contracted genital herpes.

"I was stunned," she said. "Not only because of my age, but I am an intelligent, educated person who just should have done things differently."

But Jones' predicament is less surprising given the changing landscape of sexual activity among people 50 years and older.

Revolution Revealed

A hidden revolution inside America was uncovered by the American Association of Retired Persons (AARP) in 2004. The movement involved no threats against the government or terrorist plots. The only thing toppled was the conventional wisdom about the sexual behaviors and attitudes of America's older population.

AARP's study revealed many people 45 years and older place significant importance on their sex life and are more willing to talk about it. AARP's researchers dubbed this change a "revolution."

But the quest for sexual fulfillment is also perilous. Genital herpes, syphilis, chlamydia, HIV/AIDS, and other sexually transmitted diseases know no age limits.

AARP conducted a similar study in 1999. In comparison, the new study showed more older Americans use sexual performance drugs and 60% said they consider sexual activity a critical part of a good relationship.

"We used to think people over 50 didn't have sex," Jones said. "But age isn't always a factor. There are the young elderly who are vibrant, healthy, and still have sex. Other people who might be in their 40s have health problems and don't."

Older Americans Are More Willing to Consult Health Professionals

"Midlife and older adults are more willing to discuss sex as a health issue with their health professionals," said Linda Fisher, AARP's research director. "Professionals have long known that sexual dysfunction is not only a major problem for relationships and mental health, but can be a marker of life-threatening physical health issues, especially heart disease."

The report described attitudes toward sex as "progressive." Traditional moral standard remained; 95% of the respondents said they did not approve of infidelity.

Lurking Dangers

Rick Watson, associate medical director of Texas HealthSpring, said people 50 and older represent only a tiny percentage of sexually transmitted disease (STD) cases—perhaps 1 or 2%.

"It's still a very small number of reported cases," Watson said. "So senior citizens are often not thought of in the group (that is in danger). But I suspect there are a number of cases that go unreported, are misdiagnosed, or are undetected."

Many sexually transmitted diseases are on the rise. The Centers for Disease Control and Prevention reported the national syphilis rate has increased every year since 2000. CDC's preliminary statistics indicate the disease rose by 12% in 2007 from 2006, reaching 3.7 cases per 100,000 people.

Seniors are not exempt from the diseases. The CDC estimated that people 50 and older account for 15% of new HIV/AIDS diagnoses.

Though the AARP report indicates seniors more readily consult health professionals about sex, Watson said embarrassment or doubt that they have a sexually transmitted disease make some seniors reluctant to seek help.

"When seniors were growing up, it was a different time," Watson explained. "If there is any question, they need to see a physician as quickly as possible and be tested for their health and to prevent the spread of disease."

Jones admitted to being embarrassed about her genital herpes and has told only a few people about it. Still, she was determined not to spread the disease. If she is in a relationship moving beyond friendship, she tells her partner about her condition.

"It's contagious and there is no cure," Jones said. "Most men appreciate my honesty. And most go away and find someone else. But that's OK. I don't like dealing with it either."

But not all go away. Jones has been in a relationship with a man for almost a year.

Protection Key

Condoms are essential for anyone engaging in sexual activity. Watson said some seniors who don't need to worry about birth control forego using condoms.

"No matter how well they know a person, when they begin to engage in sexual activity with a new partner, protection must be kept in the forefront of their thinking."

Jones said she didn't use a condom when she got genital herpes. But she does now. Her partner doesn't have the virus but she said they hope condoms will protect him.

"He knows and is willing to take the risk. (A reassuring factor) is he is in the relationship for me, not just for the sex."

While symptoms of these diseases often show within a couple of weeks, some are tricky. Genital herpes can have symptoms such as blisters on the genitals and rectum that turn into sores lasting two to four weeks. In many cases, people experience few or no symptoms.

Watson said seniors should take the initiative.

"They may want to consider having a new partner tested before engaging in sexual activity," Watson said. "Patients should also bring up testing with their doctors."

The good news is once detected, many STDs can be treated effectively with medication. A doctor should always be consulted to determine which medication is a good fit. Although some STDs can be cured, others can only be controlled. Jones said her doctor prescribed medication to relieve the initial genital herpes attack. Later she also tried acupuncture and traditional Chinese herbal brews that she said reduced outbreaks.

Casualties often accompany revolutions. Jones said she hoped her story would prevent others from falling prey to sexually transmitted diseases. She seems convinced people are never too old to learn.

Section 7.2

HIV, AIDS, and Older People

"HIV, AIDS, and Older People," National Institute on Aging (www.nia.nih.gov), March 31, 2008.

Grace was dating again. George, a close family friend she had known for a long time, was starting to stay overnight more and more often. Because she was past childbearing age, Grace didn't think about using condoms. And because she had known George for so long, she didn't think to ask him about his sexual history. So, Grace was shocked when she tested positive for HIV.

What Is HIV? What Is AIDS?

Like most people, you probably have heard a lot about HIV and AIDS. You may have thought that these diseases weren't your problem and that only younger people have to worry about them. But anyone at any age can get HIV/AIDS.

HIV (short for human immunodeficiency virus) is a virus that damages the immune system—the system your body uses to fight off diseases. HIV infection leads to a much more serious disease called AIDS (acquired immunodeficiency syndrome). When the HIV infection gets in your body, your immune system can weaken. This puts you in danger of getting other life-threatening diseases, infections, and cancers. When that happens, you have AIDS. AIDS is the last stage of HIV infection. If you think you may have HIV, it is very important to get tested. Today there are drugs that can help your body keep the HIV in check and fight against AIDS.

What Are the Symptoms of HIV/AIDS?

Many people have no symptoms when they first become infected with HIV. It can take as little as a few weeks for minor, flu-like symptoms to show up, or more than 10 years for more serious symptoms to appear. Signs of HIV include headache, cough, diarrhea, swollen glands, lack of energy, loss of appetite and weight loss, fevers and sweats, repeated yeast infections, skin rashes, pelvic and abdominal cramps, sores in the mouth or on certain parts of the body, or short-term memory loss.

Getting Tested for HIV/AIDS

- It can take as long as three to six months after the infection for the virus to show up in your blood.
- Your health care provider can test your blood for HIV/AIDS. If you don't have a health care provider, check your local phone book for the phone number of a hospital or health center where you can get a list of test sites.
- Many health care providers who test for HIV also can provide counseling.
- In most states the tests are private, and you can choose to take the test without giving your name.

You can now also test your blood at home. The "Home Access Express HIV-1 Test System" is made by the Home Access Health Corporation. You can buy it at the drug store. It is the only HIV home test system approved by the Food and Drug Administration (FDA) and legally sold in the United States. Other HIV home test systems and kits you might see on the Internet or in magazines or newspapers have not been approved by FDA and may not always give correct results.

How Do People Get HIV and AIDS?

Anyone, at any age, can get HIV and AIDS. HIV usually comes from having unprotected sex or sharing needles with an infected person, or through contact with HIV-infected blood. No matter your age, you may be at risk if any of the following are true:

- You are sexually active and do not use a latex or polyurethane condom. You can get HIV/AIDS from having sex with someone who has HIV. The virus passes from the infected person to his or her partner in blood, semen, and vaginal fluid. During sex, HIV can get into your body through any opening, such as a tear or cut in the lining of the vagina, vulva, penis, rectum, or mouth. Latex condoms can help prevent an infected person from transferring the HIV virus to you. (Natural condoms do not protect against HIV/AIDS as well as the latex and polyurethane types.)

- You do not know your partner's drug and sexual history. What you don't know can hurt you. Even though it may be hard to do, it's very important to ask your partner about his or her sexual history and drug use. Here are some questions to ask: Has your partner been tested for HIV/AIDS? Has he or she had a number of different sex partners? Has your partner ever had unprotected sex with someone who has shared needles? Has he or she injected drugs or shared needles with someone else? Drug users are not the only people who might share needles. For example, people with diabetes who inject insulin or draw blood to test glucose levels might share needles.
- You have had a blood transfusion or operation in a developing country at any time.
- You had a blood transfusion in the United States between 1978 and 1985.

Is HIV/AIDS Different in Older People?

A growing number of older people now have HIV/AIDS. About 19% of all people with HIV/AIDS in this country are age 50 and older. This is because doctors are finding HIV more often than ever before in older people, and because improved treatments are helping people with the disease live longer.

But there may even be many more cases than we know about. Why? One reason may be that doctors do not always test older people for HIV/AIDS and so may miss some cases during routine check-ups. Another may be that older people often mistake signs of HIV/AIDS for the aches and pains of normal aging, so they are less likely than younger people to get tested for the disease. Also, they may be ashamed or afraid of being tested. People age 50 and older may have the virus for years before being tested. By the time they are diagnosed with HIV/AIDS, the virus may be in the late stages.

The number of HIV/AIDS cases among older people is growing every year because of the following reasons:

- Older Americans know less about HIV/AIDS than younger people. They do not always know how it spreads or the importance of using condoms, not sharing needles, getting tested for HIV, and talking about it with their doctor.
- Health care workers and educators often do not talk with middle-age and older people about HIV/AIDS prevention.

- Older people are less likely than younger people to talk about their sex lives or drug use with their doctors.
- Doctors may not ask older patients about their sex lives or drug use, or talk to them about risky behaviors.

Facts about HIV/AIDS

You may have read or heard things that are not true about how you get HIV/AIDS. The following are the FACTS about HIV transmission:

- You cannot get HIV through casual contact such as shaking hands or hugging a person with HIV/AIDS.
- You cannot get HIV from using a public telephone, drinking fountain, restroom, swimming pool, Jacuzzi, or hot tub.
- You cannot get HIV from sharing a drink.
- You cannot get HIV from being coughed or sneezed on by a person with HIV/AIDS.
- You cannot get HIV from giving blood.
- You cannot get HIV from a mosquito bite.

Anyone facing a serious disease like HIV/AIDS may become very depressed. This is a special problem for older people, who may have no strong network of friends or family who can help. At the same time, they also may be coping with other diseases common to aging such as high blood pressure, diabetes, or heart problems. As the HIV/AIDS gets worse, many will need help getting around and caring for themselves. Older people with HIV/AIDS need support and understanding from their doctors, family, and friends.

HIV/AIDS can affect older people in yet another way. Many younger people who are infected turn to their parents and grandparents for financial support and nursing care. Older people who are not themselves infected by the virus may find they have to care for their own children with HIV/AIDS and then sometimes for their orphaned or HIV-infected grandchildren. Taking care of others can be mentally, physically, and financially draining. This is especially true for older caregivers. The problem becomes even worse when older caregivers have AIDS or other serious health problems. Remember, it is important to get tested for HIV/AIDS early. Early treatment increases the chances of living longer.

HIV/AIDS in People of Color and Women

The number of HIV/AIDS cases is rising in people of color across the country. About half of all people with HIV/AIDS are African American or Hispanic.

The number of cases of HIV/AIDS for women has also been growing over the past few years. The rise in the number of cases in women of color age 50 and older has been especially steep. Most got the virus from sex with infected partners. Many others got HIV through shared needles. Because women may live longer than men, and because of the rising divorce rate, many widowed, divorced, and separated women are dating these days. Like older men, many older women may be at risk because they do not know how HIV/AIDS is spread. Women who no longer worry about getting pregnant may be less likely to use a condom and to practice safe sex. Also, vaginal dryness and thinning often occurs as women age; when that happens, sexual activity can lead to small cuts and tears that raise the risk for HIV/AIDS.

Treatment and Prevention

There is no cure for HIV/AIDS. But if you become infected, there are drugs that help keep the HIV virus in check and slow the spread of HIV in the body. Doctors are now using a combination of drugs called HAART (highly active antiretroviral therapy) to treat HIV/AIDS. Although it is not a cure, HAART is greatly reducing the number of deaths from AIDS in this country.

Prevention: Remember, there are things you can do to keep from getting HIV/AIDS. Practice the steps below to lower your risk:

- If you are having sex, make sure your partner has been tested and is free of HIV. Use male or female condoms (latex or polyurethane) during sexual intercourse.
- Do not share needles or any other equipment used to inject drugs.
- Get tested if you or your partner had a blood transfusion between 1978 and 1985.
- Get tested if you or your partner has had an operation or blood transfusion in a developing country at any time.

Section 7.3

Statistics and Concerns about AIDS in Older Patients

"HIV Disease in Individuals Ages Fifty and Above," U.S. Department of Human Services Health Resources and Services Administration (http://www.hrsa.gov), February 2001. Full references for this document are available at ftp://ftp.hrsa.gov/hab/hrsa2-01.pdf. Updated by David A. Cooke, M.D., February 2009.

Twelve percent of AIDS cases reported in the United States have been among individuals ages 50 and above. With highly active antiretroviral therapy (HAART) extending lives much beyond what was hoped for just five years ago, more individuals are living into their sixth decade and beyond. Simultaneously, changes in demographic patterns and social norms may be increasing the risk for HIV among people in their 40s, 50s, and 60s. The convergence of these factors warrants increased attention to the impact of HIV disease among older Americans.

Demographic Trends

The population is becoming older with the maturing of the "baby-boomer" generation. Social norms about divorce, sex, and dating in America are changing, and drugs like Viagra are facilitating a more active sex life. Consequently, the risk of exposure to HIV for older Americans is increasing.

Yet, little in the public dialogue acknowledges the risk for HIV infection after youth has passed, or that individuals have sexual relationships throughout their lives, or that the threat of substance abuse is not necessarily mitigated by the aging process. A study from the National Institute on Aging substantiates concerns that HIV/AIDS education programs are overlooking older people. Dr. Isaac Montoya, an HIV researcher with Affiliated Systems Research of Houston, confirms that the public discourse about sexually transmitted diseases, HIV infection, and substance abuse tends to focus on young people in their teens, twenties, and thirties. Few programs target older Americans.

A Chicago study has attempted to measure the risk for HIV among older men who have sex with men. Researchers compared sexual behaviors among 432 self-identified gay men in an age range of 25–77. Forty-four percent of men older than 60 reported multiple partners, virtually equal to the number in the 30–39 age group (45%). Younger men were more likely to have participated in a wider range of sexual activities, including receptive anal intercourse, while fewer of the older men were in long-term relationships with other men.

Older women in particular appear to be uninformed about HIV transmission and risks. In an analysis of trends in the incidence of sexually transmitted diseases may indicate growing risk for HIV among older Americans. Most STDs occur among individuals under 35, but the incidence of gonorrhea among individuals ages 45 and over increased from 27% in 2003 to 30% in 2007, an 11% increase. The increase was only 4.7% in the general population. In contrast to infections among younger Americans, most infections in individuals ages 45 and over are among men.

Jane Fowler, age 64, of Kansas City, contracted HIV in the mid-1980s. Motivated to warn other seniors about the risks of HIV, Fowler founded the National Association of HIV Over 50, which can be found on the Web at www.hivoverfifty.org. Fowler and Nathan Linsk, PhD, of the Chicago AIDS and Aging Project at the Midwest AIDS Education and Training Center (AETC), co-chair the organization's national steering committee. A video called "It Can Happen to Men," produced by the American Association of Retired Persons, also educates people over 50 about their risk for HIV infection.

Surveillance

AIDS Prevalence

In 2006, it was estimated that there are 280,000 HIV cases in the United States among individuals ages 50 and above. This accounts for about 25% of the total population of HIV-infected individuals in the U.S.

The primary exposure category for HIV in older Americans who have been diagnosed with AIDS is men who have sex with men. But, heterosexual contact is a growing factor, as is injection drug use. Blood transfusion is a significant factor among this population, as many older Americans received transfusions prior to the screening of the blood supply, which began in 1985.

HIV Incidence

HIV incidence data reported by the 33 states with HIV reporting systems indicate that nearly 15% of infections in those states were in individuals ages 50 and older. These data are not representative of the national epidemic as they do not include some states with large populations of individuals living with HIV disease, and they do not include individuals who are HIV positive but unaware of their serostatus.

AIDS Mortality

With HIV-positive individuals living longer, a growing proportion of deaths from AIDS is occurring among older individuals. In 1994, one in four deaths from AIDS occurred among people ages 45 years and older. In 1998, two years after the wide-scale introduction of HAART, the proportion had risen to one in three. Rates remained similar in the 2006 surveys, underscoring need for systems of care and support that respond to the needs of an aging HIV-positive population.

Care Challenges

Treating HIV disease in concert with conditions often associated with the aging process is complex. Doctors may have difficulty distinguishing HIV-related illnesses from those related to aging. For example, Pneumocystis pneumonia may be mistaken for congestive heart failure in individuals with chronic heart disease; HIV-related dementia may mimic Alzheimer's or Parkinson's disease.

Dr. Linsk, who teaches at the Midwest AETC, points out that while symptoms of HIV may resemble other diseases associated with aging, all health care providers should know that symptoms like fatigue, shortness of breath, chronic pain, weight loss, and rashes are often associated with HIV disease.

Some research indicates that as people age, they are at higher risk for progression to AIDS than are younger people. T-cell counts appear to fall to lower levels more rapidly in older infected persons. Among people with low T-cell counts, there is also greater risk of progression to AIDS among older people.

There has been little clinical research among people over 60. While theoretically admitted to clinical drug trials in the United States since 1993, certain criteria regarding renal or liver function can effectively exclude a disproportionate number of older people from participation. Other barriers include lack of information and fear of stigma associated with the loss of anonymity.

Older as well as younger Americans with HIV face myriad psychosocial issues in dealing with their illness, including fear, changes in self-image, depression, isolation, disclosure, homophobia, and other forms of discrimination. As Jane Fowler of the National Association on HIV Over 50 told *USA Today* in October, "Older people with HIV suffer two stigmas. One is the stigma of living with a disease that is transmitted sexually or through drug abuse. The second is the stigma of being older."

Fowler recounts the story of a high school student's response to a speech she gave: "We're all going to die sometime. You're old. What's the big deal?"

"I'd like to live another two decades," Fowler said. "That's the big deal."

Chapter 8

Substance Abuse and STDs

Chapter Contents

Section 8.1

Facts about Substance Abuse and Risky Sexual Behavior

"Public Service Announcements—Keep Your Body Healthy: Facts about Substance Abuse and Risky Sexual Behavior," National Institute on Drug Abuse (www.drugabuse.gov), January 2, 2008.

Adolescents and other young adults who use drugs and alcohol often take risks that endanger their health and the health of others. One of the most harmful risks is that of engaging in risky sexual activities. Scientific research has demonstrated that the use of alcohol and drugs is related to the occurrence of unsafe sexual behavior that places adolescents at risk for pregnancy or contracting sexually transmitted diseases (STDs), such as HIV/AIDS. Young people need to recognize the deadly consequences of HIV/AIDS, and that they are potential targets for infection.

- Adolescents are at high behavioral risk for contracting most STDs, and teens account for one-quarter of the 15 million new cases of STDs diagnosed each year. STD infection may result in infertility, birth defects, and the transmission of HIV.*
- It has been estimated that at least half of all new HIV infections in the United States are among people under age 25, and the majority of young people are infected sexually.*
- Since the HIV/AIDS epidemic began, injection drug use has directly and indirectly accounted for 36% of AIDS cases in the United States. Racial and ethnic minority populations in the United States are most heavily affected by injection drug use–associated AIDS.*
- From 1999 to 2000, the use of Ecstasy (MDMA) increased among 8th-, 10th-, and 12th-grade levels. For 10th and 12th graders, this is the second consecutive year MDMA use has increased. Past-year use of Ecstasy among 8th graders increased from 1.7% in 1999 to 3.1% in 2000; from 4.4% to 5.45% among

10th graders; and from 5.6% to 8.2% among 12th graders. Also among 12th graders, the perceived availability of Ecstasy rose from 40.1% in 1999 to 51.4% in 2000 (not measured for 8th and 10th graders).**

- White and Hispanic students show considerably higher rates of Ecstasy use than African American students. For example, past-year use among African American 12th graders is 1.3%, compared to 7.6% for white and 10.6% for Hispanic 12th graders.**
- Past-year use of steroids among 10th graders increased from 1.7% in 1999 to 2.2% in 2000. In addition, a decrease was noted among 12th graders in the perceived risk of harm from using steroids.**
- Since 1999, marijuana use has remained stable in all three grades.**
- Among 12th graders, past-year heroin use rose from 1.1% in 1999 to 1.5% in 2000, resulting in one of the highest reported rates of heroin use among seniors. This trend may reflect the increasing availability of high-purity heroin in smokable and snortable form.**

References

*Centers for Disease Control and Prevention

**National Institute on Drug Abuse

Section 8.2

Substance Abuse and HIV/AIDS

"Drug Use and HIV," Fact Sheet #154, © 2008 AIDS InfoNet. Reprinted with permission. Fact Sheets are regularly updated. Check http://www.aidsinfonet.org for the most recent information.

How Does Drug Use Relate to HIV?

Drug use is a major factor in the spread of HIV infection. Shared equipment for using drugs can carry HIV and hepatitis, and drug use is linked with unsafe sexual activity.

Drug and alcohol use can also be dangerous for people who are taking antiretroviral medications (ARVs). Drug users are less likely to take all of their medications, and street drugs may have dangerous interactions with ARVs.

Injection and Infection

HIV infection spreads easily when people share equipment to use drugs. Sharing equipment also spreads hepatitis B, hepatitis C, and other serious diseases.

Infected blood can be drawn up into a syringe and then get injected along with the drug by the next user of the syringe. This is the easiest way to transmit HIV during drug use because infected blood goes directly into someone's bloodstream.

Even small amounts of blood on your hands, cookers, filters, tourniquets, or in rinse water can be enough to infect another user.

To reduce the risk of HIV and hepatitis infection, never share any equipment used with drugs, and keep washing your hands. Carefully clean your cookers and the site you will use for injection.

A recent study showed that HIV can survive in a used syringe for at least four weeks. If you have to re-use equipment, you can reduce the risk of infection by cleaning it between users. If possible, re-use your own syringe. It still should be cleaned because bacteria can grow in it.

The most effective way to clean a syringe is to use water first, then bleach and a final water rinse. Try to get all blood out of the syringe by shaking vigorously for 30 seconds. Use cold water because hot water can make the blood form clots. To kill most HIV and hepatitis C virus, leave bleach in the syringe for two full minutes. Cleaning does not always kill HIV or hepatitis. Always use a new syringe if possible.

Needle Exchange Programs

Some communities have started needle exchange programs to give free, clean syringes to people so they won't need to share. These programs are controversial because some people think they promote drug use. However, research on needle exchange shows that this is not true. Rates of HIV infection go down where there are needle exchange programs, and more drug users sign up for treatment programs.

The North American Syringe Exchange Network has a web page listing several needle exchange programs at http://www.nasen.org/.

Drug Use and Unsafe Sex

For a lot of people, drugs and sex go together. Drug users might trade sex for drugs or for money to buy drugs. Some people connect having unsafe sex with their drug use.

Drug use, including methamphetamine or alcohol, increases the chance that people will not protect themselves during sexual activity. Someone who is trading sex for drugs might find it difficult to set limits on what they are willing to do. Drug use can reduce a person's commitment to use condoms and practice safer sex.

Often, substance users have multiple sexual partners. This increases their risk of becoming infected with HIV or another sexually transmitted disease. Also, substance users may have an increased risk of carrying sexually transmitted diseases. This can increase their risk of becoming infected with HIV, or of transmitting HIV infection.

Medications and Drugs

It is very important to take every dose of ARVs. People who are not adherent (miss doses) are more likely to have higher levels of HIV in their blood, and to develop resistance to their medications. Drug use is linked with poor adherence, which can lead to treatment failure.

Some street drugs interact with medications. The liver breaks down some medications used to fight HIV, especially the protease inhibitors and the non-nucleoside reverse transcriptase inhibitors. It also breaks down some recreational drugs, including alcohol. When drugs and medications are both "in line" to use the liver, they might both be processed much more slowly. This can lead to a serious overdose of the medication or of the recreational drug.

An overdose of a medication can cause serious side effects. An overdose of a recreational drug can be deadly. At least one death of a person with HIV has been blamed on mixing a protease inhibitor with the recreational drug Ecstasy.

Some ARVs can change the amount of methadone in the bloodstream. It may be necessary to adjust the dosage of methadone in some cases. See the fact sheets for each of the medications you are taking, and discuss your HIV medications with your methadone counselor.

The Bottom Line

Drug use is a major cause of new HIV infections. Shared equipment can spread HIV, hepatitis, and other diseases. Alcohol and drug use, even when just used recreationally, contribute to unsafe sexual activities.

To protect yourself from infection, never re-use any equipment for using drugs. Even if you re-use your own syringes, clean them thoroughly between times. Cleaning is only partly effective.

In some communities, needle exchange programs provide free, new syringes. These programs reduce the rate of new HIV infections.

Drug use can lead to missed doses of ARVs. This increases the chances of treatment failure and resistance to medications.

Mixing recreational drugs and ARVs can be dangerous. Drug interactions can cause serious side effects or dangerous overdoses.

Section 8.3

HIV Prevention in Drug-Using Populations

"Principles of HIV Prevention in Drug-Using Populations: Frequently Asked Questions 1," National Institute on Drug Abuse (www.drugabuse.gov), January 2, 2008.

How can drug users reduce their risks for HIV/AIDS?

Drug users should be advised that stopping all drug use, including drug injection, is the most effective way to reduce their risks for contracting HIV/AIDS and other blood-borne diseases, including hepatitis B and hepatitis C. However, not every drug user is ready to stop using drugs, and many of those who stop may relapse.

A variety of HIV/AIDS prevention strategies to protect against becoming infected are available for individuals who may be considering or already injecting drugs. These are described in the following hierarchy of HIV/AIDS risk-reduction messages, beginning with the most effective behavioral changes that drug users can make:

- Stop using and injecting drugs.
- Enter and complete drug abuse treatment, including relapse prevention.
- If you continue to inject drugs, take the following steps to reduce personal and public health risks:
  - Never reuse or "share" syringes, water, or drug preparation equipment.
  - Use only sterile syringes obtained from a reliable source (e.g., a pharmacy or a syringe access program).
  - Always use a new, sterile syringe to prepare and inject drugs.
  - If possible, use sterile water to prepare drugs; otherwise use clean water from a reliable source (e.g., fresh tap water).
  - Always use a new or disinfected container ("cooker") and a new filter ("cotton") to prepare drugs.

- Clean the injection site with a new alcohol swab before injecting drugs.
- Safely dispose of syringes after one use.

As the hierarchy shows, drug injectors can best reduce their risks by stopping all drug use. If they inject drugs, they should always use sterile supplies and never share them. When this is not possible, cleaning and disinfecting techniques should be considered. Full-strength bleach is the most effective disinfectant when safer options are not available. However, sterile, unused injection equipment is safer than previously used injection equipment disinfected with bleach. Drug users should never share their other injection equipment, such as cookers, cottons, rinse water, and drug solutions prepared for injection. Sharing these materials presents an important but often overlooked HIV transmission risk.

In addition to learning how to make the behavioral changes described in the hierarchy, drug users and their sex partners should be counseled about sexual risks for HIV and other STDs and the importance of avoiding unprotected sex.

Community-based outreach workers, treatment providers, and other public health professionals should use any contact with a drug user as an opportunity to convey these important HIV/AIDS risk-reduction messages. The messages should be delivered along with referrals for testing and counseling services for HIV and other blood-borne infections, drug abuse—treatment programs, and other services.

What is the best HIV/AIDS prevention strategy for drug users?

Given the diversity of drug users and their sex partners, no single HIV/AIDS prevention strategy will work effectively for everyone. A comprehensive approach is the most effective strategy for preventing HIV/AIDS and other blood-borne infections in drug-using populations and their communities. A comprehensive approach readily adapts and responds to changing patterns of drug use and HIV/AIDS risk behaviors, to the characteristics of the local setting, and to the varied service needs of drug users and their sex partners. At every contact with a drug user, outreach workers, interventionists, and counselors deliver drug- and sex-related risk-reduction messages and provide the means to reduce or eliminate their risks for transmitting HIV and other blood-borne infections.

What are the components of a comprehensive HIV/AIDS prevention approach?

The comprehensive HIV/AIDS prevention approach for drug users includes three complementary approaches: community-based outreach, drug abuse treatment, and sterile syringe access programs. Each of these also includes HIV testing and counseling.

Community-based outreach is an effective approach for contacting drug users in their local neighborhoods to provide them with the means to change their risky drug- and sex-related behaviors. This approach relies on outreach workers who typically reside in the local community and are familiar with its drug use subculture. As a result, they are in a unique position to educate and influence their peers to stop using drugs and reduce their risks for HIV and other blood-borne infections. Outreach workers distribute HIV/AIDS educational information, bleach kits for disinfecting injection equipment when sterile equipment is not available, and condoms for safer sex. They also provide drug users with referrals for drug treatment, syringe access and exchange programs, and HIV, HBV, and HCV testing and counseling.

Drug abuse treatment is HIV prevention. Drug users who enter and continue in treatment are more likely than those who remain out of treatment to reduce risky activities, such as sharing needles and injection equipment or engaging in unprotected sex. Drug abuse treatment can be conducted in a variety of settings (e.g., inpatient, outpatient, residential) and often involves various approaches, including behavioral therapy, medications, or a combination of both. The best treatment programs offer their clients HIV testing and counseling and referral to other services.

Sterile syringe access programs complement community-based outreach and drug abuse treatment by providing drug users who will not or cannot seek treatment, or who are in treatment but continue to inject drugs, with access to sterile syringes and other services. These programs help remove potentially contaminated needles from circulation. They also serve as a bridge to active and out-of-treatment drug users by providing them with HIV/AIDS information and materials (e.g., bleach kits and condoms) to reduce their risks, by offering opportunities for HIV testing and counseling, and by providing referrals for drug abuse treatment and other social services. Hence, it is important that drug abuse treatment and other services are available and accessible to drug users referred by sterile syringe access programs.

Testing and Counseling Services for HIV and Other Blood-Borne Infections

HIV testing and counseling services are an important part of comprehensive HIV prevention programs. These services are most effective when a range of anonymous and confidential testing options are available in diverse, accessible settings (e.g., mobile clinics) and at nontraditional times. The most current, rapid testing technologies can be especially useful. These allow drug users and others at risk to learn their test results as soon as they are available, plan a course of action to stop using drugs and reduce their risk of transmitting HIV to others, and get a referral to appropriate drug abuse treatment and other health services. HIV testing and counseling staff also can inform drug users about their potential risks for contracting HBV and HCV and explain why it is important to be tested for these and other blood-borne and sexually transmitted infections. Staff are trained to help people who test positive for HIV and/or other infections to inform their drug use and sex partners about their potential risks for infection and the importance of getting testing and counseling.

Part Two

Preventing Sexually Transmitted Diseases

Chapter 9

Safer Sex Reduces the Risk of STDs

Safer Sex ("Safe Sex") at a Glance

- Reduces our risk of getting a sexually transmitted infection.
- Using condoms makes vaginal or anal intercourse safer sex.
- Using condoms or other barriers makes oral sex safer sex.
- Having sex play without intercourse can be even safer sex.
- Safer sex can be very pleasurable and exciting.

We all care about protecting ourselves and the ones we love. For sexually active people that means practicing safer sex. We can use it to reduce our risk of getting a sexually transmitted disease (STD). It lets us protect ourselves—and our partners—while we enjoy sex play with them. Safer sex is for responsible people who care about their and their partners' pleasure and health.

What Is Safer Sex?

Safer sex is anything we do during sex play to reduce our risk of getting a sexually transmitted infection. Even though a lot of people say "safe sex" instead of "safer sex," there is no kind of skin-to-skin sex play with a partner that is totally risk-free. But being "safer" is something all of us can do.

"Safer Sex ('Safe Sex')," Reprinted with permission from Planned Parenthood ® Federation of America, Inc.

These are the most important ways to practice safer sex:

- Understand and be honest about the risks we take.
- Keep our blood, pre-cum, semen, or vaginal fluids out of each other's bodies.
- Always use latex or female condoms for anal or vaginal intercourse.
- Don't have sex play when we have a sore caused by a sexually transmitted infection.
- Find ways to make safer sex as pleasurable as possible.

How Can I Lower My Risk Using Safer Sex?

One way to have safer sex is to only have one partner who has no sexually transmitted infections and no other partners than you.

But, this isn't always the safest kind of safer sex. That's because most people don't know when they have infections. They are very likely to pass them on without knowing it.

Another other reason is that some people aren't as honest as they should be. In fact, about one out of three people will say they don't have an infection when they know they do, just to have sex. So most of us have to find other ways to practice safer sex.

Another way to practice safer sex is to only have sex play that has no risk—or a lower risk—of passing STDs. This means no vaginal or anal intercourse. Many of us find that great sex is about a lot more than a penis going in a vagina or anus. It is about exploring the many other ways you and your partner can turn each other on. Not only is it a way to discover new sexual pleasures, it's also safer.

No-risk safer sex play includes:

- masturbation;
- mutual masturbation;
- cybersex;
- phone sex;
- sharing fantasies.

Low-risk safer sex play includes:

- kissing;
- fondling—manual stimulation of one another;

- sexy massage;
- body-to-body rubbing—frottage, "grinding," or "dry humping";
- oral sex (even safer with a condom or other barrier);
- playing with sex toys—alone or with a partner.

The highest risk kinds of sex play are:

- vaginal intercourse;
- anal intercourse.

Luckily, we can use condoms during vaginal and anal intercourse to make them safer.

Condoms for Safer Sex

Condoms work by forming a barrier between the penis and anus, vagina, or mouth. The barrier keeps one partner's fluids from getting into or on the other. And condoms reduce the amount of skin-to-skin contact. There are two main kinds of condoms—latex condoms and female condoms.

- Latex condoms are great safer sex tools for anal or vaginal intercourse. They are easy to get at a pharmacy, grocery store, or at a Planned Parenthood health center. They are cheap. And they come in a variety of shapes, sizes, and textures. People with latex allergies can use condoms made of polyurethane. They also make sex safer, but they are not as widely available as latex condoms.
- Female condoms reduce your risk of infection, too. Female condoms aren't quite as easy to find as latex condoms, but they are available in some drugstores and many Planned Parenthood health centers. You can also order them online if you can't find them in your neighborhood. Follow the instructions on the package for using female condoms correctly.

How Different Sexually Transmitted Infections Get Passed Along

Not all sexually transmitted infections are passed in the same way. Here are the basics:

Unprotected Vaginal or Anal Intercourse—High Risk for Passing:

- chancroid;
- chlamydia;
- cytomegalovirus (CMV);
- gonorrhea;
- hepatitis B;
- herpes;
- human immunodeficiency virus (HIV);
- human papilloma virus (HPV);
- pelvic inflammatory disease (PID);
- pubic lice;
- scabies;
- syphilis;
- trichomoniasis.

Unprotected Oral Sex—High Risk for Passing:

- CMV;
- gonorrhea;
- hepatitis B;
- herpes;
- syphilis.

Skin-to-Skin Sex Play without Sexual Intercourse—Risky for Passing:

- CMV;
- herpes;
- HPV;
- pubic lice;
- scabies.

Lots of other infections, from the flu to mononucleosis, can also be passed during sex play.

Is Oral Sex Safer Sex?

When it comes to HIV, oral sex is safer sex than vaginal or anal intercourse. But other infections, like herpes, syphilis, and hepatitis B, can be passed by oral sex. Condoms or other barriers can also be used to make oral sex even safer.

How Can I Use Sheer Glyde or Dental Dams to Make Oral Sex Safer?

Dental dams are small, thin, square pieces of latex used to protect the throat during certain kinds of dental work. They can also be placed on the vulva or the anus when the mouth, lips, or tongue are used to sexually arouse a partner. Like the condom, dams keep partners' body fluids out of each other's bodies. They also prevent skin-to-skin contact. A special kind of dam, the Sheer Glyde dam, has been approved by the FDA especially for safer sex. Like dental dams, Sheer Glyde dams are available online, in some drugstores, and at many Planned Parenthood health centers.

If Sheer Glyde dams or dental dams aren't handy, you can use plastic wrap or a cut-open condom.

How Can I Have Safer Sex with My Sex Toys?

Many people like to spice up sex play with sex toys—dildos, vibrators, strap-ons, butt plugs, and more. These toys need special care, too, when used alone or with partners. Unless they are kept clean between uses, they can build up bacteria, which can cause an infection. And if they are shared between partners, they can pass along sexually transmitted infections.

The best way to keep sex toys clean and safe is to protect them with a latex condom. The condom should be changed whenever the toy is passed from partner to partner or from one body opening to another—mouth, anus, or vagina.

If you don't use condoms to keep a sex toy clean, it's important to clean it before and after every use. Sex toys are made of many different materials—silicone, jelly rubber, vinyl, stainless steel, acrylic, etc. They all may have to be cleaned different ways. Some toys can be soaked in water—and some cannot. Please read the instructions on the package carefully. Never use breakable household objects, like glass bottles, as sex toys.

Keeping your sex toys clean will help them last longer, and they'll give you pleasure instead of infections!

How Can I Use Lubricant for Safer Sex?

A good lubricant can go a long way in making sure that safer sex is pleasurable and fun. Lubricant is important in safer sex because it also makes condoms and dams slippery and less likely to break. Lubricants make safer sex feel better by cutting down on the dry kind of friction that a lot of people find irritating.

When buying a bottle of lube, it's important to find the right kind—one that works for you and one that works for your condom. Never use oil-based lube with a latex condom—it can break down latex. Use only water- or silicone-based lube with latex. Read the package insert if you have any questions about what you can use.

What about Safer Sex and Drugs and Alcohol?

Alcohol and other drugs can make you forget you promised yourself to have safer sex. The use of too much alcohol or any amount of drugs often leads to high-risk sex.

How Does Safer Sex Make Sex Feel Better?

Worrying about sexually transmitted infections can make sex less satisfying. Safer sex can reduce that worry. Practicing safer sex can also help you and your partner:

- add variety to sexual pleasure;
- make sex play last longer by postponing orgasms;
- increase intimacy and trust;
- strengthen relationships;
- improve communication—verbal and nonverbal.

The bottom line is that safer sex can be fun. It is a great way to explore who we are sexually, express our feelings, bond with others, and have a good time. Practicing safer sex can enhance our pleasure—and who doesn't want more pleasure?

Am I Ready for Safer Sex?

Which of the following statements are true for you?

- I am ready to let my partner know where and how I like to be touched.

- I am ready to buy condoms, even if it's embarrassing.
- If I decide I want to use sex toys, I'm ready to keep them clean.
- I am ready to let my partner know my limits when it comes to taking risks.
- I am ready to say no to sex when I don't want to have it.
- I am ready to have regular physical exams and tests for sexually transmitted infections.
- I am ready to talk with my health care provider about my sex life.
- I am ready to enjoy sex without having to get high.

If you answered "True" to more than half of these questions, you are well on your way to being ready for safer sex. Congratulations!

Chapter 10

Barrier Methods, Contraceptives, and STD Prevention

Chapter Contents

Section 10.1

Condoms and Female Condoms

"What Is the Role of Male Condoms in HIV Prevention?" reprinted with permission from the Center for AIDS Prevention Studies, University of California – San Francisco.

Do condoms work?

Yes. The condom is one of the only widely available and highly effective HIV prevention tools in the U.S.[1] When used consistently and correctly, latex male condoms can reduce the risk of pregnancy and many sexually transmitted infections (STIs), including HIV, by about 80–90%.[1–6] Condoms, including female condoms, are the only contraceptive method that is effective at reducing the risk of both STIs and pregnancy.

When placed on the penis before any sexual contact, the male condom prevents direct contact with semen, sores on the head and shaft of the penis, and discharges from the penis and vagina. Condoms thus should effectively reduce the transmission of STIs that are transmitted primarily through genital secretions such as gonorrhea, trichomoniasis, chlamydia, hepatitis B, and HIV.[1–6] Because condoms only cover the penis, they provide less protection from STIs primarily transmitted through skin-to-skin contact such as genital herpes, syphilis, chancroid, and genital warts.

Abstinence, mutual monogamy between uninfected partners, reducing the number of sexual partners, and correctly and consistently using condoms during intercourse are all essential to slowing the spread of HIV/STIs.[7]

Condom effectiveness depends heavily on the skill level and experience of the user. Appropriate education, counseling, and training on partner negotiation skills can greatly increase the ability of a person to use a condom correctly and consistently.[2]

What are the advantages?

Accessibility: Using condoms does not require medical examination, prescription, or fitting. Condoms can be bought at drug stores, grocery stores, vending machines, gas stations, bars, and the internet, and are distributed free at many STI and HIV clinics.

Sexual enhancement: Using condoms can help delay premature ejaculation. Lubricated condoms can make intercourse easier and more pleasurable for women. And condoms do away with the "wet spot" left by semen leakage after sex. Using condoms helps reduce anxiety and fears of pregnancy and STIs so that men and women can enjoy sex more.

Protect fertility: Some STIs can affect a woman's ability to get pregnant; condoms can protect against some STIs and therefore help reduce the risk of infertility.[8]

What are the disadvantages?

Lack of cooperation: Women cannot directly control whether a condom is used and have to rely upon male cooperation. When men refuse, condom use may be impossible.

Physical problems: Many men and their partners complain that condoms reduce sensitivity. Proper condom use requires an erect penis. Some men cannot consistently maintain an erection so condom use becomes difficult. Trying different kinds of condoms (such as thinner condoms) and using water-based lubricant can help increase sensation.

Embarrassment: Some men and women may be embarrassed to buy condoms at a store, or take free condoms from a clinic. Others may be embarrassed to suggest or initiate using condoms because they perceive condom use implies a lack of trust or intimacy.[9]

How are they used?

The most important key messages for condom use are quite simple: 1) Use a new condom every time, with every act of intercourse, if there is a risk of pregnancy or STIs. 2) Before penetration, carefully unroll the condom onto the erect penis, all the way to the base. Put it on before the penis comes in contact with the partner's vagina or anus. 3) After ejaculation (while the penis is still erect), hold the rim of the condom against the base of the penis during withdrawal.[2,10]

Even with adequate training and access to condoms, people won't always use condoms perfectly. In the real world, people may fall in love, or make mistakes, or get drunk or simply decide not to use condoms. Having sex under the influence of alcohol and/or drugs greatly increases the chances of condom non-use, misuse, and failure.[11]

What are concerns?

Condom education/distribution in schools: Although schools can be an important source of information on HIV/STIs,[12] only 2% of public schools have school-based health centers, and only 28% of those make condoms available to students.[13] In 2000, persons aged 15–24 had 9.1 million new cases of STIs and made up almost half of all new STI cases in the U.S.[14] 47% of U.S. high school students have had sexual intercourse.[15]

Condom breakage and slippage (condom failure): Condom quality has been improving[16] and for most users condom failure is relatively rare. About 4% of condoms break or slip off.[2] However some persons report much higher rates. In one study, gay men who were unemployed and reported amphetamine and/or heavy alcohol use were more likely to report condom failure. Men who were frequent users of condoms and used lubricant reported less failure.[11] Counseling and education on condom use can greatly reduce condom failure.[2]

Effectiveness of N-9: Condoms lubricated with the spermicide nonoxynol-9 (N-9) often cost more, have no proven protective advantage over condoms without N-9, have a shorter shelf life, and might be harmful if used excessively. Many manufacturers have discontinued N-9 condoms.[2,16]

What works?

The following programs have been documented as effective by the Centers for Disease Control and Prevention, and are currently being replicated nationwide.[17]

Training on condom use and negotiation: The SISTA Project is a social skills training intervention for African American women designed to increase their comfort with and use of condoms. In small group sessions, women learn sexual assertion skills and proper condom use and discuss cultural and gender triggers that affect condom negotiation. Homework activities involve their male partners. Participants reported more condom use.[18]

Changing community norms: The Mpowerment Project is a community-level program developed by and for young gay men that increases peer support and acceptance for safer sex. Peer-led M-groups use a gay-positive and sex-positive approach to teach men negotiation and condom use and train and motivate them to conduct informal outreach with their friends. Participants reported decreased rates of unprotected anal intercourse.[19]

Combining HIV prevention with STI and unintended pregnancy prevention: The VOICES/VOCES program was implemented in an STI clinic and uses culturally-specific videos and skills building to increase condom use and negotiation among African American and Latino/a heterosexuals. The program is bilingual and includes education about different types of condoms and condom distribution. Participants reported more condom use and fewer repeat STIs.[20]

What needs to be done?

Better marketing and increased accessibility to condoms is needed in the U.S. Although condom use has increased in the past decade, there are still unacceptably high rates of STIs among sexually active adolescents and young adults and among gay men, two populations that are also at increased risk for HIV. New approaches to condom promotion are needed, ideally before the onset of sexual activity. For adolescents to use them, condoms must be easily and anonymously accessible, widely available, and low cost. Distributing free condoms can also help increase condom use.[21]

To effectively address HIV prevention, all persons should have accurate and complete information about different prevention options. But the emphasis needs to be different for different groups. For example, while young people who have not started sexual activity need information and access to condoms, the first priority should be to encourage abstinence and delay of sexual intercourse. When targeting those at highest risk for HIV, the first priority should be to encourage correct and consistent condom use along with avoiding high-risk behaviors and partners.[7]

Are condoms foolproof? No. Neither are seat belts, helmets, abstinence pledges, or vaccines. But in the real world we drive to work, vaccinate our children, and hope to get through the day unscathed. No public health strategy can guarantee perfect protection. The real question is not are condoms 100% effective, but how can we more effectively use condoms and other approaches to help reduce the risk of disease.

Says who?

1. Scientific evidence on condom effectiveness for STD prevention. Report from the NIAID. July 2001.
2. Warner L, Hatcher RA, Steiner MJ. Male Condoms. In: Hatcher RA, Trussel J, Stewart F, et al, editors. Contraceptive Technology. New York: Ardent Media Inc. 2004:331–353.
3. Holmes KK, Levine R, Weaver M. Effectiveness of condoms in preventing sexually transmitted infections. Bulletin of the World Health Organization. 2004;82:454–461.
4. Weller S, Davis K. Condom effectiveness in reducing heterosexual HIV transmission. *Cochrane Database Systematic Review.* 2002;(1):CD003255.
5. Hearst N, Chen S. Condom promotion for AIDS prevention in the developing world: is it working? *Studies in Family Planning*. 2004;35:39–47.
6. CDC. Male latex condoms and STDs.
7. Halperin DT, Steiner MJ, Cassell MM, et al. The time has come for common ground on preventing sexual transmission of HIV. *Lancet*. 2004;364:1913–1915.
8. Ness RB, Randall H, Richter HE, et al. Condom use and the risk of recurrent pelvic inflammatory disease, chronic pelvic pain, or infertility following an episode of pelvic inflammatory disease. *American Journal of Public Health*. 2004;94:1327–1329.
9. Miller LC, Murphy ST, Clark LF, et al. Hierarchical messages for introducing multiple HIV prevention options: promise and pitfalls. *AIDS Education and Prevention*. 2004;16:509–25.
10. ASHA. The right way to use a male condom. 1/30/05.
11. Stone E, Heagerty P, Vittinghoff E, et al. Correlates of condom failure in a sexually active cohort of men who have sex with men. *Journal of AIDS*. 1999;20:495–501.
12. McElderry DH, Omar HA. Sex education in the schools: what role does it play? *International Journal of Adolescent Medical Health*. 2003;15:3–9.

13. Santelli JS, Nystrom RJ, Brindis C, et al. Reproductive health in school-based health centers: findings from the 1998–99 census of school-based health centers. *Journal of Adolescent Health*. 2003;32:443–451.

14. Weinstock H, Berman S, Cates W. Sexually transmitted diseases among American youth: incidence and prevalence estimates, 2000. *Perspectives in Sexual and Reproductive Health*. 2004;36:6–10.

15. Youth risk behavior surveillance—U.S., 2003. *Morbidity and Mortality Weekly Report*. 2004;53:1–98.

16. Condoms: extra protection. *Consumer Reports*. Feb 2005.

17. www.effectiveinterventions.org

18. DiClemente RJ, Wingood GM. A randomized controlled trial of an HIV sexual risk reduction intervention for young African-American women. *Journal of the American Medical Association*. 1995;274:271–276.

19. Kegeles SM, Hays RB, Pollack LM, et al. Mobilizing young gay and bisexual men for HIV prevention: a two-community study. *AIDS*. 1999;13: 1753–1762.

20. O'Donnell CR, O'Donnell L, San Doval A, et al. Reductions in STD infections subsequent to an STD clinic visit: using video-based patient education to supplement provider interactions. *Sexually Transmitted Diseases*. 1998;25:161–168.

21. Cohen DA, Farley TA. Social marketing of condoms is great, but we need more free condoms. *Lancet*. 2004;364:13.

Section 10.2

Other Contraceptives and STDs

"Contraceptive Choices and Their Role in STD Prevention," by David A. Cooke, M.D. © 2009 Omnigraphics.

The term "contraception" means "prevention." Usually, this means prevention of unintended pregnancy. However, sexually transmitted diseases are another hazard of sexual relationships, and some contraceptives can help prevent them.

Contraceptives are medications, devices, or behaviors intended to prevent undesired consequences. In same-sex relationships, unplanned pregnancy is not a consideration, but sexually transmitted diseases (STDs) are a risk for same-sex and different sex couples alike.

Sexual behavior is usually the largest factor in STD risk. Higher numbers of sexual partners bring higher risks of STDs. Keep in mind that this includes past sexual partners, as well as current ones. It has been said that when you have sex, you are also having sex with all of your partner's prior partners; there is some truth to this. Additionally, certain sexual practices, such as anal insertive sex, have a higher risk of transmitting some diseases because they may damage the skin.

Medical testing can be helpful to determine the risk each partner brings to the relationship. This can help exclude some infections at the start of a relationship, but this still has limitations. Reliable tests are not available for some STDs, and a negative test now does not prevent risky behavior by a partner in the future. Partner selection is critical.

There has been a long and heated debate about whether sexual behavior is influenced by the choice of contraceptive. Does an easy and reliable form of birth control give a false sense of security, and lead to higher-risk sexual behavior? This question is beyond the scope of this section, and there is no generally agreed upon answer. Instead, discussion here will focus on the odds of transmission if one partner carries an STD and the other does not.

Contraceptives can be divided into three basic categories: barrier, hormonal, and miscellaneous. It's important to understand how a contraceptive method affects the risk of transmitting STDs.

Currently Available Forms of Contraception

Barrier Methods

Barrier methods physically prevent contact with sexual fluids. They include male condoms, female condoms, diaphragms, cervical caps, and spermicides.

Condoms (male and female): Condoms work by preventing direct contact between the genital tissues, and preventing mixing of fluids. However, they are more effective at blocking contact with male fluids than female fluids, due to the differing anatomy. There are varieties that fit over the penis (male condoms) and some that fit inside the vagina (female condoms). Dental dams, thin square pieces of latex, can be used for oral sex.

Diaphragms and cervical caps: These are latex devices designed to fit over the opening of a woman's cervix. After an initial fitting, they can be placed and removed by the woman. Both are usually used in combination with a spermicide.

Spermicides: Spermicides are chemicals that kill sperm cells. They are usually placed in the vagina, and are available in several forms, including jellies, foams, and a spermicide-soaked sponge. Some condoms are coated with a lubricant that contains a spermicide. Some spermicides can also kill bacteria or viruses that cause STDs, but they don't seem to be protective against them in practice.

Hormonal Methods

Hormonal contraceptives alter levels of various hormones in a woman's body, preventing ovulation, making the uterus inhospitable to pregnancy, or both. At present, there are no hormonal contraceptives available for men.

Oral contraceptives ("The Pill"): These are pills taken daily that contain a combination of the female hormones estrogen and progesterone, or just progesterone alone. The hormones prevent a woman from ovulating, and make it difficult for a fertilized egg to take root and grow in the uterus. Many different formulations and variations are available. Hormone-releasing skin patches and intravaginal rings exist, but they are otherwise pretty similar to the oral drugs. All require regular use to be reliable.

Injectable contraceptives: These consist of female hormones, and work similarly to oral contraceptives. However, they are given by injection into muscle, and are slowly released over time. Depo-medroxyprogesterone (Depo Provera™) is the most commonly used form, and is given every three months. They are highly reliable, as long as the injection schedule is kept.

Miscellaneous Methods:

This encompasses several different approaches that do not work through barrier or hormonal means.

Intrauterine devices (IUDs): An IUD is a small metal and plastic device that is inserted into a woman's uterus by a physician, and left there for months or years at a time. Some are designed to slowly release hormones over time, while others have no hormonal effects. It's not completely understood how IUDs prevent pregnancy, but it is believed that they prevent a fertilized egg from implanting in the uterine lining

Behavioral: Withdrawal is perhaps the oldest method of contraception. It requires the male to pull out prior to ejaculation, in order to prevent semen from entering the vagina. This can be difficult in practice, because it requires considerable control, and some semen may be released prior to ejaculation.

There are several methods that involve avoiding sex during the times of the month when a woman is expected to be fertile. They are often referred to as "rhythm" or "natural" methods. They do not tend to work well for women who have irregular menstrual cycles.

Surgical sterilization: These procedures involve minor surgery to interrupt the passage of sperm out of the testicles (vasectomy) or the egg from the ovaries (tubal ligation). They are recommended only for individuals who want permanent loss of fertility, as they are very difficult to reverse.

Effectiveness of Different Contraceptives

It is important to understand that while pregnancy and STDs may both be considerations in a relationship, methods that protect against one may not protect against the other.

Barrier Methods

Barrier methods are very dependent on how they are used. Protection is generally good if they are used properly and with every sexual contact. Many studies have found that men and women who say they use barrier contraceptives, in fact, do not use them all of the time. Because of this, they tend not to be as reliable in practice as they could be if they were used perfectly.

Condoms are quite effective for prevention of sexually transmitted diseases as well as pregnancy, because they prevent direct contact between the genital tissues. Of these, male and female condoms appear to be most effective, and have been reported to reduce the risk of pregnancy, transmission of HIV, and other STDs by 80–95% in some studies. As noted above, protection is much better if they are used properly and every single time.

Unfortunately, even when used very carefully, condoms are not foolproof. They can leak, slip off, or break, allowing direct contact. Additionally, they do not cover the entire genital area, so some skin will still come into contact.

The risk of disease transmission is somewhat different depending upon whether the infected partner is male or female. In general, a partner who receives sexual fluids (i.e., receiving vaginal sex, anal sex, or oral sex) is at higher risk of contracting an infection. Condoms impact on this, but not equally. An infected woman is more likely to transmit an STD despite a condom because condoms do not prevent contact with her genital fluids. By contrast, an infected man is less likely to transmit an infection if he uses a condom, because this prevents exposure to his semen.

Diaphragms and cervical caps are generally less effective for prevention of sexually transmitted diseases than they are for pregnancy, because they do not create as complete a barrier as condoms. Still, they do modestly reduce the risk of STDs, compared to non-barrier methods.

Spermicides alone tend to have disappointing effectiveness against pregnancy. However, they are often used in combination with other forms of contraception, and this greatly increases their reliability. For prevention of STDs, they appear to have little, if any, benefit. Some spermicides, particularly nonoxynol-9, have been suspected to increase the risk of STD transmission because they can irritate skin and create breaks that bacteria or viruses can penetrate.

On the whole, condoms are the most reliable method for prevention of STDs, short of abstinence.

Hormonal Methods

In general, hormonal methods are highly effective for prevention of pregnancy, provided they are used as recommended. In fact, they are the most reliable approaches for pregnancy prevention, short of abstinence or surgical sterilization.

Unfortunately, they provide essentially no protection against sexually transmitted diseases. The hormonal effects that prevent pregnancy do not interfere with disease transmission. In fact, there is limited evidence that suggests that they may increase the risk for women becoming infected with certain diseases, due to changes they cause in the vaginal and cervical lining. For example, there have been conflicting data on whether oral contraceptives may increase the risk of acquiring chlamydia.

Overall, hormonal contraceptives are very effective for prevention of pregnancy, but they are inadequate when disease transmission is a concern.

Miscellaneous Methods

The effectiveness of these methods for pregnancy prevention range from excellent (IUDs) to fair (withdrawal). However, none of them protect against sexually transmitted diseases, because they do not block infectious particles from passing between partners. Of note, IUDs are generally recommended for women in stable monogamous relationships, because the devices can become infected if exposed to partners with STDs.

Which Contraceptive to Choose?

Unfortunately, there is no contraceptive available that is highly effective against both pregnancy and STDs. Methods that work very well against pregnancy (e.g., hormonal contraceptives, IUDs, and surgical sterilization) offer no protection against STDs. Barrier methods give fairly good protection against STDs and pregnancy, but even a low risk of failure may not be good enough in some situations.

As discussed above, careful partner selection and STD testing are probably the most important factors in avoiding STDs. If one partner is known to have an STD, proper treatment can prevent infecting the other. For those STDs that cannot be cured, both partners need to know about the risk of transmitting the infection so they can make decisions about the level of risk they are willing to accept.

Use of condoms will provide at least some safety margin for almost all sexually transmitted diseases, and probably should be used in all but the lowest risk situations. Cervical caps or diaphragms are the next best choice, but condoms are definitely more effective.

If pregnancy is a possibility, a combination approach to contraceptives may be the best option. Use of a barrier method (e.g., condom) along with a second method (e.g., hormonal contraceptive) gives the highest level of protection against unintended pregnancy, and the barrier element reduces the risk of sexually transmitted diseases.

Section 10.3

Hormonal Contraception and STD Risk

"New Research: Depo Provera and STD Risk," © 2004 Reproductive Health Technologies Project (www.rhtp.org). Reprinted with permission. Reviewed in January 2009 by Dr. David A. Cooke, M.D., Diplomate, American Board of Internal Medicine.

A recent study compared rates of chlamydia and gonorrhea infection among women choosing Depo Provera or oral contraceptives with those not using hormonal contraception at two clinics in Baltimore, Maryland.[1] A total of 819 women participated in the four-year study, which was conducted at two sites—an inner-city facility with a largely minority clientele and a suburban clinic serving primarily white, college-educated women. Participants were interviewed, given physical exams, and tested for chlamydia and gonorrhea at three, six, and twelve months after enrollment. Women who chose to enroll in the study received standard contraceptive counseling, which includes information on protection against both pregnancy and STDs.

What was the purpose of the Baltimore study?

The study sought to determine whether there is a connection between using hormonal contraceptives and acquiring bacterial sexually transmitted infections (STDs). Researchers explored whether women using the quarterly progesterone shot Depo Provera or daily oral contraceptive pills containing estrogen and progestin were more likely than women choosing not to use a hormonal contraceptive to contract chlamydia or gonorrhea, two of the most common, curable bacterial STDs. Researchers were also interested in finding out whether any increased rates of chlamydia or gonorrhea among hormonal contraceptive users could be explained by cervical ectopy—a condition that occurs when the thinner, glandular layer of cells typically found inside the cervical canal appear on the outside of the cervix, possibly making it more susceptible to infection.

What did the study find?

Women who chose Depo Provera for their method of contraception had higher rates of chlamydia and gonorrhea over the course of a year, when compared to those who did not use a hormonal birth control method. The findings suggest that women who chose to use Depo Provera experienced a three-fold increase in the risk of acquiring these two STDs. Researchers did not find a statistically significant increase in the risk of infection among women using the Pill, although the study did not rule out the possibility that such a connection might exist. The study also found that rates of cervical ectopy were not different among Depo Provera users when compared to non-hormonal contraception users.

Does this study show that Depo Provera causes chlamydia or gonorrhea?

No. No method of contraception—including Depo Provera—causes these infections, which cannot occur unless specific types of bacteria are present. Although researchers in this study found higher rates of infection among women using Depo Provera, they could not confirm a direct link—or "cause and effect" relationship—between the two. In fact, researchers do not yet know why these women were more likely to contract chlamydia or gonorrhea.

Are there other factors that could account for the higher rates of STDs among women using Depo Provera?

Yes. The study authors found that there were other, independent risk factors associated with chlamydia or gonorrhea infection, including younger age, being of a nonwhite ethnicity, obtaining services at the inner-city facility, and having multiple sex partners. The authors also note that women with cervical ectopy could have an independent risk of becoming infected. While researchers found higher rates of infection among Depo Provera users even after they accounted for these factors, it is still possible this association could be explained by some other factor or characteristic not measured in the study.

Isn't a study that reports a three-fold increase in the risk of acquiring an STD a cause for concern?

Ultimately, a woman's risk of infection is based on her exposure to the STD in question. A woman who is in a mutually faithful, monogamous relationship with an uninfected partner is not at increased risk if she uses Depo Provera. There is also little chance of infection for a woman who relies on Depo Provera to prevent pregnancy, but also uses condoms consistently and correctly. In other words, this study is an important reminder that if a woman chooses a contraceptive other than condoms as her primary means of preventing pregnancy, she needs to honestly evaluate her STD risk and assess how best to protect herself against infection.

Should women at risk for STDs stop using Depo Provera?

Not necessarily. Depo Provera is still an important option for many women who need reliable, long-term birth control that leaves little room for mistakes or accidents to happen (such as missing a Pill). However, women at risk for STDs who use Depo Provera and other hormonal contraceptives to prevent pregnancy should consider other ways to reduce their exposure to these infections—such as using condoms correctly and consistently and limiting the number of their sexual partners. Women who are not able to take these measures—or do not have access to STD screening and treatment—may want to consider choosing a contraceptive method that is not associated with increased rates of infection.

Should health care providers restrict Depo Provera use to women who are not at risk for STDs?

No. The findings of this study do not justify preventing a woman from choosing this safe, highly effective contraceptive method if she determines it is her best option to prevent pregnancy. Health care providers should be sure to remind women that Depo Provera—like any contraceptive method other than condoms—does not protect against STDs. And a woman who is sexually active—but not in a monogamous relationship with an uninfected partner—should continue to be educated about the importance of using condoms, getting tested and treated for STDs, and limiting the number of partners to reduce her risk of infection, regardless of which birth control method she is using.

What were the strengths of the Baltimore study?

This was a prospective study, designed specifically to evaluate the association between hormonal contraception and cervical infection over a one-year follow up period. Only women initiating use of Depo Provera or oral contraceptives (rather than existing users) were eligible to participate, and researchers enrolled large numbers from a diverse population seeking reproductive health services. The study also used careful measures to gauge contraceptive use—monthly self-reports compared against clinic records—and highly sensitive tests for infection as well as cervical ectopy.

What were the limitations of this study?

Researchers noted that ethical and practical considerations prevented them from using a randomized, case-control design, which is considered the research "gold standard." The women enrolled in the study came to the clinics seeking birth control—usually with a particular method in mind. Evidence shows women who are given their first choice in birth control method are more likely to use it. Participants were allowed to choose their contraceptive method, rather than being randomly assigned one of the three methods being studied. Because the women who chose Depo Provera may differ from women who chose the alternate methods, other characteristics—as yet unidentified—may place Depo Provera users at a higher risk of contracting chlamydia or gonorrhea.

1. Morrison, Charles S et al., "Hormonal Contraceptive Use, Cervical Ectopy, and the Acquisition of Cervical Infections," *Sexually Transmitted Diseases*, September 2004 Vol. 31, No. 9, p. 561-567.

Chapter 11

Oral Sex: Does It Prevent STDs?

Can I get HIV from oral sex?

Yes, it is possible for either partner to become infected with HIV through performing or receiving oral sex. There have been a few cases of HIV transmission from performing oral sex on a person infected with HIV. While no one knows exactly what the degree of risk is, evidence suggests that the risk is less than that of unprotected anal or vaginal sex.

If the person performing oral sex has HIV, blood from their mouth may enter the body of the person receiving oral sex through the following means:

- The lining of the urethra (the opening at the tip of the penis)
- The lining of the vagina or cervix
- The lining of the anus
- Directly into the body through small cuts or open sores

If the person receiving oral sex has HIV, their blood, semen (cum), pre-seminal fluid (pre-cum), or vaginal fluid may contain the virus. Cells lining the mouth of the person performing oral sex may allow HIV to enter their body.

The risk of HIV transmission increases under these conditions:

"Can I Get HIV from Oral Sex?" Centers for Disease Control and Prevention (www.cdc.gov), October 20, 2006.

- If the person performing oral sex has cuts or sores around or in their mouth or throat
- If the person receiving oral sex ejaculates in the mouth of the person performing oral sex
- If the person receiving oral sex has another sexually transmitted disease (STD)

Not having (abstaining from) sex is the most effective way to avoid HIV.

If you choose to perform oral sex, and your partner is male, these practices may help you avoid HIV transmission:

- Use a latex condom on the penis.
- If you or your partner is allergic to latex, plastic (polyurethane) condoms can be used.

Studies have shown that latex condoms are very effective, though not perfect, in preventing HIV transmission when used correctly and consistently. If either partner is allergic to latex, plastic (polyurethane) condoms for either the male or female can be used.

If you choose to have oral sex, and your partner is female, this practice may help you to avoid HIV transmission:

- Use a latex barrier (such as a natural rubber latex sheet, a dental dam, or a cut-open condom that makes a square) between your mouth and the vagina. A latex barrier such as a dental dam reduces the risk of blood or vaginal fluids entering your mouth. Plastic food wrap also can be used as a barrier.

If you choose to perform oral sex with either a male or female partner and this sex includes oral contact with your partners anus (anilingus or rimming), the following practice may help you avoid HIV transmission:

- Use a latex barrier (such as a natural rubber latex sheet, a dental dam, or a cut-open condom that makes a square) between your mouth and the anus. Plastic food wrap also can be used as a barrier.

If you choose to share sex toys with your partner, such as dildos or vibrators, these guidelines may help you to avoid HIV transmission:

- Each partner should use a new condom on the sex toy.
- Be sure to clean sex toys between each use.

Chapter 12

HIV and AIDS Prevention

Chapter Contents

Section 12.1

Sex and Prevention Concerns for People Who Are HIV Positive

"Sex and Prevention Concerns for Positive People," © 2002 Project Inform. Reprinted with permission. For more information, contact the National HIV/AIDS Treatment Hotline, 1-800-822-7422, or visit our website at www.projectinform.org. Reviewed in January 2009 by Dr. David A. Cooke, M.D., Diplomate, American Board of Internal Medicine.

Safer sex and prevention messages are often targeted solely to HIV-negative people. Yet, preventing HIV and other infections remains an important issue for people living with HIV as well. Whether your partner is HIV-positive, HIV-negative, female, male, or transgendered, there are many reasons to be concerned about safer sex and prevention. This section explores some of the most common sexual transmission concerns for people living with HIV.

What Are the Risks of Passing HIV to My HIV-Negative Partner?

A concern of many people living with HIV is passing HIV to their uninfected partner(s). While much evidence suggests that men transmit HIV more easily than women, women can still pass HIV to uninfected partners—both male and female. This is because HIV is present in blood (including menstrual blood), vaginal secretions, and in cells in the vaginal and anal walls. In fact, high levels of HIV can be found in these areas even if there's a low amount of HIV in your blood.

For women, HIV levels in vaginal fluids greatly increase when you have gynecological (GYN) conditions, like yeast infections or inflammation. Several studies in test tubes show that some sexually transmitted diseases (STDs), like chlamydia, increase HIV reproduction. Vaginal inflammation, a common symptom of these infections, causes tiny scrapes and cuts on the delicate skin of the vaginal area that can then harbor HIV. HIV levels can also temporarily increase after treating some of these conditions.

Likewise, men with active STDs, especially active herpes lesions, etc., are more likely to both acquire and transmit HIV. Less is known about whether HIV levels are actually higher in blood and semen during an active STD infection in men, but certainly any infection that causes a lesion, like herpes, provides a portal for HIV to pass through and makes transmission more likely. Studies do show that even when a man has undetectable levels of HIV in his blood, there are sometimes detectable HIV levels in semen and pre-cum fluid. HIV transmission from men with undetectable HIV levels in their blood has been documented several times.

In short, if you're not practicing safer sex, there's no way to know when you're more or less likely to pass HIV to your partner(s). Exposure to vaginal or anal secretions, semen, or other blood with high levels of HIV increases your risk of transmission. The risk further increases when one's partner has an infection or inflammation. It's also possible to have active infections or GYN conditions without having symptoms or knowing it.

Finally, a number of known cases have shown multi-drug resistant HIV being passed from people living with HIV to their partners. What this means is that the newly infected partners have a form of the virus difficult to treat with anti-HIV drugs, leaving them with limited options to treat their infections.

What Kinds of Infections Can I Protect Myself from Getting?

Prevention isn't just about protecting someone else from getting HIV; it's also about protecting yourself from other harmful infections. You can do something about many common and serious infections. The risks of unsafe sex are numerous because many STDs can cause serious harm in people living with HIV.

Cytomegalovirus (CMV) is such a condition. While most adults are infected with CMV, it doesn't cause disease in healthy, HIV-negative people. Therefore, most people carry the virus but don't have active CMV disease. However, once CMV becomes an active infection, it's the leading cause of blindness and among the major causes of death in people with AIDS. Ways to prevent CMV infection include practicing safer sex.

CMV prevention is probably much more relevant to women than to men, particularly adult gay men. The rate of CMV infection among women is generally lower (40% among women living with HIV) than what's seen among adult gay men (80–90% of whom are already infected with CMV, regardless of HIV status). The bottom line is that if you're not infected with CMV, safer sex remains a potent tool in helping to prevent CMV disease.

Like CMV, human papilloma virus (HPV) is another STD. HPV is the virus that causes genital warts in some people. These warts may or may not be visible by external examination, yet might be present in the anus or cervix. As one of the major causes of anal and cervical cancer, HPV is common and difficult to treat among people living with HIV. Some types of HPV are more likely to develop into cancer than other types.

Both men and women are at risk for anal cancer associated with HPV. Some studies suggest that a woman living with HIV is more at risk of developing anal cancer as opposed to cervical cancer associated with HPV infection. Unlike other conditions associated with HIV disease, the rate of anal and cervical cancer associated with HPV infection does not appear to be dramatically declining with increased use of anti-HIV therapy. Unfortunately, condom and other barrier protections may not protect you from HPV infection and transmission, but they might decrease the risk of transmission.

Hepatitis, cryptosporidiosis, parasites, and other infections can also be passed during sexual activity. Every condition described above can be deadly in anyone living with HIV, especially with a weakened immune system.

It's important for people living with HIV to protect themselves from these unwanted and possibly dangerous infections. Lab tests can detect these infections, but your medical coverage may not pay for them. You can ask your doctor about possibly getting these tests. Then, use the results to build a prevention plan that helps protect you from getting new infections.

Transmission of Multi-Drug Resistant HIV

There is increasing concern over the transmission of drug-resistant virus and multi-drug resistant HIV. People infected with multi-drug resistant HIV are unlikely to optimally benefit from most, if not all, of the available anti-HIV therapies. While many known cases of azidothymidine (AZT)-resistant HIV transmission have occurred in the past, transmission of multi-drug resistant virus is being seen increasingly. These observations underscore the importance of including safer sex in your life, even when you and your partner(s) are both living with HIV.

We're Both Positive: What Are Our Concerns?

For people whose partner(s) also live with HIV, prevention messages and reasons to practice safer sex sometimes become unclear. A common question is: "If I'm positive and my partner is positive, then why do we have to practice safer sex?" Simply put, safer sex remains important among positive partners. This is because in addition to preventing new infections as discussed above, other factors place positive sex partners at risk.

One of these factors is re-infection with HIV. While the issue of re-infection remains unclear, some new evidence shows that it can and does happen. If you're on therapy that HIV has become resistant to, it's possible for you to transmit the drug-resistant strain to your partner, possibly crippling the benefits of those therapies for your partner. On the other hand, if your partner is on anti-HIV therapy, you could become infected with his or her drug-resistant strain(s) and have decreased benefits from therapy.

Finally, it's important to remember that your partner's viral load (amount of HIV in blood) may not relate to the level of virus in semen or vaginal or anal fluids. Therefore, while HIV levels in blood may be undetectable by a lab test, they still may be present in high levels elsewhere. (Note: Standard viral load tests do not measure HIV in semen or vaginal or anal fluids. Also, in studies, even when viral load tests of semen came back undetectable, HIV-infected cells could still be found in the semen. These cells are believed important for passing HIV from person to person.)

When both partners live with HIV, consider these points when discussing safer sex:

- Infections like CMV, HPV, herpes, hepatitis (B and C), among others, remain major concerns. All these are potentially deadly infections in people living with HIV, but they can be prevented, to some degree, through practicing safer sex.
- Re-infection with drug-resistant or more aggressive strains of HIV remains a theoretical possibility. It must be considered when negotiating safer sex between positive partners.

HIV and STDs: Woman-to-Woman

Woman-to-woman sexual activity has generally been associated with a lower risk of passing HIV, although a number of cases have been reported. The risk of passing HIV and other STDs between women has not been thoroughly studied. But the few studies to date note that many women who have sex with women engage in a number of high-risk behaviors that may increase their risks of both getting and passing HIV and other STDs (including the types of HPV associated with cervical and anal cancer). So in the meantime, it's best to play safe and refrain from making easy assumptions about HIV and STD transmission during woman-to-woman sex.

The Reality of Safer Sex

You put yourself at risk for infections through unprotected sex with a partner—activities that expose you to your partner's blood, blood products, urine, feces, semen, or vaginal or anal fluids. In some cases these infections may never harm your partner, but they might be life-threatening to you should your immune system weaken as a result of HIV.

If your partner(s) is also living with HIV, neither of you is immune to new infections. Be aware of both the real and theoretical risks as you discuss and negotiate safer sex. Every sexual behavior or activity carries some level of infection risk. It's generally believed that some activities are less risky than others, but low risk obviously doesn't mean no risk.

Negotiating safer sex and using risk reduction to prevent passing or getting HIV or other infections is not easy. Safer sex requires the involvement of willing partners. This is especially difficult for women because safe and low-cost woman-initiated methods of HIV prevention do not currently exist. For people in situations where domestic violence occurs, this willing involvement can be almost impossible. In this case, seeking family violence prevention services is probably the safest and smartest plan of action.

Safer Sex Guidelines

In addition to protecting from HIV infection and transmission, practicing safer sex also reduces the risk of passing or contracting other diseases, like chlamydia, gonorrhea, herpes, and hepatitis. These can be especially troublesome in people with weakened immune systems. A few tips on how to protect yourself and your partner during sex are found below.

One word: Plastics! Use latex condoms and plenty of water-based lubricant (K-Y Jelly, Astroglide, Probe) for vaginal and anal sex. If you're sensitive (allergic) to latex, try polyurethane condoms (Avanti). The female condom (Reality) is also made of polyurethane. However, polyurethane condoms may have higher breakage problem than latex.

Protect the environment and your condoms! Don't use oil-containing lubricants like Crisco, Vaseline, baby oil, lotion, or whipped cream as they can destroy latex. (Note: Oil-based lubes can be safely used with polyurethane condoms). Good water-based lubricants last longer and often feel better anyway.

Read the label! Many people avoid products with the spermicide, Nonoxynol-9. Some studies now show it can cause irritation that may promote STD infections, including HIV.

Wrap it to go! For oral sex with a man, it's safest to use a condom. For oral sex with a woman or oral-anal sex (rimming), it's safest to use a dental dam (latex square), plastic food wrap, or a condom or latex glove cut to make a flat sheet.

Try a breath mint instead! Avoid brushing or flossing your teeth up to two hours before or after oral sex to minimize small cuts. Be aware of bleeding gums, cuts or sores on or in the mouth.

Let your fingers do the walking! Use latex gloves for hand jobs (sex with your hands) or fisting. Try powder-free latex or polyurethane gloves for folks who are sensitive to latex.

Good clean fun! If you share sex toys (like dildos or vibrators), put on a fresh condom for each user and/or when going to or from the anus and vagina. Clean toys with bleach, alcohol, or soap and water between uses.

On the wild side! Avoid contact with blood, semen, and vaginal and anal fluids. Sex toys like whips or knives can break the skin and should not be used on another person until they're disinfected with bleach or cleaning solution.

Preventing Your Risk of Infections

People living with HIV must consider taking precautions to avoid exposing themselves to common infections, which are possibly deadly in people with a weakened immune system. Although safer sex is usually thought of in regards to preventing HIV infection, exposure to many major infections and STDs can be reduced if safer sex is followed. Avoiding oral-anal contact can greatly reduce the risk of getting parasites that can cause diarrhea and other symptoms. (Examples of parasites include tape worms, scabies, and more common among people with HIV are toxoplasma and cryptosporidium.)

Safer sex is not the only way to prevent exposure to infections, however. There are a number of things you can do to decrease your risk of potentially harmful infections.

In general, people with HIV should not eat raw or undercooked meats, poultry or seafood. Avoid unpasteurized dairy products, which may contain parasites, bacteria, or viruses that in turn can cause severe illness. For example, eating raw shellfish can result in hepatitis A infection. Risks can be reduced further by following guidelines for "safer" food preparation. For more information, read "Food Safety" at http://www.projectinform.org/info/food/index.shtml.

You Can Prevent Common Infections at Home

Bartonella (cat scratch fever): A bacterial infection that can cause fevers, headaches, and a marked reduction in red blood cells (anemia).

Put on the flea collar!

- Avoid adopting kittens or cats under one year old.
- Avoid cat scratches or allowing cats to lick open cuts or wounds.
- Promptly wash all cat scratches or wounds.
- Use flea control for cats.

Campylobacter: A bacterial infection that can cause diarrhea, abdominal pain, and vomiting.

When Fluffy has the runs, run!

- Avoid contact with animals that have diarrhea.
- In general, get someone else to handle potty duties for pets.

Coccidioidomycosis (valley fever): A fungal infection that causes fevers, difficulty in breathing, and night sweats.

On your next archeological dig, bring Endust!

- Although there are areas of the country such as the deserts of the Southwest where it may be impossible to avoid exposure to this pest, you can still reduce the risk of exposure by avoiding excavation sites and dust storms.
- For more information, read the publication, "Valley Fever," at http://www.projectinform.org/info/vfever/index.shtml.

Cryptococcosis: A fungal infection that primarily infects the brain resulting in headaches, fevers, and altered mental behavior.

Don't feed the birds!

- Avoid areas that may be heavily contaminated with the pest that causes the infection (called cryptococcus), including areas with a lot of pigeon droppings. Avoid handling birds, even those kept as pets.

Cryptosporidiosis: A parasite that can cause diarrhea.

Put down the baby, and move away from the goat!

- Wash hands after fecal contact (like after changing a baby's diaper) and after gardening or other contact with soil.
- Avoid contact with young farm animals or animals with diarrhea (including pet stores and animal shelters).
- Wash hands after handling pets and avoid contact with pet feces.
- Boil water for at least one minute. If possible, install a water filter system that can filter out cryptosporidium.
- Avoid swimming in water that may be contaminated by cryptosporidia. Some lakes, rivers, swimming pools, and salt water beaches may be contaminated with human or animal waste that contains cryptosporidia.
- For more information on preventing infection with crypto, call Project Inform's Hotline at 1-800-822-7422.
- For more information, read the publication, "Cryptosporidiosis," at http://www.projectinform.org/info/cryptos/index.shtml.

Cytomegalovirus (CMV): A virus that infects the entire body. (Left untreated, CMV can cause diarrhea, blindness, inflammation of the brain, etc.)

Safer sex is hot sex (and it's not just about HIV infection).

- Wash hands after fecal contact.
- Follow safer sex practices.
- If blood transfusions are required, only CMV antibody negative or leukocyte-reduced blood products should be used.
- For more information, read Project Inform's publication, "Cytomegalovirus," at http://www.projectinform.org/info/cmv/index.shtml.

Hepatitis A, B, and C Virus (HAV, HBV, and HCV): Viral infections that can cause liver damage, failure, and sometimes cancer.

- Talk to your doctor about the appropriateness of vaccination (for HAV and HBV).
- Follow safer sex practices.
- Learn about particular risks for HAV and traveling in areas where threat for exposure is great and vaccination prior to travel highly recommended.
- For more information, read Project Inform's publications, "Hepatitis A" (http://www.projectinform.org/info/hepa/index.shtml), "Hepatitis B" (http://www.projectinform.org/info/hepb/index.shtml), and "Hepatitis C" (http://www.projectinform.org/info/hepc/index.shtml).

Herpes: A viral infection that can cause ulcer lesions around the mouth, genitals, and rectum.

- Follow safer sex practices.
- For more information, read the publication, "Oral and Genital Herpes," at http://www.projectinform.org/info/herpes/index.shtml.

Histoplasmosis: A fungal infection that can cause fevers, reduction in red blood cells, and difficulty in breathing.

Put down the mop and move away from the chicken coop!

- Although it may be impossible to avoid exposure to this organism in areas of the country like the Midwest river valleys, people can still reduce their risk by not cleaning chicken coops, disturbing soil under bird roosting sites, or exploring caves.
- For more information, read the publication, "Histoplasmosis," at http://www.projectinform.org/info/histo/index.shtml.

Human papillomavirus: A viral infection that can cause warts, which can become cancerous.

- Follow safer sex practices. Condoms cannot wholly prevent HPV transmission.

Listeriosis: A bacterial infection that can cause meningitis, an inflammation in the brain.

- Avoid eating any non-pasteurized dairy products, such as soft cheeses like Brie and goat cheese.
- Heat ready-to-eat foods like hot dogs and ensure that they're steaming hot before eating them.

Microsporidiosis: A parasite that can cause diarrhea.

- Wash hands frequently and follow other good personal hygiene measures.

Salmonella: A bacterial infection that can cause food poisoning and diarrhea.

- Avoid Caesar salads or anything that may contain raw eggs.
- Avoid eating under-cooked eggs and poultry.
- Avoid contact with animals that have diarrhea.
- Avoid contact with reptiles like snakes, lizards, iguanas, and turtles.

Toxoplasmosis: A parasite that mostly infects the brain resulting in confusion and delusional behavior.

These recommendations only apply to people who are NOT antibody positive to toxoplasma.

- Avoid eating raw or under-cooked meats. (Cook to an internal temperature of 150° F or 65.5° C.)
- Wash hands after contact with raw meat and after gardening or other contact with soil.
- Wash fruits and vegetables in filtered water or in a 0.05% bleach solution before eating raw.
- Wash hands after changing a cat's litter box or preferably have an HIV-negative person change it.
- Cats should be kept indoors and be fed canned or dried commercial cat food and not raw or undercooked meats.
- For more information, read the publication, "Toxoplasmosis," at http://www.projectinform.org/info/toxo/index.shtml.

Tuberculosis: Primarily infects the lungs and can cause cough, weight loss, and fatigue.

- If possible, avoid working or volunteering in facilities considered high risk for tuberculosis, such as healthcare and correctional facilities and homeless shelters.
- For more information, read Project Inform's publication, "Tuberculosis and HIV Disease," at http://www.projectinform.org/info/tb/index.shtml.

Varicella-Zoster: A viral infection commonly known as chicken pox and shingles.

- People who have NOT had chicken pox or shingles should avoid direct contact with people with active chicken pox or shingles.

Section 12.2

Preventing Mother-to-Child Transmission

"Mother-to-Child (Perinatal) HIV Transmission and Prevention," Centers for Disease Control and Prevention (www.cdc.gov), October 16, 2007.

HIV transmission from mother to child during pregnancy, labor and delivery, or breastfeeding is called perinatal transmission. Research published in 1994 showed that zidovudine (ZDV) given to pregnant women infected with HIV and their newborns reduced the risk for this type of HIV transmission.[1] Since then, the testing of pregnant women and treatment for those who are infected have resulted in a dramatic decline in the number of children perinatally infected with HIV. However, much work remains to be done: About 100–200 infants in the United States are infected with HIV annually. Many of these infections involve women who were not tested early enough in pregnancy or who did not receive prevention services.

Perinatal HIV transmission is the most common route of HIV infection in children and is now the source of almost all AIDS cases in children in the United States. Most of the children with AIDS are members of minority races/ethnicities.[2]

Statistics

HIV/AIDS in 2005

The following bullets are data from the 33 states with long-term, confidential name-based HIV reporting.

- HIV/AIDS was diagnosed for an estimated 142 children less than 13 years old who had been infected with HIV perinatally.[2]
- An estimated 6,051 persons who had been infected with HIV perinatally were living with HIV/AIDS at the end of 2005.[2]
- Of the perinatally infected persons living with HIV/AIDS at the end of 2005, an estimated 66% were black (not Hispanic or Latino), and an estimated 20% were Hispanic/Latino.[2]

AIDS in 2005

- Of the estimated 68 children for whom AIDS was diagnosed during 2005, an estimated 67 had been infected with HIV perinatally.[2]
- An estimated 46 persons with AIDS who had been infected with HIV perinatally died in 2005.[2]
- Since the beginning of the epidemic, AIDS has been diagnosed for an estimated 8,460 children who were infected perinatally. Of those, an estimated 4,800 (57%) had died.[2]
- Over the course of the epidemic, the number of AIDS cases associated with perinatal transmission has decreased dramatically. This decrease is largely due to the increased identification of women infected with HIV and timely interventions to prevent perinatal transmission.[3]

Risk Factors and Barriers to Prevention

Lack of Awareness of HIV Serostatus

The main risk factor, which is also a barrier to the prevention of perinatal HIV transmission, is lack of awareness of HIV status among pregnant women.

- Because approximately 25% of all people infected with HIV do not know their HIV status,[4] many women who are infected with

HIV may not know they are infected. This is why CDC has recommended routine, opt-out* HIV testing for all pregnant women.[5] If women are tested early in their pregnancy, those who are infected can be given therapy to improve their own health and reduce the risk of transmitting HIV to the baby.

- In the United States, without antiretroviral therapy, approximately 25% of pregnant women infected with HIV will transmit the virus to their child.[1]

Uneven HIV Testing Rates

Recent CDC studies found that HIV testing rates for pregnant women varied widely and that a relatively high proportion of women of childbearing age were unaware that treatment is available to reduce the risk for perinatal transmission.[6,7] In a 2002 study of HIV testing in the United States, 31% of the 748 women who had recently been pregnant reported that they had not been tested during prenatal care.[8] Continued efforts are needed to ensure that all women know their HIV status as early as possible in pregnancy.

- Because of prenatal testing, most HIV-infected women know they are infected before they give birth.[3] Still, testing rates in the United States remain uneven: 18% of the women in another study were not tested until after childbirth.[9]
- State HIV testing rates differ, depending on the testing approach used. For example, rates for states using the opt-in** approach ranged from 25% to 69%. The opt-out approach results in higher testing rates.[6] CDC recommends the opt-out approach,[5] but in many prenatal settings, it has not been implemented. CDC is working with state and local health departments and national organizations to increase the rates of HIV testing among pregnant women.

Prevention

To reduce further the incidence of HIV infection, CDC announced a new initiative, Advancing HIV Prevention (AHP), in 2003.[10] This initiative comprises four strategies: making HIV testing a routine part of medical care, implementing new models for diagnosing HIV infections outside medical settings, preventing new infections by working with HIV-infected persons and their partners, and further decreasing perinatal HIV transmission.

In 2006, CDC published "Revised Recommendations for HIV Testing of Adults, Adolescents, and Pregnant Women in Health-Care Settings."[5] To further reduce the number of children who are infected with HIV perinatally, these recommendations called for routine opt-out HIV screening for all pregnant women, with repeat HIV screening in the third trimester for women who meet one or more of four criteria (for example, women at high risk and women who receive health care in jurisdictions with elevated rates of HIV infection among women). Women whose HIV status is unknown at the time of labor should be offered opt-out screening with a rapid HIV test.

In support of these recommendations, CDC developed a social marketing campaign—One Test. Two Lives.—with the goal of ensuring that all women are tested for HIV early in their pregnancy. The campaign provides quick access to a variety of resources for health care providers, along with materials for their patients, to encourage universal voluntary prenatal testing for HIV. Information on this campaign can be found at http://www.cdc.gov/1test2lives.

Already, perinatal HIV prevention has saved lives.

- The number of children with a diagnosis of AIDS who had been perinatally exposed to HIV declined from 118 in 2001 to 67 in 2005.[2] The number of infants infected with HIV through perinatal transmission decreased from an estimated peak of 1,650 HIV-infected infants born in 1991[3] to 96–186 infants born in 2004.[11]
- Antiretroviral therapy administered to the mother during pregnancy, labor and delivery, and then to the newborn, as well as elective cesarean section for women with high viral loads (more than 1,000 copies/ml), can reduce the rate of perinatal HIV transmission to 2% or less.[12] If medications are started during labor and delivery, the rate of perinatal transmission can still be decreased to less than 10%.[13]

CDC funds 15 state and local health departments to conduct perinatal HIV prevention programs. The following are examples of CDC-funded perinatal HIV prevention programs:

- Comprehensive social marketing campaigns in New York to encourage women to be tested for HIV and to get early prenatal care.[14]
- Tracking and surveillance programs in Louisiana to identify HIV-infected pregnant women who are not receiving medical care and connect these women to health care resources.[15]

- Outreach programs in Florida for women in nontraditional settings, including jails.[15]
- Intensive provider education programs in New Jersey to disseminate the state standard of care for perinatal HIV prevention, educate providers about interventions for perinatal prevention, and implement rapid HIV testing for women whose HIV status is unknown at the time of labor and delivery
- Technical assistance to hospitals in Illinois to increase readiness and compliance with the Illinois Perinatal HIV Prevention Act.[16]
- Regional strategic planning workshops supported by CDC-funded national organizations to help hospitals implement rapid HIV testing for women in labor whose HIV status is unknown.[17]

*Opt-out HIV testing: Women are told that an HIV test will be included in the standard group of prenatal tests but that they may decline HIV testing.

**Opt-in HIV testing: Women are provided pretest counseling and must specifically consent to an HIV test.

References

1. Connor EM, Sperling RS, Gelber R, et al. Reduction of maternal-infant transmission of human immunodeficiency virus type with zidovudine treatment. *New England Journal of Medicine* 1994;331:1173–1180.
2. CDC. HIV/AIDS Surveillance Report, 2005. Vol. 17. Rev. ed. Atlanta: US Department of Health and Human Services, CDC; 2007:1–54.
3. Lindegren ML, Byers RH, Thomas P, et al. Trends in perinatal transmission of HIV/AIDS in the United States. *JAMA* 1999; 282:531–538.
4. Marks G, Crepaz N, Janssen RS. Estimating sexual transmission of HIV from persons aware and unaware that they are infected with the virus in the USA. *AIDS* 2006;20(10):1447–1450.
5. CDC. Revised recommendations for HIV testing of adults, adolescents, and pregnant women in health-care settings. *MMWR* 2006;55(RR-14):1–17.

6. CDC. HIV testing among pregnant women—United States and Canada, 1998–2001. *MMWR* 2002;51:1013–1016.

7. Anderson JE, Ebrahim S, Sansom S. Women's knowledge about treatment to prevent mother-to-child human immunodeficiency virus transmission. *Obstetrics and Gynecology* 2004;103:165–168.

8. Anderson JE, Sansom S. HIV testing among U.S. women during prenatal care: findings from the 2002 National Survey of Family Growth. *Maternal and Child Health Journal* 2006;10(5):413–417.

9. Aynalem G, Mendoza P, Mascola L, Frederick T. Trends and associated factors in timing of maternal HIV status identification: implications for preventing perinatal HIV/AIDS infection. National HIV Prevention Conference; August 2003; Atlanta. Abstract M2-B0303.

10. CDC. Advancing HIV Prevention: New Strategies for a Changing Epidemic—United States, 2003. *MMWR* 2003;52(15):329–332.

11. McKenna MT, Hu X. Recent trends in the incidence and morbidity associated with perinatal human immunodeficiency virus infection in the United States. *American Journal of Obstetrics and Gynecology* 2007;197(3)(suppl 1):S10–S16.

12. Cooper ER, Charurat M, Mofenson LM, et al. Combination antiretroviral strategies for the treatment of pregnant HIV-1–infected women and prevention of perinatal HIV-1 transmission. *Journal of Acquired Immune Deficiency Syndromes* 2002;29(5):484–494.

13. Wade NA, Birkhead GS, Warren BL, et al. Abbreviated regimens of zidovudine prophylaxis and perinatal transmission of the human immunodeficiency virus. *New England Journal of Medicine* 1998;339(20):1409–1414

14. Doyle PA, Rogers P, Gerka M, et al. Implementation of a comprehensive model for recruiting pregnant women at risk for HIV and late or no prenatal care. National HIV Prevention Conference; August 2003; Atlanta. Abstract T1-C1002.

15. Clark J, Sansom S, Simpson BJ, et al. Promising strategies for preventing perinatal HIV transmission: model programs from

three states. *Maternal and Child Health Journal* 2006;10(4):367–373.

16. Bryant Borders AE, Eary RL, Olszewski Y, et al. Ready or not—intrapartum prevention of perinatal HIV transmission in Illinois. *Maternal and Child Health Journal* 2007;11(5):485–493.

17. Burr CK, Lampe MA, Gross E, Clark J, Jones R. A strategic planning approach to influencing hospital practice regarding rapid HIV testing in labor and delivery. Annual Meeting of the American Public Health Association; 2007; Washington DC. Abstract 161680.

Section 12.3

Preventing HIV Transmission among Injection Drug Users

"Access to Sterile Syringes," Centers for Disease Control and Prevention (www.cdc.gov), December 26, 2007.

- If injection drug users who continue to inject use a new sterile syringe for every drug injection, it can substantially reduce their risks of acquiring and transmitting blood-borne viral infections.

More than 20 years into the AIDS epidemic, roughly one million Americans (estimated range between 1,039,000 and 1,185,000) are now living with HIV and about 40,000 new infections occur every year. Approximately 1.25 million Americans are chronically infected with hepatitis B; 2.7 million Americans are chronically infected with hepatitis C.[1,2,3]

As of 2004, injection drug use accounted for about one-fifth of all HIV infections and most hepatitis C infections in the United States.[1,3] Injection drug users (IDUs) become infected and transmit the viruses to others through sharing contaminated syringes and other drug injection equipment and through high-risk sexual behaviors. Women who become infected with HIV through sharing needles or having sex with an infected IDU can also transmit the virus to their babies before or during birth or through breastfeeding.

To effectively reduce the transmission of HIV and other blood-borne infections, programs must consider a comprehensive approach to working with IDUs. Such an approach includes a range of pragmatic strategies that address both drug use and sexual risk behaviors. One of the most important of these strategies is ensuring that IDUs who cannot or will not stop injecting drugs have access to sterile syringes. The U.S. Public Health Service and several institutions and governmental bodies have recommended use of sterile syringes as an important risk-reduction strategy.[4] In supporting this position, the Institute of Medicine of the National Academy of Sciences has said: "For injection drug users who cannot or will not stop injecting drugs, the once-only use of sterile needles and syringes remains the safest, most effective approach for limiting HIV transmission."[5]

Why Are Sterile Syringes Necessary for Injection Drug Users?

The process of preparing and injecting drugs provides many opportunities for transmitting HIV and viral hepatitis. Before injecting intravenously, an IDU determines whether the needle is in a vein by pulling back on the syringe plunger. If blood enters the syringe, the needle is in a vein and the IDU will inject the drug. After injecting, the IDU rinses the syringe with water. This water is often used to later prepare drugs for injection. If the IDU has HIV or viral hepatitis, his or her blood will contaminate the entire syringe and the preparation equipment with the virus, which can remain viable for several weeks.[5]

Transmission can occur directly, when an infected IDU shares a syringe with others, or indirectly, when an infected injector shares injection paraphernalia such as water, cookers, cottons, and spoons, or when he or she jointly prepares and shares drugs with other IDUs. Given the efficiency with which HIV and other blood-borne viruses can be transmitted through injection practices, ensuring that IDUs who continue to inject have access to sterile syringes is a vitally important strategy to prevent disease transmission. Ensuring access to sterile syringes does not increase the number of persons who inject drugs or the number of drug injections.[5,6,7] It does reduce the sharing and reuse of syringes.[8,9]

How Do IDUs Obtain Syringes?

IDUs get their syringes in several ways, including the following:[10]

- Through illegal or "black market" sources, such as street drug dealers, needle dealers, or shooting galleries or from friends, injection partners, or diabetics—these syringes may not be sterile and may have been used and contaminated with blood; used syringes are sometimes repackaged and sold as new.
- By buying them from pharmacies—this ensures that the syringes are sterile.
- From syringe exchange programs (SEPs)—this ensures that the syringes are sterile and provides an avenue for safe disposal of used syringes.

Why Is Access to Sterile Syringes a Critical Issue?

It is estimated that an individual IDU injects about 1,000 times a year.[11] This adds up to millions of injections, requiring millions of syringes every year. Most IDUs who continue to inject are currently unable to obtain a sufficient number of sterile syringes to effectively reduce their risks of acquiring and transmitting blood-borne viral infections.[12]

What Factors Limit IDUs' Access to Sterile Syringes?

- Most states have legal restrictions on the sale and distribution of sterile syringes[12]: 47 states have drug paraphernalia laws and 8 states have syringe prescription laws. These restrictions present significant barriers to the sale of syringes to IDUs by pharmacists, the prescription of sterile syringes to IDUs by physicians, and the operation of SEPs.
- Twenty-three states have pharmacy regulations or practice guidelines that limit the pharmacy sale of sterile syringes to IDUs. For example, pharmacy practice regulations that require purchasers to show identification, sign a register of syringe purchasers, or state the purpose for the purchase, reduce IDUs' ability or willingness to buy syringes. Even in states that have repealed laws and regulations banning the sale of sterile syringes to IDUs, these sales may be hampered by specific pharmacy store policies and the personal reluctance of some

pharmacy managers or pharmacists to sell syringes to customers who may be IDUs.

- The fear and negative attitudes about drug use and IDUs felt by the general public, police, policy makers, and community leaders contribute to strong opposition to initiatives that might increase opportunities for IDUs to obtain sterile syringes.
- IDUs' own attitudes and circumstances also limit access. These include fear of arrest, lack of money to buy sterile syringes, reluctance to self-identify as an IDU by going to a SEP or a physician to obtain a prescription for syringes, or lack of readily available sources of sterile syringes when needed.

What Have States and Communities Done to Increase Access to Sterile Syringes?

Three types of interventions are now being carried out in the U.S. to increase IDUs' access to sterile syringes.

- Several states and municipalities are engaged in policy efforts to change existing syringe laws and regulations to allow increased pharmacy sales of syringes, remove criminal penalties for possessing syringes, and permit SEP operation.
- State and community-sponsored initiatives with pharmacists and physicians to increase syringe prescriptions and sales also are underway to provide education about public health approaches to HIV prevention, including the role of sterile syringes in reducing the transmission of blood-borne pathogens, to address concerns and questions about syringe prescription sales and disposal, and to encourage changes in policies and practice.
- Many cities and states are pursuing efforts to support syringe exchange programs, which provide IDUs with free sterile syringes and a way to safely dispose of blood-contaminated used syringes. Many SEPs also provide other services, such as links to substance abuse treatment, education and counseling, and health services.
- In communities throughout the United States, law enforcement officials, medical and pharmacy organizations, public health professionals, policy makers, community-based organizations, and providers have worked together to examine the legal, policy,

and social circumstances regarding obtaining sterile syringes for IDUs who continue injecting drugs. Community leaders have educated their states and communities about the facts of injection-related transmission of blood-borne infection and the public health benefits of improving access to sterile syringes as part of a comprehensive public health approach. They also have educated IDUs about substance abuse treatment and the importance of using sterile syringes, addressed concerns about safe syringe disposal, and developed initiatives that improve IDUs' access to this and other vital prevention strategies.

Safe Disposal of Used Syringes: An Integral Element of the Access Issue

Ensuring that IDUs who continue to inject can obtain a sufficient number of sterile syringes is only part of the equation; counseling, health education, and access to substance abuse treatment are equally important. Safe disposal of used syringes is another important consideration, both to reduce the chances that an IDU will reuse a blood-contaminated syringe and to respond to community and pharmacist fears about the risks of discarded syringes in neighborhoods.

References

1. Glynn M, Rhodes P. Estimated HIV prevalence in the United States at the end of 2003. 2005 National HIV Prevention Conference; June 12–15, 2005. Atlanta, GA. Abstract 595.
2. Centers for Disease Control and Prevention (CDC). Hepatitis B fact sheet. Accessed December 22, 2005 from http://www.cdc.gov/ncidod/diseases/hepatitis/b/fact.htm.
3. Centers for Disease Control and Prevention (CDC). Hepatitis C fact sheet. Accessed December 22, 2005 from http://www.cdc.gov/ncidod/diseases/hepatitis/c/fact.htm.
4. Centers for Disease Control and Prevention, Health Resources and Services Administration, National Institute on Drug Abuse and Substance Abuse and Mental Health Services Administration. HIV prevention bulletin: Medical advice for persons who inject illicit drugs. May 9, 1997.
5. Normand J, Vlahov D, Moses LE, eds. Preventing HIV transmission: the role of sterile needles and bleach. Washington

(DC): National Academy Press, 1995. Accessed December 23, 2005 from http://www.nap.edu/books/0309052963/html/

6. Guydish J, Bucardo, J, Young M, Woods W, Grinstead O, Clark W. Evaluating needle exchange: are there negative effects? *AIDS* 1993;7:871–876.

7. Needle RH, Coyle SL, Normand J, Lambert E, Cesari H. HIV prevention with drug-using populations—current status and future prospects: introduction and overview. *Public Health Reports* 1998;113(Suppl 1):4–18.

8. Gleghorn AA, Wright-De Agüero L, Flynn C. Feasibility of one-time use of sterile syringes: a study of active injection drug users in seven United States metropolitan areas. *Journal of Acquired Immune Deficiency Syndromes and Human Retrovirology* 1998;18(Suppl 1):S30–S36.

9. Heimer R, Khoshnood K, Bigg D, Guydish J, Junge B. Syringe use and reuse: effects of syringe exchange programs in four cities. *Journal of Acquired Immune Deficiency Syndromes and Human Retrovirology* 1998;18(Suppl 1):S37–S44.

10. Gleghorn AA, Jones TS, Doherty MC, Celentano DD, Vlahov D. Acquisition and use of needles and syringes by injecting drug users in Baltimore, Maryland. *Journal of Acquired Immune Deficiency Syndromes and Human Retrovirology* 1995;10:97–103.

11. Lurie P, Jones TS, Foley J. A sterile syringe for every drug user injection: how many injections take place annually, and how might pharmacists contribute to syringe distribution? *Journal of Acquired Immune Deficiency Syndromes and Human Retrovirology* 1998;18(Suppl 1):S45–S51.

12. Gostin LO, Lazzarini Z, Flaherty K, Jones TS. Prevention of HIV/AIDS and other blood-borne diseases among injection drug users: A national survey on the regulation of syringes and needles. *JAMA* 1997;277(1):53–62.

Section 12.4

Post-Exposure HIV Prevention

If you are reading this because you've had a possible exposure to HIV within the last 72 hours and you are considering nPEP [non-occupational post-exposure prophylaxis], call your doctor, an nPEP study site or other resources (like a hospital emergency room), immediately. Take this paper to your doctor and use it to help you both in making decisions.

If it has already been longer than 72 hours since your exposure, nPEP is not a viable option for you. If you have waited longer than 72 hours before starting nPEP, there's little chance that the treatments will be able to block the establishment of HIV infection. In this case, seek out information about your HIV screening options (read Project Inform's publication, "Ways to Test for HIV" [http://www.projectinform.org/info/npep/test.shtml]) and seek HIV prevention and risk reduction counseling. Even if you have had a possible HIV exposure, you might not be infected. HIV screening is the only way you will be able to know if you have become infected.

Post-exposure prophylaxis (PEP) is starting HIV drugs within 72 hours (three days) of a suspected exposure to HIV, the virus that causes AIDS. The goal of PEP is to prevent the establishment of HIV infection in a person recently exposed to the virus. PEP is not appropriate, and may be harmful, for people with early or established HIV infection. Ideally, whenever PEP is considered or undertaken, it should be coupled with counseling about HIV risk, prevention, and screening.

PEP programs for exposures to HIV during sex or injection drug use are open in a few centers in the U.S. (These are called non-occupational exposures. This publication refers to these exposures as nPEP.) Through these programs, people who believe they might have been exposed to HIV can talk with a doctor to assess their risk for HIV infection. If their risk is high, they will be offered HIV therapy (two or three drugs) after discussing the risks and potential benefits of therapy. If they choose to take therapy, they will be encouraged to take the drugs for about a month. People who participate in nPEP studies are usually given the drugs and lab testing for free.

An individual does not have to participate in a study in order to use HIV therapy in this situation. However, insurance companies and other health care reimbursement programs, like Medicaid or MediCal, may not pay for its cost and related lab work for someone who has not been shown to actually have HIV infection.

Currently, using PEP for sexual or injection drug use HIV exposure is considered experimental and has not been proven to block the establishment of HIV infection in people, even when used within 72 hours. There is some evidence that it can block infection from what are called "occupational" exposures. This is when a health care worker is stuck by a needle that has had contact with HIV, or has a cut or abrasion that makes contact with HIV-infected blood.

Why Do People Use PEP?

Interest in using anti-HIV therapy to decrease the risk of establishing HIV infection is based on three observations. One is the observation of fewer HIV infections among health care workers with occupational exposures to HIV when anti HIV therapy was used within hours of the exposure. Another are results from studies which show that therapy given to HIV-positive pregnant women during pregnancy/labor and to newborn children for their first six weeks of life reduces the risk of mother-to-child HIV transmission rates from 25% to about 8%. In this study, not all children received anti-HIV therapy for six weeks, but HIV rates were lowest among the children who did—which is perhaps the strongest argument for using PEP. There have also been animal studies where, in some cases, using PEP prevented the establishment of infection in the sexual exposure setting. These results suggest that PEP may also lower the risk of HIV infection in possible exposures in other settings, such as human sexual exposure to HIV or other needle stick exposures.

The limitations of these studies make it unclear whether these findings will apply in all HIV risk exposures. For example, in the health care worker setting, PEP is given within four hours of an exposure. It is unknown if starting PEP after four hours will have the same kind of effect in other settings.

How HIV establishes itself may be very different in a needlestick accident compared to sexual exposure. In sexual exposure, different cell types may be the first targets of HIV transmission and infection. Thus it might be easier for HIV to get into cells and hide from the effects of anti-HIV therapy in the vaginal or anal cell walls. Success with PEP in the needlestick setting might not translate into success for sexual exposure to HIV.

Finally, the dynamics of the virus in animals may be very different in humans. The exposures in the animal studies were artificial and controlled, so they might not apply to humans.

In other words, no one knows if PEP is effective in the non-occupational setting or even in occupational exposures after four hours. Even if PEP does one day prove to be effective in other types of exposure, it's unlikely to be effective 100% of the time. So even if you choose nPEP and follow through on anti-HIV therapy as prescribed, you may still develop HIV infection.

Occupational Vs. Non-Occupational Exposure

Occupational exposure to HIV refers to needlestick and other accidents that happen in the health care worker setting, like a hospital. The most common occupational exposure to HIV happens when a health care worker accidentally sticks himself or herself with a needle that has been used for giving an injection or starting an IV (intravenous line) in a person living with HIV.

Non-occupational exposure to HIV includes pretty much all other HIV exposures. Some examples of possible non-occupational exposures include:

- being stuck with a used syringe (accidentally or on purpose);
- sharing needles or other injection drug equipment;
- being the victim of sexual assault;
- having a condom break or not using a condom during insertive or receptive anal or vaginal sex;
- sharing sex toys, without cleaning them between use; or
- having unprotected oral sex.

This is not an exhaustive list, nor does it reflect a priority in terms of which situation is more or less likely to expose someone to HIV.

How Do You Assess Your Risk of Exposure?

HIV cannot be passed through casual contact. The following casual contact scenarios are not considered a risk for HIV exposure and transmission. If you fear a possible HIV exposure because of an incident similar to any of these described below, you're not at risk for HIV infection and PEP would definitely not be warranted.

- Holding hands, touching, hugging, or kissing someone living with HIV.
- Being in the same room as someone living with HIV who coughs.
- Drinking from the same glass, eating off the same plate, or sharing eating utensils with someone living with HIV.
- Using a telephone that was just used by someone living with HIV.

You can only become infected with HIV by being exposed to the blood or blood products, including vaginal fluids or semen, of someone living with HIV. The following chart describes the level of risk from various activities. In all the scenarios described, the HIV status of the "source" (e.g., person whose blood you were exposed to) is important in determining the risk of possible HIV exposure. The following factors mask for HIV infection:

- The amount of blood or blood products you were exposed to
- Violence or abrasion associated with the activity that might have caused open wounds or bleeding
- The presence of other active sexually transmitted diseases and/or genital ulcers, either in yourself or in the person who is the suspected source of HIV
- The stage or status of HIV infection in the source or that person's anti-HIV treatment status
- The number of these factors present in the situation

Different methods of contact with HIV also have varying levels of risk associated with them. These risks, in turn, may be influenced by the factors listed above.

The risks for HIV transmission and infection from other activities, like oral sex, are generally considered to be lower than any of these listed above and not well enough documented to permit making

Table 12.1. Level of risk for HIV infection (risk per 10,000 exposures to an infected source)

Type of activity	Estimated risk of infection/transmission
Blood transfusion with HIV-contaminated blood	9,000 (nearly 1 in 1) 90%
Needle sharing injection drug use	67 (.67% or 2/3 of 1%)
Receptive anal sex	50 (.50% or 1/2 of 1%)
Needlestick accident with HIV-contaminated needle (occupational exposure)	30 (.30% or less than 1/3 of 1%)
Receptive penile-vaginal sex	10 (.10% or 1/10 of 1%)
Insertive anal sex	6.5 (.065 % or less than 1/10 of 1%)
Insertive penile-vaginal sex	5 (.05% or less than 1/10 of 1%)
Receptive oral sex	1 (.01 % or 1/100 of 1%)
Insertive oral sex	0.5 (.005% or less than 1/100 of 1%)

These figures are estimates. All sexual risks above assume no condom use. Last two options are moderate to high risk; others are highest risk.

numerical estimates. Risk from such activities need to be assessed on an individual basis. If you have participated in one or more of these activities, assess the risk of each by talking to a health care provider.

What Are Your Options?

If the incident that you believe put you at risk for HIV exposure/infection took place within the last 72 hours, and you are able to access nPEP within that 72 hours, generally you have two options:

Option One (consider this option whether your risk assessment suggests you are at high, moderate, or low risk for HIV exposure/infection)

Consider prevention counseling and seek support resources. Consider your HIV screening options. Work with an HIV prevention counselor to develop a comprehensive HIV prevention/risk reduction strategy that fits your lifestyle.

Screen for HIV using a standard HIV antibody test at six weeks, six months, and then yearly after the incident. Re-evaluate your prevention/risk reduction strategy yearly.

Option Two (consider this option if your risk assessment suggests that you are at high risk for HIV exposure/infection)

Screen for HIV using a standard HIV antibody test to rule out preexisting HIV infection. Start nPEP. This means you will start taking anti-HIV therapy within 72 hours of the possible exposure. Preferably you will start nPEP within 24 to 36 hours of the incident. Generally you will take therapy for 28 days.

Consider prevention counseling and seek support resources. Work with an HIV prevention counselor to develop a comprehensive HIV prevention/risk reduction strategy that fits your lifestyle.

Monitor for side effects associated with using anti-HIV therapy and use periodic screening for HIV (See Suggested Follow-up Schedule for nPEP at http://www.projectinform.org/info/npep/doctor_04.shtml).

What Are the Reasons to Not Use nPEP?

The reason to choose nPEP is the hope that using anti-HIV drugs within 72 hours of an exposure to HIV might block the establishment of HIV infection. The following is a list of reasons why you might choose not to use nPEP, despite having a high-risk exposure.

One: If you have repeated high-risk exposures to HIV and can be expected to continue doing so, nPEP is generally discouraged. In this setting, side effects of anti-HIV therapies could be hard on your body, weaken your natural immune defenses, and actually increase your risk of infection from repeated exposures.

Two: All anti-HIV therapies have possible side effects. Some, like nausea, are at their worst during the first few weeks of use. Whether or not you will have these side effects is unknown, but it's wise to assume that this may happen. If you are not prepared to manage or put up with them, you may choose not to use nPEP.

Three: If you don't think you can take the drugs routinely or have a great deal of anxiety about taking the drugs for the recommended 28 days, you might be better off not using nPEP. If you are in fact infected with HIV, taking the medications haphazardly and not strictly adhering to the prescribed regimen will almost certainly not work and could have negative long-term consequences for your future HIV treatment options.

Choosing an nPEP Regimen—Which One?

There is no agreement as to which regimen is the best to use in this setting. Generally speaking, an nPEP regimen includes using two or three drugs. Currently there are six classes of approved HIV therapy. They include NRTIs (nucleoside analogue reverse transcriptase inhibitors), NNRTIs (non-nucleoside reverse transcriptase inhibitors), protease inhibitors, fusion inhibitors, integrase inhibitors, and entry inhibitors.

Each type of drug acts against HIV in a slightly different way. Essentially all the drugs work by trying to cripple HIV's ability to reproduce (see Drug Dosing Chart at http://www.projectinform.org/info/chart.shtml). A chart from the Federal Guidelines for non-occupational PEP, including a cost analysis and side effects, is listed on pages 10 and 11 of www.ucsf.edu/hivcntr/Clinical_Resources/Guidelines/PDFs/NE_012105.pdf.

In choosing an nPEP regimen that's right for you, it's important to consider:

- the potency of the regimen;
- the potential side effects of each drug (some regimens may have side effects that concern you more or less than others);
- possible drug interactions between the drugs you're already taking and those in the nPEP regimen;
- how complex the regimen is (e.g., if it requires that you take many pills at specific times, you may have difficulty taking them according to the time schedule required); and
- the HIV therapy history of the source (if known), because a person may transmit virus that is already resistant to certain drugs and those particular drugs are then less likely to work for you.

An nPEP regimen will include, at a minimum, two NRTIs. Some regimens will include three drugs—two NRTIs and one NNRTI or protease inhibitor. As treatments advance, it's likely research will experiment with one-drug approaches as well. Currently both two- and three-drug regimens have been formulated into a single pill. What that means is that it's now possible to be on a three-drug HIV regimen that is one pill taken once daily.

Table 12.2. Antiretroviral regimens for nPEP of HIV infection

Preferred regimens	
NNRTI*-based	Efavirenz† + (lamivudine or emtricitabine) + (zidovudine or tenofovir)
PI*-based	Lopinavir/ritonavir (Kaletra) + (lamivudine or emtricitabine) + zidovudine
Alternative regimens	
NNRTI-based	Efavirenz + (lamivudine or emtricitabine) + abacavir or didanosine or stavudine§
PI-based	Atazanavir + (lamivudine or emtricitabine) + (zidovudine or stavudine or abacavir or didanosine) or (tenofovir + ritonavir [100 mg/day])
	Fosamprenavir + (lamivudine or emtricitabine) + (zidovudine or stavudine) or (abacavir or tenofovir or didanosine)
	Fosamprenavir/ritonavir‡ + (lamivudine or emtricitabine) + (zidovudine or stavudine or abacavir or tenofovir or didanosine)
	Lopinavir/ritonavir‡ + (lamivudine or emtricitabine) + (zidovudine or stavudine or abacavir or tenofovir or didanosine)
	Lopinavir/ritonavir‡ + (lamivudine or emtricitabine) + (stavudine or abacavir or tenofovir or didanosine)
	Nelfinavir + (lamivudine or emtricitabine) + (zidovudine or stavudine or abacavir or tenofovir or didanosine)
	Saquinavir/ritonavir + (lamivudine or emtricitabine) + (zidovudine or stavudine or abacavir or tenofovir or didanosine)
Triple NRTI	Abacavir + lamivudine + zidovudine (only when an NNRTI- or PI-based regimen cannot or should not be used)

* NNRTI = non-nucleoside reverse transcriptase inhibitor; PI = protease inhibitor; NRTI = nucleoside reverse transcriptase inhibitor; hgc = hard-gel capsule (Invirase).

† Efavirenz should be avoided in pregnant and women of child-bearing potential.

§ Higher incidence of lipoatrophy, hyperlipidemia, and mitochondrial toxicities associated with stavudine than with other NRTIs.

‡ Low-dose (100–400 mg) ritonavir.

** Use of ritonavir with indinavir might increase risk for renal adverse events.

Source: U.S. Department of Health & Human Services. Guidelines for the Use of Antiretroviral Agents in HIV-Infected Adults & Adolescents, November 3, 2008 revision. Available at www.aidsinfo.nih.gov. This document is updated periodically; refer to website for updated versions.

Which Two NRTIs Should You Consider?

Abacavir (Ziagen), while possibly one of the more potent drugs of this type, has a potentially life-threatening side effect that occurs in 3–5% of people taking it. Generally abacavir, or single pill combinations that include abacavir (like Trizivir or Epzicom), would not be considered as part of an nPEP regimen because of this side effect.

NRTI regimens for nPEP include any combination of AZT (Retrovir), ddI (Videx), d4T (Zerit), FTC (Emtriva), tenofovir (Viread) or 3TC (Epivir). Most of these can be safely combined with one another, except for AZT and d4T. The combination of ddI and d4T is generally discouraged. Also the drugs FTC and 3TC are very similar and rarely used together. It is assumed that any combination of these drugs is roughly equivalent. Generally speaking, if you choose a two NRTIs for nPEP, research sites would probably encourage either an AZT + 3TC (Combivir) or FTC + tenofovir (Truvada) combination, simply because the drugs are co-formulated to include two drugs in a single pill and are easy to use. The major issues to consider when choosing a regimen are side effects and ease of use. It's likely these two combination pills are equally potent when used in this setting.

AZT is the oldest drug in this class and also the most researched. Both AZT and 3TC are made by the same company and are combined into a single pill called Combivir. Thus, by taking one Combivir, twice daily, you may take a two-drug regimen that only requires taking one pill every 12 hours (total of two pills daily). FTC and tenofovir are also made by the same company and combined into a single pill called Truvada. This two-drug regimen requires a single pill, once daily. Either two-drug pill is fairly easy to use. The most common short-term side effects, either of AZT or the Combivir combination pill, are headaches, nausea, and vomiting, which tend to diminish with longer use. Nausea, vomiting, diarrhea, and flatulence (intestinal gas) are the most likely short-term side effects of Truvada. Other side effects are possible in long-term use, but these are generally not a concern in PEP because of the short duration of treatment.

Which NNRTI Or Protease Inhibitor to Consider?

Some nPEP sites routinely prescribe only two NRTIs. Others believe that if nPEP is going to be used, the best and most potent shot we have is to use three drugs. These three-drug regimens are the standard of care for people with HIV infection, and they have proven to be much more potent than two-drug regimens. For people who choose a more aggressive nPEP regimen, typically they would use two NRTIs and a protease inhibitor (PI).

In general, NNRTIs are not used in nPEP regimens. While Viramune (nevirapine) is the more widely studied drug in this class, severe rash associated with its use makes it somewhat unpalatable for nPEP. Risk of developing a severe rash may be greater than the actual chance of HIV infection due to an exposure to HIV. The other NNRTI, Sustiva (efavirenz), has been associated with a high level of side effects, especially in its first month of use, and should not be used by pregnant women or nursing mothers because of possible harmful effects to their children. Rescriptor (delavirdine) is considered the least potent NNRTI. It is not a widely used HIV drug, so an nPEP regimen with an NNRTI as a third drug is highly unusual.

If one added a PI to make a three-drug regimen, the least likely drug to use is full dose Norvir (ritonavir) because it has a high rate of side effects compared to any of the others. In terms of short-term side effects, there's little reason to choose one vs. another of the other protease inhibitors: Reyataz (atazanavir), Lexiva (fosamprenavir), Aptivus (tipranavir), Crixivan (indinavir), Invirase (saquinavir), Prezista (darunavir), Viracept (nelfinavir), or Kaletra (lopinavir + ritonavir). However, some are considerably easier to use than others. Some require twice daily dosing, such as Kaletra, Viracept, Lexiva, and Prezista. Some require a booster of a second drug (low doses of ritonavir) in order to be effective against HIV. It's unclear if this is also true when used as part of nPEP regimens. One protease inhibitor, Reyataz, can be taken once daily. Another factor to consider is the number of pills that must be taken each time the drug is used. Both Kaletra (because of its potency) and Reyataz (because of its ease of use) are often among the first choices considered for nPEP regimens.

Over the past decade, several HIV drugs have been approved, greatly expanding the options in the fight against AIDS. Some cannot be used with other drugs (including non-HIV drugs), and/or their dose must be adjusted when combining them. For example, if Reyataz is combined with Viread (tenofovir) or a single pill formulation that includes tenofovir (such as Truvada), it must be used with a low dose of the protease inhibitor ritonavir to help boost its potency. The bottom line is that constructing a PEP regimen should be done with the guidance of someone familiar with anti-HIV drugs and how to combine them. The doctor you see might not be an HIV specialist, but professional support is available to help your doctor, through the national PEPline (888-448-4911), in selecting and monitoring an nPEP regimen. This line is intended for use by health care professionals only.

In nPEP, where drugs are only taken for 28 days, it's fair to assume that both two- and three-drug regimens are roughly equal or at least adequate. The true differences in these approaches and among the different drugs probably rest in their ability to suppress HIV replication over a long period of time. In the short-term, for a 28-day nPEP regimen, either approach should be adequate.

NNRTIs are generally better tolerated than any of the PIs, which may make them more desirable for nPEP. Moreover, some PIs have more drug interactions than NNRTIs.

How The Anti-HIV Therapy History of The Source Factors In

It is not always possible or comfortable to ask the "source" their current and/or past use of HIV medications. Yet, this information may help you make a better decision about your nPEP regimen.

If, for example, the person has never taken HIV drugs, the choices of therapies to use will be easiest, as worrying about resistant virus is less of a concern. In this setting, some nPEP programs choose to use two drugs for nPEP, though no one knows if a two- or three-drug regimen is best.

On the other hand, if the person had used many different HIV drugs, it's possible that they have developed resistance to many of the medications. (Resistance happens when the HIV in their body mutates to evade the effects of the HIV drugs.) If this is the case, then using a combination of drugs that the person had not used before as your nPEP regimen might be the most effective approach. The more you know about the source's HIV therapy history, the better informed you and your doctor will be at making the best nPEP choice for you.

Where Can You Get nPEP?

Federal Recommendations on using nPEP for non-occupational exposure to HIV were published in January 2005. These are available at www.ucsf.edu.

Currently nPEP is not routinely available at public health clinics or through federal reimbursement programs, like Medicaid. Only one state (Arizona) covers the cost of nPEP through its AIDS Drug Assistance Program (ADAP). In all other states, ADAPs only cover the cost of therapies to manage HIV disease, for people living with HIV, who are uninsured and underinsured and who do not qualify for Medicaid. Some health departments throughout the country support nPEP programs. (For more information about your state's ADAP, contact your local or state Department of Public Health, or contact the Access Project at 800-734-7104 or visit their website at www.aidsinfonyc.org. Contact your local health department for information about nPEP programs in your area. Not all areas will have programs in place or guidelines.)

Currently, some people can get their insurance to cover the cost of nPEP and related lab tests. Because nPEP is considered experimental, a person's ability to access it may vary dramatically. The kinds of factors that might influence a provider's willingness to prescribe nPEP might include their knowledge about HIV and comfort level in prescribing and monitoring the effects of HIV medications. The cost of 28-day nPEP regimens range from $300–$1,800, depending on the regimen, not including costs for lab work and follow-up visits to your doctor.

These sites make nPEP available:

San Francisco, CA and Bay Area: Together with the SF Department of Public Health, San Francisco General Hospital's nPEP program has led the way in defining the issues about nPEP and making information available (415-487-5538). The San Francisco program also includes extensive HIV prevention counseling. nPEP and related lab work is provided free of charge to those who qualify.

Boston, MA: The Fenway Community Health Center (617-267-0900) has been providing nPEP to those seeking the option for several years and they are currently in the process of establishing a statewide nPEP registry. These sites provide nPEP and related lab work free of charge to those who qualify.

Other non-occupational HIV PEP programs may be available through emergency rooms or local clinics. Your city or state department of public health may have more information about HIV nPEP programs in your area. This list merely reflects formal programs that we are aware of at the time of publication.

Commentary on nPEP

The decision to use nPEP is a difficult one. Even if you participated in an activity that put you at high risk for HIV infection, the difficulties of taking nPEP, the risk of side effects from the regimen, and the many unknowns about the value of nPEP may provide enough reason not to use nPEP. The bottom line is that nPEP is not right for everyone.

The Centers for Disease Control and Prevention issued recommendations regarding the use of nPEP in January 2005. The document provides extensive data on the rationale behind using nPEP as well as guidance for those who might best benefit from intervention. It's available through the University of California – San Francisco (www.ucsf.edu) in a PDF format, or directly through the CDC at www.cdc.gov. It also offers guidance on treating and monitoring people seeking nPEP. Moreover, the CDC has established a national nPEP surveillance registry that accepts voluntary reports by clinicians. Information about the registry is available from the Non-occupational HIV PEP Registry: 877-448-1737 (toll-free 24 hours) or www.HIVpepregistry.org.

An activity called pre-exposure prophylaxis (PrEP) is also becoming increasingly popular among young people and people at high risk for HIV infection. This involves taking HIV medications before a night on the town, of risky sex, and/or needle sharing. Taking HIV drugs as a way to prevent HIV infection is currently being studied and is possibly harmful. Theoretically, it's possible that these drugs may weaken the immune system when used in this way and might actually increase the risk of HIV infection if an exposure occurs. Some of the HIV medications should not be used with alcohol and others have potentially lethal drug interactions when used with "street drugs." At this time, there's no information to support the use of HIV drugs for PrEP.

While you may be concerned about HIV exposure or infection after a risky activity, the truth is that many other infectious diseases are passed much easier and may have serious health consequences. Hepatitis, for example, is much more easily passed than HIV. Needle-sharing, needlestick accidents, and unsafe sex all are transmission risks for hepatitis B and C. Exposure to fecal matter and urine not only carries a hepatitis transmission risk but also a risk of exposure to cryptosporidium and parasites. Sexually transmitted infections, including chlamydia, gonorrhea, syphilis, herpes, and warts (HPV), are of equal concern. Some are readily treatable and they should all be monitored for and treated should they occur. If risk of hepatitis exposure is considered high, explore PEP for hepatitis. If you have not been exposed to hepatitis B, strongly consider getting hepatitis B vaccination.

Many people considering nPEP are people who have experienced sexual assault or are the victims of domestic violence. Seeking support from rape crisis counselors is strongly encouraged. For people in relationships where domestic violence is an issue, there are resources available to you. No one deserves to be abused and it's important that you reflect on what is happening to you and remember that it is wrong. An important fact: your risk of HIV infection is greater if the perpetrator of rape or violence is someone you know, rather than a stranger.

The best way to prevent HIV infection is to develop a comprehensive prevention plan that you can live with. For some people this might include gradually improving your HIV risk reduction approaches. For others, it might be easy to eliminate all HIV risk activities or behaviors from your life. It's important that whatever strategy you use, it's one that is reasonable and fits your life. nPEP is not a long-term solution; HIV prevention is.

Finally, if you find out that you are HIV-positive, there are things you can do. You are not dying and you are not alone. Project Inform can help you learn about HIV disease, therapies to treat it, and provide you with publications on developing a relationship with a health care provider and a long-term strategy for managing HIV disease.

Project Inform has publications on new developments in HIV research and treatments, available free of charge to all those who need them. We also have a toll-free hotline at 800-822-7422 or you can fill out a form (at http://www.projectinform.org/hotline/form.shtml) to send in your questions.

Chapter 13

Preventing HIV and Hepatitis Transmission

Chapter Contents

Section 13.1

What Health Care Workers Need to Know about Exposure to Blood

This section excerpted from "Exposure to Blood: What Healthcare Personnel Need to Know," Centers for Disease Control and Prevention (www.cdc.gov), July 2003. Reviewed in January 2009 by Dr. David A. Cooke, M.D., Diplomate, American Board of Internal Medicine.

Occupational Exposures to Blood

Healthcare personnel are at risk for occupational exposure to bloodborne pathogens, including hepatitis B virus (HBV), hepatitis C virus (HCV), and human immunodeficiency virus (HIV). Exposures occur through needlesticks or cuts from other sharp instruments contaminated with an infected patient's blood or through contact of the eye, nose, mouth, or skin with a patient's blood. Important factors that influence the overall risk for occupational exposures to bloodborne pathogens include the number of infected individuals in the patient population and the type and number of blood contacts. Most exposures do not result in infection. Following a specific exposure, the risk of infection may vary with factors such as the following:

- The pathogen involved
- The type of exposure
- The amount of blood involved in the exposure
- The amount of virus in the patient's blood at the time of exposure

Your employer should have in place a system for reporting exposures in order to quickly evaluate the risk of infection, inform you about treatments available to help prevent infection, monitor you for side effects of treatments, and determine if infection occurs. This may involve testing your blood and that of the source patient and offering appropriate postexposure treatment.

How can occupational exposures be prevented?

Many needlesticks and other cuts can be prevented by using safer techniques (for example, not recapping needles by hand), disposing of used needles in appropriate sharps disposal containers, and using medical devices with safety features designed to prevent injuries. Using appropriate barriers such as gloves, eye and face protection, or gowns when contact with blood is expected can prevent many exposures to the eyes, nose, mouth, or skin.

If an Exposure Occurs

What should I do if I am exposed to the blood of a patient?

1. Do the following immediately following an exposure to blood:

   - Wash needlesticks and cuts with soap and water
   - Flush splashes to the nose, mouth, or skin with water
   - Irrigate eyes with clean water, saline, or sterile irrigants

No scientific evidence shows that using antiseptics or squeezing the wound will reduce the risk of transmission of a bloodborne pathogen. Using a caustic agent such as bleach is not recommended.

2. Report the exposure to the department (e.g., occupational health, infection control) responsible for managing exposures. Prompt reporting is essential because, in some cases, postexposure treatment may be recommended and it should be started as soon as possible. Discuss the possible risks of acquiring HBV, HCV, and HIV and the need for postexposure treatment with the provider managing your exposure. You should have already received hepatitis B vaccine, which is extremely safe and effective in preventing HBV infection.

Risk of Infection after Exposure

What is the risk of infection after an occupational exposure?

HBV: Healthcare personnel who have received hepatitis B vaccine and developed immunity to the virus are at virtually no risk for infection. For a susceptible person, the risk from a single needlestick or cut exposure to HBV-infected blood ranges from 6–30% and depends on the hepatitis B e antigen (HBeAg) status of the source individual. Hepatitis B surface antigen (HBsAg)-positive individuals who are HBeAg positive have more virus in their blood and are more likely to transmit HBV than those who are HBeAg negative. While there is a risk for HBV infection from exposures of mucous membranes or nonintact skin, there is no known risk for HBV infection from exposure to intact skin.

HCV: The average risk for infection after a needlestick or cut exposure to HCV infected blood is approximately 1.8%. The risk following a blood exposure to the eye, nose, or mouth is unknown, but is believed to be very small; however, HCV infection from blood splash to the eye has been reported. There also has been a report of HCV transmission that may have resulted from exposure to nonintact skin, but no known risk from exposure to intact skin.

HIV:

- The average risk of HIV infection after a needlestick or cut exposure to HIV-infected blood is 0.3% (i.e., three-tenths of one percent, or about 1 in 300). Stated another way, 99.7% of needlestick/cut exposures do not lead to infection.
- The risk after exposure of the eye, nose, or mouth to HIV-infected blood is estimated to be, on average, 0.1% (1 in 1,000).
- The risk after exposure of non-intact skin to HIV-infected blood is estimated to be less than 0.1%. A small amount of blood on intact skin probably poses no risk at all. There have been no documented cases of HIV transmission due to an exposure involving a small amount of blood on intact skin (a few drops of blood on skin for a short period of time).

Treatment for the Exposure

Is vaccine or treatment available to prevent infections with bloodborne pathogens?

HBV: As mentioned above, hepatitis B vaccine has been available since 1982 to prevent HBV infection. All healthcare personnel who have a reasonable chance of exposure to blood or body fluids should receive hepatitis B vaccine. Vaccination ideally should occur during the healthcare worker's training period. Workers should be tested 1–2 months after the vaccine series is complete to make sure that vaccination has provided immunity to HBV infection. Hepatitis B immune globulin (HBIG) alone or in combination with vaccine (if not previously vaccinated) is effective in preventing HBV infection after an exposure. The decision to begin treatment is based on several factors, such as the following:

- Whether the source individual is positive for hepatitis B surface antigen
- Whether you have been vaccinated
- Whether the vaccine provided you immunity

HCV: There is no vaccine against hepatitis C and no treatment after an exposure that will prevent infection. Neither immune globulin nor antiviral therapy is recommended after exposure. For these reasons, following recommended infection control practices to prevent percutaneous injuries is imperative.

HIV: There is no vaccine against HIV. However, results from a small number of studies suggest that the use of some antiretroviral drugs after certain occupational exposures may reduce the chance of HIV transmission. Postexposure prophylaxis (PEP) is recommended for certain occupational exposures that pose a risk of transmission. However, for those exposures without risk of HIV infection, PEP is not recommended because the drugs used to prevent infection may have serious side effects. You should discuss the risks and side effects with your healthcare provider before starting PEP for HIV.

How are exposures to blood from an individual whose infection status is unknown handled?

HBV–HCV–HIV: If the source individual cannot be identified or tested, decisions regarding follow-up should be based on the exposure risk and whether the source is likely to be infected with a bloodborne pathogen. Follow-up testing should be available to all personnel who are concerned about possible infection through occupational exposure.

What specific drugs are recommended for postexposure treatment?

HBV: If you have not been vaccinated, then hepatitis B vaccination is recommended for any exposure regardless of the source person's

HBV status. HBIG and/or hepatitis B vaccine may be recommended depending on the source person's infection status, your vaccination status and, if vaccinated, your response to the vaccine.

HCV: There is no postexposure treatment that will prevent HCV infection.

HIV: The Public Health Service recommends a four-week course of a combination of either two antiretroviral drugs for most HIV exposures, or three antiretroviral drugs for exposures that may pose a greater risk for transmitting HIV (such as those involving a larger volume of blood with a larger amount of HIV or a concern about drug-resistant HIV). Differences in side effects associated with the use of these drugs may influence which drugs are selected in a specific situation. These recommendations are intended to provide guidance to clinicians and may be modified on a case-by-case basis. Determining which drugs and how many drugs to use or when to change a treatment regimen is largely a matter of judgment. Whenever possible, consulting an expert with experience in the use of antiviral drugs is advised, especially if a recommended drug is not available, if the source patient's virus is likely to be resistant to one or more recommended drugs, or if the drugs are poorly tolerated.

How soon after exposure to a bloodborne pathogen should treatment start?

HBV: Postexposure treatment should begin as soon as possible after exposure, preferably within 24 hours, and no later than seven days.

HIV: Treatment should be started as soon as possible, preferably within hours as opposed to days, after the exposure. Although animal studies suggest that treatment is less effective when started more than 24–36 hours after exposure, the time frame after which no benefit is gained in humans is not known. Starting treatment after a longer period (e.g., one week) may be considered for exposures that represent an increased risk of transmission.

What is known about the safety and side effects of these drugs?

HBV: Hepatitis B vaccine and HBIG are very safe. There is no information that the vaccine causes any chronic illnesses. Most illnesses reported after a hepatitis B vaccination are related to other causes and not the vaccine. However, you should report to your healthcare provider any unusual reaction after a hepatitis B vaccination.

HIV: All of the antiviral drugs for treatment of HIV have been associated with side effects. The most common side effects include upset stomach (nausea, vomiting, diarrhea), tiredness, or headache. The few serious side effects that have been reported in healthcare personnel using combinations of antiviral drugs after exposure have included kidney stones, hepatitis, and suppressed blood cell production. Protease inhibitors (e.g., indinavir and nelfinavir) may interact with other medicines and cause serious side effects and should not be taken in combination with certain other drugs, such as non-sedating antihistamines, e.g., Claritin®. If you need to take antiviral drugs for an HIV exposure, it is important to tell the healthcare provider managing your exposure about any medications you are currently taking.

Follow-Up after an Exposure

What follow-up should be done after an exposure?

HBV: Because postexposure treatment is highly effective in preventing HBV infection, CDC does not recommend routine follow-up after treatment. However, any symptoms suggesting hepatitis (e.g., yellow eyes or skin, loss of appetite, nausea, vomiting, fever, stomach or joint pain, extreme tiredness) should be reported to your healthcare provider. If you receive hepatitis B vaccine, you should be tested one to two months after completing the vaccine series to determine if you have responded to the vaccine and are protected against HBV infection.

HCV: You should be tested for HCV antibody and liver enzyme levels (alanine aminotransferase or ALT) as soon as possible after the exposure (baseline) and at four to six months after the exposure. To check for infection earlier, you can be tested for the virus (HCV RNA) four to six weeks after the exposure. Report any symptoms suggesting hepatitis (mentioned above) to your healthcare provider.

HIV: You should be tested for HIV antibody as soon as possible after exposure (baseline) and periodically for at least six months after the exposure (e.g., at 6 weeks, 12 weeks, and 6 months). If you take antiviral drugs for postexposure treatment, you should be checked for drug toxicity by having a complete blood count and kidney and liver function tests just before starting treatment and two weeks after starting treatment. You should report any sudden or severe flu-like illness that occurs during the follow-up period, especially if it involves fever, rash, muscle aches, tiredness, malaise, or swollen glands. Any of these may suggest HIV infection, drug reaction, or other medical conditions. You should contact the healthcare provider managing your exposure if you have any questions or problems during the follow-up period.

What precautions should be taken during the follow-up period?

HBV: If you are exposed to HBV and receive postexposure treatment, it is unlikely that you will become infected and pass the infection on to others. No precautions are recommended.

HCV: Because the risk of becoming infected and passing the infection on to others after an exposure to HCV is low, no precautions are recommended.

HIV: During the follow-up period, especially the first 6–12 weeks when most infected persons are expected to show signs of infection, you should follow recommendations for preventing transmission of HIV. These include not donating blood, semen, or organs and not having sexual intercourse. If you choose to have sexual intercourse, using a condom consistently and correctly may reduce the risk of HIV transmission. In addition, women should consider not breast-feeding infants during the follow-up period to prevent the possibility of exposing their infants to HIV that may be in breast milk.

Prevention of Occupational Infections with HBV, HCV, or HIV

Hepatitis B virus is largely preventable through vaccination. For HBV, HCV, and HIV, however, preventing occupational exposures to blood can prevent occupational infections with HBV, HCV, and HIV. This includes using appropriate barriers such as gown, gloves and eye protection as appropriate, safely handling needles and other sharp instruments, and using devices with safety features.

Section 13.2

Tattoo Safety

This section includes "Can I get HIV from getting a tattoo or through body piercing?" November 27, 2006, and "Health and Safety of Tattoo Artists, Body Piercers, and Their Clients," January 21, 2008, Centers for Disease Control and Prevention (www.cdc.gov).

Can I Get HIV from Getting a Tattoo or through Body Piercing?

A risk of HIV transmission does exist if instruments contaminated with blood are either not sterilized or disinfected or are used inappropriately between clients. CDC recommends that single-use instruments intended to penetrate the skin be used once, then disposed of. Reusable instruments or devices that penetrate the skin and/or contact a client's blood should be thoroughly cleaned and sterilized between clients.

Personal service workers who do tattooing or body piercing should be educated about how HIV is transmitted and take precautions to prevent transmission of HIV and other bloodborne infections in their settings.

If you are considering getting a tattoo or having your body pierced, ask staff at the establishment what procedures they use to prevent the spread of HIV and other bloodborne infections, such as the hepatitis B virus. You also may call the local health department to find out what sterilization procedures are in place in the local area for these types of establishments.

Health and Safety of Tattoo Artists, Body Piercers, and Their Clients

Tattoo artists and body piercers should follow health and safety practices to protect themselves as well as their clients from bloodborne pathogens such as hepatitis B, hepatitis C, and/or HIV.

Body art is a popular form of self-expression. Tattoos and body piercings are typically created by professional tattoo artists and body piercers and appear on the body as permanent markings and decorative metal.

Health and safety procedures for body artists may be regulated by city, county, or state agencies. Reputable shops and tattoo parlors govern themselves and follow strict safety procedures to protect their clients—and their body artists.

Considering Body Art?

If you decide to get a tattoo or body piercing, make sure you go to a licensed facility and take time to discuss the safety procedures with the artists working at the shop or tattoo parlor. They should explain the process and clarify what they do to keep everyone safe and healthy by using sterile needles and razors, washing hands, wearing gloves, and keeping surfaces clean.

Safety Procedures

Body piercers and tattoo artists protect themselves and their clients when following safe and healthy practices, such as the following:

- Use single-use, disposable needles and razors. Disposable piercing needles, tattoo needles, and razors are used on one person and then thrown away. Reusing needles or razors is not safe.
- Safely dispose of needles and razors. Used needles and razors should be thrown away in a biohazard-labeled, disposable container to protect both the client and the person changing or handling the trash bag from getting cut.
- Wash hands before and after putting on disposable gloves. Gloves are always worn while working with equipment and clients, changed when necessary, and are not reused.
- Clean and sterilize reusable tools and equipment. Some tools and equipment can be reused when creating body art. Reusable tools and equipment should be cleaned and then sterilized to remove viruses and bacteria.
- Frequently clean surfaces and work areas. Chairs, tables, work spaces, and counters should be disinfected between procedures to protect both the health of the client and the artist. Cross-contamination (spreading bacteria and viruses from one surface to another) can occur if surfaces are not disinfected frequently

and between clients. Any disinfectant that claims to be able to eliminate the tuberculosis germ can also kill HIV, hepatitis B, and hepatitis C viruses. Use a commercial disinfectant, following the manufacturer's instructions, or a mixture of bleach and water (1 part bleach to 9 parts water).

By following safety procedures, tattoo artists and body piercers protect themselves and their clients against exposure risks such as the following:

- Viruses, germs, and bacteria that can cause infections
- Tuberculosis
- Hepatitis B
- Hepatitis C
- HIV and AIDS

Chapter 14

Sex Education and STD Prevention Efforts

Chapter Contents

Section 14.1

Discussing STDs with Your Children

"STDs," November 2008, reprinted with permission from www.kidshealth.org. Copyright © 2008 The Nemours Foundation. This information was provided by KidsHealth, one of the largest resources online for medically reviewed health information written for parents, kids, and teens. For more articles like this one, visit www.KidsHealth.org, or www.TeensHealth.org.

Sometimes it's difficult to see your child as anything but that: a child. Yet, in many ways, teens today are growing up faster than ever. They learn about violence and sex through the media and their peers, but they rarely have all the facts. That's why it's so important for you to talk to your kids about sex, particularly sexually transmitted diseases (STDs).

Teens are one of the groups most at risk for contracting STDs. You can help your kids stay safe just by talking to them and sharing some important information about STDs and prevention. Before you tackle this sensitive subject, however, it's important to make sure you not only know what to say, but how and when to say it.

Timing Is Everything

It's never too late to talk to your kids about STDs, even if they're already teens. A late talk is better than no talk at all. But the best time to start having these discussions is some time during the preteen years.

Of course, the exact age varies from child to child: Some kids are more aware of sex at age 9 than others are at age 11. You'll need to read your child's cues.

No matter how old your child is, if he or she starts having questions about sex, it's a good time to talk about STDs.

Questions are a good starting point for a discussion. When kids are curious, they're more open to hearing what their parents have to say.

But not all kids ask their parents questions about sex. One way to initiate a discussion is to use a media cue, like a TV program or an article in the paper, and ask what your child thinks about it. Another way to talk to your daughter is to use the human papillomavirus (HPV) vaccine as a starting point for a conversation. The HPV vaccine is recommended for preteen girls, and has the best chance of protecting against infection if the series of shots is given before a female becomes sexually active.

The surest way to have a healthy dialogue is to establish lines of communication early on. If parents aren't open to talking about sex or other personal subjects when their kids are young, kids will be a lot less likely to seek out mom and dad when they're older and have questions.

Spend time talking with your kids from the beginning and it'll be much easier later to broach topics like sex because they'll feel more comfortable sharing thoughts with you.

Tips for Talking

To make talking about STDs a little easier for both you and your child:

- Be informed. STDs can be a frightening and confusing subject, so it may help if you read up on STD transmission and prevention. You don't want to add any misinformation and being familiar with the topic will make you feel more comfortable.
- Ask what your child already knows about STDs and what else he or she would like to learn. Remember, though: Kids often already know more than you realize, although much of that information could be incorrect. Parents need to provide accurate information so their kids can make the right decisions and protect themselves.
- Ask what your kids think about sexual scenarios on TV and in movies and use those fictional situations as a lead into talking about safe sex and risky behavior.
- Encourage your kids to raise any fears or concerns they have.
- Make your kids feel that they're in charge of this talk, not you, by getting their opinions on whatever you discuss. If you let their questions lead the way, you'll have a much more productive talk than if you stick to an agenda.
- Explain that the only sure way to remain STD-free is to not have sex or intimate contact with anyone outside of a committed,

monogamous relationship, such as marriage. However, those who are having sex should always use condoms to protect against STDs, even when using another method of birth control. Most condoms are made of latex, but for people who may have an allergic skin reaction to latex, both male and female condoms made of polyurethane are available.

Common Questions about STDs

Depending on what your kids have heard from friends and the media, their questions will probably be fairly straightforward, such as:

- **What are STDs?** An STD is a sexually transmitted disease.
- **How does someone catch one?** These infections and diseases are spread from one individual to another during anal, oral, or vaginal sex. They can also be spread when fingers or objects are used after touching genitals or body fluids.
- **What do STDs do to a person's body?** The type of STD determines what kinds of symptoms, if any, someone has. Some STDs cause virtually no symptoms, whereas others can cause the person to have discharge from the vagina or penis, sores, or pain. If STDs are untreated, they can lead to damage to the internal organs and may cause long term health problems, like infertility or cancer.
- **Are STDs curable or do you have them forever?** Both chlamydia and gonorrhea can be cured with antibiotics, but some infections—like herpes or HIV—have no cure.
- **Are people who catch STDs somehow bad?** Getting an STD does not mean that someone is a bad person, just that they need to learn how to prevent future infections.
- **Can you tell that someone has an STD just by looking at him or her?** People often may not even know that they're infected themselves. Although there may be visible signs around the genitals with certain kinds of STDs, like genital warts and herpes, most of the time, there is no way to look at someone and know that he or she has an STD.

Answering any of these questions or others as openly as possible is the best approach. It's up to you to gently correct any misinformation your child may have learned. And always answer questions honestly without being overly dramatic.

It can be tough, but try to avoid getting too emotional or preachy. You want your kids to know that you're there to support and help, not condemn.

Finding Reliable Information

Communicating with your kids may not be simple, but it's necessary. If you're always available to talk, discussions will come easier. Literature from your doctor's office or organizations like Planned Parenthood can provide answers.

And websites like www.TeensHealth.org discuss STDs and sex in teen-friendly language. Viewing them together can help you and your kids start talking.

Your child's school can be an information resource. Find out when sexuality will be covered in health or science class and read the texts that will be taught. The PTA may even offer sessions about talking to teens where you can share tips and experiences with other parents.

And don't shy away from discussing STDs or sex out of fear that talking will make kids want to have sex. Informed teens are not more likely to have sex, but they are more likely to practice safe sex.

If you try these tactics and still don't feel comfortable talking about STDs, make sure your kids can talk to someone who will have accurate information: a doctor, counselor, teacher, or another family member.

Kids and teens need to know about STDs, and it's better that they get the facts from someone trustworthy instead of discovering them on their own.

Section 14.2

Sex Education Report

"What Works Best in Sex/HIV Education?" reprinted with permission from the Center for AIDS Prevention Studies, University of California – San Francisco. © 2006 University of California – San Francisco.

Why sex/HIV education?

Sex and HIV education programs have multiple goals: to decrease unintended pregnancy, to decrease STDs including HIV, and to improve sexual health among youth. In 2005, almost two-thirds (63%) of all high school seniors in the U.S. had engaged in sex, yet only 21% of all female students used birth control pills before their last sex and only 70% of males used a condom during their last sexual intercourse.[1] In 2000, 8.4% of 15–19 year old girls became pregnant, producing one of the highest teen pregnancy rates in the western industrial world.[2] Persons aged 15–24 had 9.1 million new cases of STDs in 2000 and made up almost half of all new STD cases in the U.S.[3]

There are numerous factors affecting adolescent sexual behavior and use of protection. Some of these factors have little to do with sex, such as growing up in disadvantaged communities, having little attachment to parents, or failing at school. Other factors are sexual in nature, such as beliefs, values, perceptions of peer norms, attitudes and skills involving sexual behavior, and using condoms or contraception.[4] It is these sexual factors that sex/HIV education programs can potentially affect, thereby impacting behavior. Sex/HIV education programs alone cannot totally reduce sexual risk-taking, but they can be an effective part of a more comprehensive initiative.

Do sex/HIV education programs work?

Yes. Some sex/HIV education programs delay initiation of intercourse, reduce the frequency of sex, reduce the number of sexual partners, and increase use of condoms or other forms of contraception. Also, research indicates that sex/HIV education programs—even those that encourage condom and contraceptive use—do not increase sexual activity. In a recent review, almost two-thirds of the programs evaluated within the U.S. significantly improved one or more of these behaviors.[5] The results were even more positive in developing countries. Thus, many programs are effective, but others may not be and communities should implement either those programs that have been demonstrated to be effective or those programs that incorporate common characteristics of effective programs.[5]

Can effective programs be replicated?

Yes. Several curricula have been implemented and evaluated up to five times in different states and consistently produced positive changes in sexual behavior when implemented as designed. One of them was even replicated in more than 80 community-based organizations (CBOs) and found to be effective.[6] However, when the curricula are greatly shortened, when condom lessons are cut, or when programs designed for the community are implemented in the classroom, they are less likely to significantly change behavior.

Which curricula are most likely to significantly change behavior?

- In a randomized trial of young women, SiHLE (sistering, informing, healing, living, and empowering) significantly increased condom use, reduced the pregnancy rate, and reduced the STD rate.[7]
- In four different studies, Reducing the Risk delayed the initiation of sex and/or increased condom use for up to 18 months.[8,9]
- In a randomized trial, Safer Choices delayed sex among some youth and increased condom and contraceptive use among sexually active youth over a 31 month period.[10]
- Finally, in multiple randomized trials, Making Proud Choices[11] and Becoming a Responsible Teen[12] increased condom use for at least one year.

These and other effective programs share [17] characteristics that contribute to their success. Characteristics are divided into development, the curriculum itself, and implementation.[5]

How are effective programs developed?

Effective programs can be developed by teams of people with backgrounds in psychosocial theory, adolescent sexual behavior, curriculum design, community culture, and/or teaching sex/HIV education. They review local data on teens' sexual behavior, pregnancy rates, and STD rates, and often conduct focus groups with teens and interviews with adults. Using a logic model framework, they identify the behaviors they want to change, the risk and protective factors affecting them, and activities that would change them. They then design activities consistent with community values and resources and finally pilot-test and revise the curricula.

What do effective curricula look like?

Effective curricula really focus on reducing unintended pregnancy, STD/HIV, or both. They do this by emphasizing the consequences of unintended pregnancy, STDs or HIV, and the risk of experiencing them; by giving a very clear message about sexual behavior; and by discussing situations that might lead to sex and how to avoid or get out of those situations.

Particularly important are the behavioral messages. Effective curricula most commonly emphasize that abstinence is the safest and best approach and encourage condom/contraceptive use for those having sex. Sometimes other values, such as being proud, being responsible, respecting yourself, sticking to your limits, and remaining in control, are also emphasized, and are clearly linked to particular behaviors.

Effective curricula incorporate activities, instructional methods, and behavioral messages that are appropriate to the youths' culture, developmental age, gender, and sexual experience. All actively involve youth to help them personalize the information.

- To increase basic knowledge about risks of teen sex and methods of avoiding intercourse or using protection, effective programs can use: short lectures, class discussions, competitive games, skits or videos, and flip charts or pamphlets.
- To address risk, programs can use: data on the incidence or prevalence of pregnancy or STD/HIV among youth and their consequences, class discussions, HIV+ speakers, and simulations such as the STD handshake.
- To change individual values and peer norms about abstinence and condom use, programs can use: clear behavioral messages, forced choice value exercises, peer surveys/voting, peer role plays, discussions of effectiveness of condoms, and visits to drug stores or clinics where condoms are sold or distributed.

- To build skills to help avoid unwanted or unprotected sex and insist on and use condoms or contraception, programs can use: role playing including describing the skills, modeling the skills, and repeated individual practice role playing the skills.
- To use condoms properly, youth can practice opening the package and putting a condom over their fingers, or talking through all the steps for using condoms.

How are effective programs implemented?

When effective programs are implemented, they typically obtain necessary support from appropriate authorities, select educators with desirable traits and train them, implement activities to recruit and retain youth if needed, and implement the curricula with fidelity. Programs can be effective with either adult or peer educators.

What needs to be done?

Policy makers should fund and encourage the implementation of sex/HIV education programs that have been demonstrated to be effective. If a new program is used, it should have the common characteristics of effective programs.[5] Untested programs should be evaluated for effectiveness. Although programs should be implemented everywhere, they especially should be implemented in the locations and among populations where youth are at highest risk for HIV, STDs, and unplanned pregnancy.

In order for evidence-based sex/HIV education programs to be implemented broadly, they should have support from appropriate authorities such as directors of youth-serving organizations, school districts, principals, and teachers. Staff or teachers conducting programs should be trained and supported to implement programs with fidelity. This includes allowing enough time in the classroom or organization to deliver the program.

Says who?

1. Centers for Disease Control and Prevention. Youth risk behavior surveillance—United States, 2005. Surveillance Summaries. June 9, 2006.
2. Alan Guttmacher Institute. U.S. teenage pregnancy statistics: Overall trends, trends by race and ethnicity and state-by-state information. New York: The Alan Guttmacher Institute, 2004.

3. Weinstock H, Berman S, Cates W. Sexually transmitted diseases among American youth: incidence and prevalence estimates, 2000. *Perspectives in Sexual and Reproductive Health*. 2004;36:6–10.

4. Kirby D, Lepore G, Ryan J. Sexual risk and protective factors: Factors affecting teen sexual behavior, pregnancy, childbearing and sexually transmitted disease: Which are important? Which can you change? Washington DC: National Campaign to Prevent Teen Pregnancy. 2005.

5. Kirby D, Laris BA, Rolleri L. Sex and HIV education programs for youth: Their impact and important characteristics. Washington DC: Family Health International, 2006.

6. Jemmott III, JB. Effectiveness of an HIV/STD risk-reduction intervention implemented by nongovernmental organizations: A randomized controlled trial among adolescents. Presented at the American Psychological Association Annual Conference. Washington DC: August, 2005.

7. DiClemente RJ, Wingood GM, Harrington KF, et al. Efficacy of an HIV prevention intervention for African American adolescent girls: a randomized controlled trial. *Journal of the American Medical Association*. 2004;292:171–179.

8. Kirby D, Barth RP, Leland N, et al. Reducing the risk: Impact of a new curriculum on sexual risk-taking. *Family Planning Perspectives*. 1991;23:253–263.

9. Hubbard BM, Giese ML, Rainey J. A replication of Reducing the Risk, a theory-based sexuality curriculum for adolescents. *Journal of School Health*. 1998;68:243–247.

10. Kirby DB, Baumler E, Coyle KK, et al. The "Safer Choices" intervention: its impact on the sexual behaviors of different subgroups of high school students. *Journal of Adolescent Health*. 2004;35:442–452.

11. Jemmott JB, Jemmott LS, Fong GT. Abstinence and safer sex: A randomized trial of HIV sexual risk-reduction interventions for young African-American adolescents. *Journal of the American Medical Association*. 1998;279:1529–1536.

12. St. Lawrence JS, Brasfield TL, Jefferson KW, et al. Cognitive-behavioral intervention to reduce African American adolescents'

risk for HIV infection. *Journal of Consulting and Clinical Psychology*. 1995;63:221–237.

*All websites accessed July 2006

Section 14.3

Impact of STD Prevention Efforts

"Return on Investment: Impact of STD Prevention Efforts," Centers for Disease Control and Prevention (www.cdc.gov), August 20, 2007.

Three CDC studies show how federally funded efforts to prevent sexually transmitted diseases have dramatically reduced STDs and their associated health costs.

The first study[1] provided evidence that funding for STD and HIV prevention has a discernible impact on new cases of STDs. The authors found that greater amounts of federal STD and HIV prevention funding in a given year are associated with reductions in reported gonorrhea rates at the state level in following years. Results suggest that each dollar of prevention funding (per capita) is associated with a later decrease in gonorrhea of up to 20%. Because gonorrhea is a marker for risky sexual behavior, the findings are likely generalizable to other STDs, including HIV.

The second study[2] examined the impact of federally funded STD prevention efforts over the past 33 years, estimating that approximately 32 million cases of gonorrhea were avoided from 1971 to 2003 as a result of prevention efforts. The study demonstrated that STD prevention programs paid for themselves. Savings realized by preventing gonorrhea exceeded the STD prevention program expenditures by more than $3.7 billion during the 33-year period. If other benefits were considered (such as the prevention of other STDs), the estimated effectiveness and cost-effectiveness of STD prevention in the United States would be even greater.

In the third study[3], researchers estimated that reductions in new cases of gonorrhea and syphilis from 1990 to 2003 saved $5.0 billion in direct medical costs. This estimate was based on reported cases of the two diseases in the United States, coupled with published estimates of direct medical costs per STD case. Authors calculated that the total direct medical cost of gonorrhea and syphilis was $3.8 billion over the 14-year period, compared to $8.9 billion if STD rates had remained at their 1990 levels. Because gonorrhea and syphilis infection are known to increase the risk of HIV transmission, a significant portion ($3.9 billion) of the total savings ($5.0 billion) reflected HIV infections that were averted due to reduced gonorrhea and syphilis rates.

References

1. Chesson HW, Harrison P, Scotton CR, and Varghese B. Does funding for HIV and sexually transmitted disease prevention matter? Evidence from panel data. *Evaluation Review* 2005; 29(1): 3–23.
2. Chesson HW. Estimated effectiveness and cost-effectiveness of federally-funded prevention efforts on gonorrhea rates in the United States, 1971–2003, under various assumptions about the impact of prevention funding. *Sexually Transmitted Diseases* 2006; 33(10): S140–S144.
3. Chesson HW, Gift TL, Pulver ALS. The economic value of reductions in gonorrhea and syphilis incidence in the United States, 1990–2003. *Preventive Medicine* 2006; 43: 411–415.

Part Three

Types of Sexually Transmitted Diseases and Their Treatments

Chapter 15

Chancroid

What is chancroid?

Though curable, chancroid is a highly contagious sexually transmitted disease (STD). It is caused by bacteria called *Haemophilus ducreyi* (or *H. ducreyi*). Chancroid causes ulcers or sores, usually on the genitals. Also, swollen, painful lymph glands in the groin area are often associated with chancroid. Left untreated, chancroid may make the transmission of HIV easier.

How common is chancroid?

Chancroid is very common in Africa and parts of Asia, and it is becoming more common in the United States.

How is chancroid transmitted?

Chancroid may be transmitted sexually through skin-to-skin contact with an open sore and non-sexually by means of autoinoculation when contact is made with the pus-like fluid from the ulcer. A person is considered infectious when ulcers or sores are present. Therefore, as long as there are chancroid sores on the body, the person can spread the infection. Good news is that there has been no reported disease in infants born to women with active chancroid at time of delivery.

What are the signs and symptoms of chancroid?

If infected, symptoms usually occur within 10 days from exposure. They rarely develop earlier than three days or later than 10 days. The ulcer or sore begins as a tender, elevated bump that becomes a pus-filled, open sore with eroded or ragged edges. The ulcers are soft to the touch and can be very painful in men. Painful lymph glands or lymph nodes may occur in the groin on one or both sides of the body. Women may not experience pain and are unaware of the infection.

What are complications of chancroid?

Chancroid is well established as a cofactor for HIV transmission. An individual infected with chancroid may be more easily infected with HIV. Someone infected with both chancroid and HIV may transmit HIV more easily to a partner who is not infected. Also, persons with HIV may experience slower healing of chancroid, even with treatment, and may need to take medications for longer time periods.

Additional complications from chancroid may include the following:

- In 50% of cases, the lymph node glands in the groin become infected within five to eight days of appearance of initial sores.
- Glands on one side become enlarged, hard, painful, and fuse together to form a bubo, an inflammation and swelling of one or more lymph nodes with overlying red skin. Surgical drainage of the bubo may be necessary to relieve pain.
- Ruptured buboes are susceptible to secondary bacterial infections.
- In uncircumcised males, new scar tissue may result in phimosis (constriction so the foreskin cannot be retracted over the glans or head of the penis). To correct this, circumcision may be required.

How does chancroid affect a pregnant woman and her baby?

No adverse effects of chancroid on pregnancy outcome are reported.

How is chancroid diagnosed?

Diagnosis is made by examining the bacteria *Haemophilus ducreyi* in a culture from a genital ulcer or sore. Because the ulcer or sore is often confused with symptoms of other STDs like syphilis or herpes, it is important that a health care provider rule out these other diseases.

What is the treatment for chancroid?

If one partner shows symptoms of chancroid, both should be examined and treated with antibiotics regardless of whether symptoms are present. A follow-up examination should be conducted three to seven days after treatment begins. If treatment is successful, ulcers usually improve within three to seven days. The time required for complete healing is related to the size of the ulcer. Large ulcers may require two weeks or longer to heal. In severe cases, scarring may result.

How can chancroid be prevented?

As with other STDs there are things people can do to reduce or eliminate the risk of infection with chancroid. These include:

- abstinence (not having sex);
- mutual monogamy (having sex with only one uninfected partner);
- avoid touching the infected area to prevent chance of autoinoculation; and
- use latex condoms for vaginal, oral, and anal sex to reduce risks. (Although using condoms may protect the penis or vagina from infection, it does not protect body parts such as the scrotum or anal area.)

Chapter 16

Chlamydia

Chapter Contents

Section 16.1

Chlamydia Overview

"Chlamydia—CDC Fact Sheet," Centers for Disease Control and Prevention (www.cdc.gov), December 20, 2007.

What is chlamydia?

Chlamydia is a common sexually transmitted disease (STD) caused by the bacterium, *Chlamydia trachomatis*, which can damage a woman's reproductive organs. Even though symptoms of chlamydia are usually mild or absent, serious complications that cause irreversible damage, including infertility, can occur "silently" before a woman ever recognizes a problem. Chlamydia also can cause discharge from the penis of an infected man.

How common is chlamydia?

Chlamydia is the most frequently reported bacterial sexually transmitted disease in the United States. In 2006, 1,030,911 chlamydial infections were reported to CDC from 50 states and the District of Columbia. Under-reporting is substantial because most people with chlamydia are not aware of their infections and do not seek testing. Also, testing is not often done if patients are treated for their symptoms. An estimated 2,291,000 non-institutionalized U.S. civilians ages 14–39 are infected with chlamydia based on the U.S. National Health and Nutrition Examination Survey. Women are frequently reinfected if their sex partners are not treated.

How do people get chlamydia?

Chlamydia can be transmitted during vaginal, anal, or oral sex. Chlamydia can also be passed from an infected mother to her baby during vaginal childbirth.

Any sexually active person can be infected with chlamydia. The greater the number of sex partners, the greater the risk of infection. Because the cervix (opening to the uterus) of teenage girls and young women is not fully matured and is probably more susceptible to infection, they are at particularly high risk for infection if sexually active. Since chlamydia can be transmitted by oral or anal sex, men who have sex with men are also at risk for chlamydial infection.

What are the symptoms of chlamydia?

Chlamydia is known as a "silent" disease because about three quarters of infected women and about half of infected men have no symptoms. If symptoms do occur, they usually appear within one to three weeks after exposure.

In women, the bacteria initially infect the cervix and the urethra (urine canal). Women who have symptoms might have an abnormal vaginal discharge or a burning sensation when urinating. When the infection spreads from the cervix to the fallopian tubes (tubes that carry fertilized eggs from the ovaries to the uterus), some women still have no signs or symptoms; others have lower abdominal pain, low back pain, nausea, fever, pain during intercourse, or bleeding between menstrual periods. Chlamydial infection of the cervix can spread to the rectum.

Men with signs or symptoms might have a discharge from their penis or a burning sensation when urinating. Men might also have burning and itching around the opening of the penis. Pain and swelling in the testicles are uncommon.

Men or women who have receptive anal intercourse may acquire chlamydial infection in the rectum, which can cause rectal pain, discharge, or bleeding. Chlamydia can also be found in the throats of women and men having oral sex with an infected partner.

What complications can result from untreated chlamydia?

If untreated, chlamydial infections can progress to serious reproductive and other health problems with both short-term and long-term consequences. Like the disease itself, the damage that chlamydia causes is often "silent."

In women, untreated infection can spread into the uterus or fallopian tubes and cause pelvic inflammatory disease (PID). This happens in up to 40% of women with untreated chlamydia. PID can cause permanent damage to the fallopian tubes, uterus, and surrounding tissues. The damage can lead to chronic pelvic pain, infertility, and potentially fatal ectopic pregnancy (pregnancy outside the uterus). Women infected with chlamydia are up to five times more likely to become infected with HIV, if exposed.

To help prevent the serious consequences of chlamydia, screening at least annually for chlamydia is recommended for all sexually active women age 25 years and younger. An annual screening test also is recommended for older women with risk factors for chlamydia (a new sex partner or multiple sex partners). All pregnant women should have a screening test for chlamydia.

Complications among men are rare. Infection sometimes spreads to the epididymis (the tube that carries sperm from the testis), causing pain, fever, and, rarely, sterility.

Rarely, genital chlamydial infection can cause arthritis that can be accompanied by skin lesions and inflammation of the eye and urethra (Reiter's syndrome).

How does chlamydia affect a pregnant woman and her baby?

In pregnant women, there is some evidence that untreated chlamydial infections can lead to premature delivery. Babies who are born to infected mothers can get chlamydial infections in their eyes and respiratory tracts. Chlamydia is a leading cause of early infant pneumonia and conjunctivitis (pink eye) in newborns.

How is chlamydia diagnosed?

There are laboratory tests to diagnose chlamydia. Some can be performed on urine, other tests require that a specimen be collected from a site such as the penis or cervix.

What is the treatment for chlamydia?

Chlamydia can be easily treated and cured with antibiotics. A single dose of azithromycin or a week of doxycycline (twice daily) are the most commonly used treatments. HIV-positive persons with chlamydia should receive the same treatment as those who are HIV negative.

All sex partners should be evaluated, tested, and treated. Persons with chlamydia should abstain from sexual intercourse until they and their sex partners have completed treatment, otherwise reinfection is possible.

Women whose sex partners have not been appropriately treated are at high risk for reinfection. Having multiple infections increases a woman's risk of serious reproductive health complications, including infertility. Retesting should be encouraged for women three to four months after treatment. This is especially true if a woman does not know if her sex partner received treatment.

How can chlamydia be prevented?

The surest way to avoid transmission of STDs is to abstain from sexual contact, or to be in a long-term mutually monogamous relationship with a partner who has been tested and is known to be uninfected.

Latex male condoms, when used consistently and correctly, can reduce the risk of transmission of chlamydia.

CDC recommends yearly chlamydia testing of all sexually active women age 25 or younger, older women with risk factors for chlamydial infections (those who have a new sex partner or multiple sex partners), and all pregnant women. An appropriate sexual risk assessment by a health care provider should always be conducted and may indicate more frequent screening for some women.

Any genital symptoms such as an unusual sore, discharge with odor, burning during urination, or bleeding between menstrual cycles could mean an STD infection. If a woman has any of these symptoms, she should stop having sex and consult a health care provider immediately. Treating STDs early can prevent PID. Women who are told they have an STD and are treated for it should notify all of their recent sex partners (sex partners within the preceding 60 days) so they can see a health care provider and be evaluated for STDs. Sexual activity should not resume until all sex partners have been examined and, if necessary, treated.

Section 16.2

Study Shows Heavy Impact of Chlamydia on U.S. Men and Women

"New Data Show Heavy Impact of Chlamydia on U.S. Men and Women, Particularly Young People," Centers for Disease Control and Prevention (www.cdc.gov), July 12, 2005.

New data show a heavy burden of chlamydia in young women and men in the United States, particularly among pregnant women attending publicly funded clinics and economically disadvantaged youth, according to the Centers for Disease Control and Prevention (CDC). Other research found that federal sexually transmitted disease prevention efforts have prevented millions of infections and saved an estimated five billion dollars in direct medical costs over the past 30 years. These new data were presented at the 16th biennial meeting of the International Society for Sexually Transmitted Diseases Research (ISSTDR), July 10–13, 2005, in Amsterdam.

"STDs often have no symptoms and therefore frequently go unrecognized and undiagnosed," said Dr. John Douglas, director of CDC's STD prevention programs. "Stepping up screening and prevention efforts is critical to ensuring that young people do not suffer the long-term effects of untreated chlamydia, including infertility."

Toll of Chlamydia Greatest among Young Women, but Men Also Bear Heavy Burden

In the first nationally representative study of chlamydia prevalence in the general adult population (ages 14–39), CDC researchers found a chlamydia prevalence of 2.2% and no significant differences between women and men overall. Nearly 1 in 20 women between the ages of 14–19 (4.6%) were infected—the highest proportion of any age group. Among men, 20- to 29-year-olds were most heavily affected, with a prevalence of 3.2%. Prevalence was higher among blacks in all age groups, at 6.4%, compared to 1.5% among whites. The findings were based on responses from participants in the National Health and Nutrition Examination Survey (NHANES) from 1999 to 2002.

Two separate analyses of economically disadvantaged young adults (16–24) enrolled in a national job training program found that roughly 1 in 10 were infected with chlamydia. Analysis of test results from more than 106,000 young women from 1998 through 2004, nearly two-thirds of whom were black or Hispanic, found that 10.9% were infected. Prevalence was highest among 16-year-old women at 13.3%.

CDC's evaluation of test results from more than 50,000 young men (63% of them black or Hispanic) in the same job training program from July 2003 to December 2004 represented the first widespread chlamydia screening among men in the U.S. The results showed 8.2% were infected with chlamydia, with the highest rate among 20- to 24-year-old men (8.8%). Only 2.4% of men with chlamydia had reported symptoms, suggesting they would have remained undiagnosed without the screening offered by this program.

Chlamydia Infection High among Pregnant Women, Particularly Minority Women

In a separate study, researchers analyzed data on more than 86,000 women ages 15–45 who were screened for chlamydia at publicly funded prenatal clinics in 18 states. Test results were positive for 5.8%, with the highest prevalence among 15- to 19-year-olds (9.7%). Prevalence among black women (11.1%) was nearly four times that of white (3.9%) and Hispanic (3.8%) women. Because chlamydia can have serious consequences for newborns, including pneumonia and conjunctivitis, study authors recommend continued emphasis on prenatal chlamydia screening.

In 2003, 877,478 cases of chlamydia were reported in the United States, making it the nation's most commonly reported STD. Chlamydia is easily cured with antibiotics but is often undiagnosed because of its lack of symptoms. Besides infertility, the disease can cause other serious health problems in women: pelvic inflammatory disease, ectopic pregnancy, and chronic pelvic pain. CDC recommends the delay of sexual initiation among teens as the only 100% effective method of STD prevention, and annual chlamydia screening for all sexually active women under age 25.

Chapter 17

Cytomegalovirus Infection

What is CMV?

CMV, or cytomegalovirus, is a common virus that infects people of all ages. Once CMV is in a person's body, it stays there for life. Most infections with CMV are "silent," meaning most people who are infected with CMV have no signs or symptoms. However, CMV can cause disease in unborn babies and in people with a weakened immune system.

CMV is a member of the herpesvirus family, which includes the herpes simplex viruses and the viruses that cause chickenpox (varicella-zoster virus) and infectious mononucleosis (Epstein-Barr virus).

Who is at risk for CMV disease?

Anyone can become infected with CMV. Most healthy adults and children who have a CMV infection will have few, if any, symptoms. However, certain groups are at higher risk of getting CMV disease. These groups include the following:

- Unborn babies who are infected during pregnancy
- People with a weakened (immunocompromised) immune system

"Frequently Asked Questions about CMV," Centers for Disease Control and Prevention (www.cdc.gov), March 28, 2006.

Risk of CMV infection is likely to be reduced by careful attention to good personal hygiene, such as hand washing.

How is CMV spread?

- Person-to-person contact (such as kissing, sexual contact, and getting saliva or urine on your hands and then touching your eyes, or the inside of your nose or mouth)
- Through the breast milk of an infected woman who is breast feeding
- Infected pregnant women can pass the virus to their unborn babies
- Blood transfusions and organ transplantations

CMV is sometimes found in body fluids, including urine, saliva (spit), breast milk, blood, tears, semen, and vaginal fluids. A person can become infected with CMV when they come in contact with infected body fluids. However, people who are CMV-positive (have been infected with CMV sometime in the past) usually do not have virus in these fluids, so the chance of getting a CMV infection from casual contact is very small.

Contact with the saliva or urine of young children is a major cause of CMV infection among pregnant women.

Women who are pregnant or planning a pregnancy should follow hygienic practices (e.g., careful hand washing) to avoid CMV infection. Because young children are more likely to have CMV in their urine or saliva (spit) than are older children or adults, pregnant women who have young children or work with young children should be especially careful.

What are the signs and symptoms of CMV?

Most healthy children and adults infected with CMV have no symptoms and may not even know that they have been infected. Others may develop a mild illness. Symptoms may include fever, sore throat, fatigue, and swollen glands. These symptoms are similar to those of other illnesses, so most people are not aware that they are infected with CMV.

Most babies born with CMV (in other words, "congenital" CMV) never develop symptoms or disabilities. When babies do have symptoms, some can go away but others can be permanent.

Examples of symptoms or disabilities caused by congenital (meaning present at birth) CMV include the following:

Temporary Symptoms

- Liver problems
- Spleen problems
- Jaundice (yellow skin and eyes)
- Purple skin splotches
- Lung problems
- Small size at birth
- Seizures

Permanent Symptoms or Disabilities

- Hearing loss
- Vision loss
- Mental disability
- Small head
- Lack of coordination
- Seizures
- Death

In some children, symptoms do not appear until months or years after birth. The most common of these late-occurring symptoms are hearing loss and vision loss. Children with congenital CMV are more likely to have permanent disabilities and symptoms that get worse if they had symptoms of CMV infection at birth. But, some children who appear healthy at birth can develop hearing or vision loss over time due to congenital CMV. For this reason, if you know your baby was born with CMV, it is important to have her or his hearing and vision tested regularly.

What health problems does CMV cause in babies?

- Hearing loss
- Vision loss
- Mental disability
- Lung problems

- Bleeding problems
- Spleen problems
- Liver problems
- Growth problems

CMV can cause symptoms when the baby is born or later in the baby's life. Most babies born with CMV never develop symptoms or disabilities. In some infants, hearing or vision loss occur months or years after birth.

How do I know if I have CMV?

Most CMV infections are not diagnosed because the infected person usually has few or no symptoms. However, persons who have been infected with CMV develop antibodies to the virus, which may stay in a person's body for their lifetime. Antibodies are immune proteins that are the body's response to infection.

A blood test can tell a person if they have CMV, but this test is not commonly performed. Laboratory tests can detect the virus in a person's body fluids (blood or urine) or by a tissue biopsy (a small piece of the body's tissue). CMV can also be detected in the body by measuring the antibodies (immune proteins) in the blood targeted against CMV. This is called serologic testing.

Congenital CMV disease is most likely to occur when a woman is infected for the first time during a pregnancy. This is known as a primary CMV infection. Primary infections occur in 1%–4% of seronegative (have no CMV antibodies) pregnant women and lead to fetal infection in one third of these pregnancies. In women who are already infected before becoming pregnant (CMV seropositive women), CMV reactivation or reinfection leads to fetal infection in less than 1% of pregnancies. Approximately 10% of congenitally infected infants have symptoms at birth, and of the 90% who have no symptoms, 10%–15% will develop symptoms over months or even years.

How do you prevent CMV during pregnancy?

No actions can eliminate all risks of becoming infected with CMV, but there are measures that can reduce spread of the disease:

- Wash hands often with soap and water, especially after changing diapers. Wash well for 15 to 20 seconds. More information on hand washing is available on the CDC Ounce of Prevention site (http://www.cdc.gov/ncidod/op/).

- Do not kiss young children under the age of five or six on the mouth or cheek. Instead, kiss them on the head or give them a big hug.
- Do not share food, drinks, or utensils (spoons or forks) with young children.

If you are pregnant and work in a day care center, reduce your risk of getting CMV by working with children who are older than 2½ years of age, especially if you are CMV seronegative (have never been infected with CMV) or are unsure if you are seronegative.

If I have a baby with congenital CMV, will my next baby also have congenital CMV?

Nearly all women who have one baby with congenital CMV will be protected from future CMV infections because they have developed immunity. There have been few reports of mothers who gave birth to more than one baby with congenital CMV. However, these cases are rare.

Is there a treatment for CMV?

Currently, no treatment is recommended for CMV infection in the healthy individual, including pregnant women. However, antiviral drugs ganciclovir and valganciclovir are being used for patients with weakened immune systems. Antiviral drugs are being tested in infants born with congenital CMV. Because of its strong side effects, ganciclovir should only be considered for infants with severe congenital CMV disease.

Vaccines for preventing CMV infection are still in the research and development stage.

Chapter 18

Epididymitis

Definition

Epididymitis is an inflammation of the epididymis, the tubular structure that connects the testicle with the vas deferens.

Causes

Acute epididymitis causes swelling of the scrotum, pain in the testicles, and sometimes a fever of up to six weeks duration or less (usually with a gradual onset over several days).

If not treated, or in some other cases, the condition can become chronic. In chronic cases, there is usually no swelling, but simply pain.

The incidence is approximately 600,000 cases per year. The highest prevalence is in young men 19 to 35 years of age. The disorder is a major cause of hospital admissions in the military (causing approximately 20% of admissions).

Epididymitis is usually caused by spread of infection from the urethra or the bladder. The most common organisms involved in the condition in young heterosexual men are gonorrhea and chlamydia. In children and older men, typical uropathogens, such as coliform organisms (*E. coli*), are much more common. This is also true in the case of homosexual men.

Mycobacterium tuberculosis (TB) can manifest also as epididymitis. "Beadlike" irregularities along vas deferens are the characteristic sign of this condition. Other bacteria (such as Ureaplasma) may also cause epididymitis.

A non-infectious cause of epididymitis is the use of anti-arrhythmic medication, amiodarone. In this case, the inflammation is limited to the head of the epididymis and does not respond to anti-microbial therapy. The treatment is dosage reduction or change of medications.

An increased risk is associated with sexually active men who are not monogamous and do not use condoms. Men who have recently had surgery or have a history of structural problems involving the genitourinary tract are also at increased risk (regardless of sexual behaviors). Other risk factors include chronic indwelling urethral catheter use and being uncircumcised.

Epididymitis may begin with a low grade fever and chills and a heavy sensation in the testicle. The testicle becomes increasingly sensitive to pressure or traction.

There may be lower abdominal discomfort or pelvic discomfort, and urination may cause burning or pain. On occasion, there may be a discharge from the urethra, blood in the semen, or pain on ejaculation. The testicle may enlarge significantly and produce severe pain.

It is important that this condition be distinguished from testicular torsion (a reduction or stoppage of the blood flow to the testicle), which requires emergency care. Testicular torsion is a surgical emergency and should be treated as soon as possible. Acute testicular pain should never be ignored.

Symptoms

- Painful scrotal swelling (testes enlarged)
- Testicular lump
- Tender, swollen testicle on affected side
- Tender, swollen groin area on affected side
- Testicle pain aggravated by bowel movement
- Fever
- Discharge from urethra (the opening at the end of the penis)
- Blood in the semen
- Groin pain

Exams and Tests

Physical examination shows a red, tender, and sometimes swollen mass on the affected hemi-scrotum. Tenderness is usually localized to a small area of the testicle where the epididymitis is attached.

Enlarged lymph nodes in the groin area (inguinal nodes) may be present. There may be a discharge from penis. A rectal examination may reveal an enlarged or tender prostate.

These tests may be performed:

- a urinalysis and culture (the provider may request several specimens including: initial stream, mid-stream, and after a prostate massage);
- tests to screen for Chlamydia and gonorrhea;
- CBC (complete blood count);
- Doppler ultrasound to rule out testicular torsion—hypoechoic region may be visible on the affected side as well as increased blood flow or scrotal abscess;
- testicular scan (nuclear medicine scan) to rule out torsion—in case of the epididymitis, increased blood flow may also be demonstrated.

Treatment

Medications to treat infection are prescribed. Sexually transmitted infections require special antibiotics, and the patient's sexual partners should also be simultaneously treated. Pain medications may be required and anti-inflammatory medications are often prescribed.

Bed rest, with elevation of the scrotum and ice packs applied to the area, is recommended. It is very important to have a follow-up visit with your health care provider to evaluate whether the infection has completely resolved.

Outlook (Prognosis)

Epididymitis usually resolves with appropriate antibiotic therapy, without any damage to prior sexual or reproductive abilities. Recurrence is fairly common.

Possible Complications

Complications include testicular infarction, scrotal abscess, cutaneous scrotal fistula, chronic epididymitis, and infertility.

Acute scrotal pain is a true medical emergency with serious consequences—immediate medical evaluation is critical.

When to Contact a Medical Professional

Call your health care provider if symptoms of epididymitis develop. Go to the emergency room or call the local emergency number (such as 911) if severe testicle pain develops suddenly or follows an injury.

Prevention

Complications from epididymitis may be prevented by early diagnosis and adequate treatment (plus reporting if applicable) of the infectious diseases associated with it. Prophylactic (preventive course) antibiotics are frequently given at the time of surgeries in which the patient is at increased risk for epididymitis. Safer sexual practices (monogamous relationships, use of barriers such as condoms and similar practices) may be helpful in preventing those cases of epididymitis associated with sexually-transmitted diseases.

Chapter 19

Gonorrhea

Chapter Contents

Section 19.1

Gonorrhea Overview

"Gonorrhea," National Institute of Allergy and Infectious Diseases (www3.niaid.nih.gov/), June 4, 2007.

Gonorrhea is a curable sexually transmitted infection (STI). It is the second most commonly reported bacterial STI in the United States following chlamydia. In 2004, 330,132 cases of gonorrhea were reported to the Centers for Disease Control and Prevention (CDC). When examining race and ethnicity, age, and gender, the highest rates of gonorrhea were found in African Americans, 15 to 24 years of age, and women, respectively.

Gonorrhea can spread into the uterus and fallopian tubes, resulting in pelvic inflammatory disease (PID). PID affects more than one million women in this country every year and can cause tubal (ectopic) pregnancy and infertility in as many as 10% of infected women. In addition to gonorrhea playing a major role in PID, some health researchers think it adds to the risk of getting HIV infection.

Cause

Gonorrhea is caused by bacteria called *Neisseria gonorrhoeae*. These bacteria can infect the genital tract, mouth, and rectum of both men and women. In women the opening to the uterus (cervix) is the first place of infection.

Transmission

You can get gonorrhea during vaginal, oral, or anal sex with an infected partner.

If you are pregnant and have gonorrhea, you may give the infection to your baby as it passes through your birth canal during delivery.

Symptoms

The bacteria are carried in semen and vaginal fluids and cause a discharge in men and women. A small number of people may be infected for several months without showing symptoms.

For women, the early symptoms of gonorrhea often are mild. Symptoms usually appear within 2 to 10 days after sexual contact with an infected partner. When women have symptoms, the first ones may include the following:

- Bleeding during vaginal intercourse
- Painful or burning sensations when urinating
- Yellow or bloody vaginal discharge

More advanced symptoms, which may indicate development of PID, include cramps and pain, bleeding between menstrual periods, vomiting, or fever.

Men have symptoms more often than women, including the following:

- White, yellow, or green pus from the penis with pain
- Burning sensations during urination that may be severe
- Swollen or painful testicles

If left untreated, men could experience prostate complications and epididymitis (inflammation of the testicles).

Symptoms of rectal infection include discharge, anal itching, and occasional painful bowel movements with fresh blood in the feces. Symptoms typically appear two to five days after infection but could appear as long as 30 days.

Diagnosis

Health care providers usually use three laboratory tests to diagnose gonorrhea.

- Staining samples directly for the bacteria
- Detecting bacterial genes or DNA in urine
- Growing the bacteria in laboratory cultures

Many providers prefer to use more than one test to increase the chance of an accurate diagnosis.

You usually can get the staining test results while in your doctor's office or in a clinic. This test is quite accurate for men but not so in women. Only one in two women with gonorrhea has a positive stain.

More often, health care providers use urine or cervical swabs for a new test that detects the genes of the bacteria. These tests are more accurate than culturing the bacteria.

The laboratory culture test involves placing a sample of the discharge onto a culture plate. The health care provider also can take a culture to detect gonorrhea in the throat. Culture also allows testing for drug-resistant bacteria.

Treatment

Health care providers usually prescribe a single dose of one of the following antibiotics to treat gonorrhea.

- Cefixime
- Ceftriaxone
- Single-dose cephalosporin regimens

If you are pregnant, or are younger than 18 years old, you should not be treated with certain types of antibiotics. Your health care provider can prescribe the best and safest antibiotic for you.

Gonorrhea and chlamydia often infect people at the same time. Therefore, health care providers usually prescribe a combination of antibiotics, which will treat both diseases.

If you have gonorrhea, all of your sexual partners should get tested and then treated if infected, whether or not they have symptoms. Health experts also recommend that you not have sex until your infected partners have been treated.

For updated information on treatment for gonorrhea, read the CDC Sexually Transmitted Diseases Treatment Guidelines.

Prevention

The surest way to avoid transmission of STIs is to abstain from sexual contact or be in a long-term mutually monogamous relationship with a partner who has been tested and is not infected.

By using latex condoms correctly and consistently during vaginal or rectal sexual activity, you can reduce your risk of getting gonorrhea and developing complications.

Complications

In untreated gonorrhea infections, the bacteria can spread up into the reproductive tract, or more rarely, can spread into the blood stream and infect the joints, heart valves, or the brain.

The most common result of untreated gonorrhea is pelvic inflammatory disease. Gonococcal PID often appears immediately after the menstrual period. PID causes scar tissue to form in the fallopian tubes. If the tube is partially scarred, the fertilized egg may not be able to pass into the uterus. If this happens, the embryo may implant in the tube causing a tubal (ectopic) pregnancy. This serious complication may result in a miscarriage and can cause death of the mother.

In men, gonorrhea causes epididymitis, a painful condition of the testicles that can lead to infertility if left untreated. Also, gonorrhea affects the prostate gland and may cause scarring in the urine canal.

Rarely, untreated gonorrhea can spread through the blood to the joints. This can cause an inflammation of the joints, which is very serious.

If you are infected with gonorrhea, your risk of getting HIV infection increases. Therefore, it is extremely important for you to either prevent yourself from getting gonorrhea or get treated early if you already are infected with it.

Complications in Newborns and Children

If you are pregnant and have gonorrhea, you may give the infection to your baby as it passes through the birth canal during delivery. A health care provider can prevent infection of your baby's eyes by applying silver nitrate or other medicine to the eyes immediately after birth.

Because of the risks from gonococcal infection to both you and your baby, health experts recommend that pregnant women have at least one test for gonorrhea during prenatal care.

When gonorrhea occurs in the genital tract, mouth, or rectum of a child, it is due most commonly to sexual abuse.

Research

The National Institute of Allergy and Infectious Diseases (NIAID) continues to support a comprehensive, multidisciplinary program of research on *N. gonorrhoeae* (gonococci). Researchers are trying to understand how gonococci infect cells while evading defenses of the human immune system. Studies are ongoing to find the following:

- How this bacterium attaches to host cells
- How it gets inside cells
- Gonococcal surface structures and how they can change
- Human response to infection by gonococci

Together, these efforts have led to, and will lead to, further improvements in diagnosis and treatment of gonorrhea. They also may lead to development of an effective vaccine against gonorrhea.

Another important area of gonorrhea research concerns antibiotic resistance. This is particularly important because strains of *N. gonorrhoeae* that are resistant to recommended antibiotic treatments have been increasing and are becoming widespread in the United States. These events add urgency to conduct research on and develop new antibiotics and to prevent antibiotic resistance from spreading.

NIAID also supports research to develop topical microbicides (preparations that can be inserted into the vagina to prevent infection) that are effective and easy for women to use.

Recently, scientists have determined the complete genome (genetic blueprint) for *N. gonorrhoeae*. They are using this information to help them better understand how the bacterium causes disease and becomes resistant to antibiotics.

Section 19.2

Gonorrhea Missed in Screening at STD Clinics

"Oral Abstract A1d: Missed Gonorrhea Infections by Anatomic Site among Asymptomatic Men Who Have Sex with Men Attending U.S. STD Clinics, 2002–2006," 2008 National STD Prevention Conference, Centers for Disease Control and Prevention (www.cdc.gov), April 7, 2008.

Gonorrhea Infections in Asymptomatic MSM Missed Due to Lack of Testing at All Exposed Anatomic Sites

New data from several STD clinics suggest that more than one third of rectal gonorrhea infections and more than a quarter of pharyngeal (throat) gonorrhea infections among asymptomatic men who have sex with men (MSM) are missed and not treated because many are not tested at all sites of reported exposure.

Led by CDC's Kristen C. Mahle, researchers evaluated asymptomatic MSM tested for gonorrhea and estimated the proportion of asymptomatic infections that were missed as a result of incomplete testing in STD clinics in eight cities between 2002 and 2006. CDC guidelines recommend that MSM be tested for gonorrhea at all exposed anatomic sites (pharyngeal, urethral, and rectal) on an annual basis, and more frequently if they engage in high-risk behaviors.

The researchers collected data on the care received during 36,926 patient visits at 10 STD clinics in eight cities (Chicago, Denver, Houston, New York City, Philadelphia, San Francisco, Seattle, and Washington, DC). Among asymptomatic patients, gonorrhea testing at the urethral site took place in 91% of patient visits in which urethral exposure was reported; pharyngeal testing took place at 74% of patient visits in which pharyngeal exposure was reported, and rectal testing in 64% of patient visits in which rectal exposure was reported. The analysis also found that asymptomatic MSM were tested for gonorrhea at all exposed anatomic sites in 52% of patient visits.

Based upon the percent of positive tests among those men, researchers estimated that 35% of rectal infections, 25% of pharyngeal infections, and 9% of urethral infections went undiagnosed, with large variations occurring across clinics.

In considering possible reasons that providers do not screen at all exposed anatomic sites, the researchers noted that nucleic acid amplification tests (NAATs) are only FDA-approved for use on specimens from the urethra but not for use on specimens from the pharynx or the rectum. NAATs are frequently the only tests available to diagnose gonorrhea. They are not constrained by strict specimen transport conditions required for bacterial culture tests, which must be used for testing non-genital sites. Furthermore, the urethra may be the only site that is typically associated with symptoms when infection is present. The researchers said that rectal and pharyngeal testing rates may also be lower because the tests require a specimen that is more difficult to collect, the culture tests needed may not be available, and a patient who has no symptoms may be less willing to undergo an uncomfortable test.

Researchers emphasize that these data point to the need for providers to screen for gonorrhea based on reported exposure, rather than symptoms only, since the majority of gonorrhea infections at non-genital sites are asymptomatic. They encourage increased education to ensure that providers are aware of the STD Treatment Guidelines and the prevalence of asymptomatic rectal and pharyngeal gonococcal infection. Providers must also consult with local laboratory directors to determine if gonorrhea culture is available or if the laboratory has taken the necessary regulatory steps to use NAATs for off-label specimen testing.

Section 19.3

Increase in Resistant Gonorrhea Prompts New Treatment Guidelines

This section excerpted from "Update to CDC's Sexually Transmitted Diseases Treatment Guidelines, 2006: Fluoroquinolones No Longer Recommended for Treatment of Gonococcal Infections," *Morbidity and Mortality Weekly Report* April 13, 2007, 56(14);332–336. Full references are available online at http://www.cdc.gov/mmwr/preview/mmwrhtml/mm5614a3.htm?s_cid=mm5614a3_e.

In the United States, gonorrhea is the second most commonly reported notifiable disease, with 339,593 cases documented in 2005. Since 1993, fluoroquinolones (i.e., ciprofloxacin, ofloxacin, or levofloxacin) have been used frequently in the treatment of gonorrhea because of their high efficacy, ready availability, and convenience as a single-dose, oral therapy. However, prevalence of fluoroquinolone resistance in *Neisseria gonorrhoeae* has been increasing and is becoming widespread in the United States, necessitating changes in treatment regimens. Beginning in 2000, fluoroquinolones were no longer recommended for gonorrhea treatment in persons who acquired their infections in Asia or the Pacific Islands (including Hawaii); in 2002, this recommendation was extended to California. In 2004, CDC recommended that fluoroquinolones not be used in the United States to treat gonorrhea in MSM. This report, based on data from the Gonococcal Isolate Surveillance Project (GISP), summarizes data on fluoroquinolone-resistant *N. gonorrhoeae* (QRNG) in heterosexual males and in MSM throughout the United States. This report also updates CDC's Sexually Transmitted Diseases Treatment Guidelines, 2006 regarding the treatment of infections caused by *N. gonorrhoeae*. On the basis of the most recent evidence, CDC no longer recommends the use of fluoroquinolones for the treatment of gonococcal infections and associated conditions such as pelvic inflammatory disease. Consequently, only one class of drugs, the cephalosporins, is still recommended and available for the treatment of gonorrhea.

GISP is a CDC-sponsored sentinel surveillance system that has been monitoring antimicrobial susceptibilities of *N. gonorrhoeae* in the United States since 1986. Annually, GISP collects approximately 6,000 urethral gonococcal isolates from males attending 26 to 30 sexually transmitted disease (STD) clinics throughout the country and provides national data to guide treatment. QRNG isolates demonstrate ciprofloxacin minimum inhibitory concentrations (MICs) of >1.0 µg/mL; isolates with intermediate resistance to fluoroquinolones demonstrate ciprofloxacin MICs of 0.125–0.500 µg/mL.

GISP began susceptibility testing for ciprofloxacin in 1990. Overall, QRNG prevalence remained <1% during 1990–2001 but increased to 2.2% in 2002, to 4.1% in 2003, and to 6.8% in 2004. In 2005, of 6,199 isolates collected by GISP, 9.4% were resistant to ciprofloxacin, and during January–June 2006, 13.3% of 3,005 isolates collected were resistant. Excluding isolates from Hawaii and California (areas that discontinued fluoroquinolone treatment in 2000 and 2002, respectively), 6.1% and 8.6% of isolates were QRNG in 2005 and 2006, respectively. Intermediate resistance to ciprofloxacin has remained stable, ranging from 0.4% to 1.1% from 1990 to 2006.

In addition, since 2001, GISP has observed QRNG increases among isolates from MSM, and more recently, from heterosexual males. In 2001, QRNG prevalence was 1.6% and 0.6% among MSM and heterosexual males, respectively. The QRNG prevalence among isolates from MSM increased to 7.2% in 2002, to 15% in 2003, to 23.8% in 2004, and to 29% in 2005. Among heterosexual males, the prevalence increased more slowly, from 0.9% in 2002 to 1.5% in 2003, to 2.9% in 2004, and to 3.8% in 2005. Preliminary data from January–June 2006 indicate that QRNG prevalence increased to 38.3% among MSM and 6.7% among heterosexual males. For isolates from sites outside of California and Hawaii, QRNG prevalence was 24.3% in MSM and 2.7% in heterosexual males in 2005; in the first six months of 2006, it was 30.7% and 5.1%, respectively.

Available data from GISP for 2005 and preliminary data from 2006 have demonstrated that QRNG has continued to increase among heterosexual males and is present in all regions of the country. Several cities outside California and Hawaii have seen substantial increases in QRNG prevalence among heterosexual males from 2004 to 2006; for example, in Philadelphia, QRNG prevalence increased from 1.2% in 2004 to 9.9% in 2005 and to 26.6% in 2006, and in Miami, prevalence increased from 2.1% in 2004 to 4.5% in 2005 and to 15.3% in 2006.

Chapter 20

Viral Hepatitis Infections

Chapter Contents

Section 20.1

Overview of Hepatitis A through E

"Viral Hepatitis: A through E and Beyond," National Digestive Diseases Information Clearinghouse (digestive.niddk.nih.gov), February 2008.

What is viral hepatitis?

Viral hepatitis is inflammation of the liver caused by a virus. Several different viruses, named the hepatitis A, B, C, D, and E viruses, cause viral hepatitis.

All of these viruses cause acute, or short-term, viral hepatitis. The hepatitis B, C, and D viruses can also cause chronic hepatitis, in which the infection is prolonged, sometimes lifelong. Chronic hepatitis can lead to cirrhosis, liver failure, and liver cancer.

Researchers are looking for other viruses that may cause hepatitis, but none have been identified with certainty. Other viruses that less often affect the liver include cytomegalovirus; Epstein-Barr virus, also called infectious mononucleosis; herpesvirus; parvovirus; and adenovirus.

What are the symptoms of viral hepatitis?

Symptoms include the following:

- Jaundice, which causes a yellowing of the skin and eyes
- Fatigue
- Abdominal pain
- Loss of appetite
- Nausea
- Vomiting
- Diarrhea
- Low-grade fever
- Headache

However, some people do not have symptoms.

Hepatitis A

How is hepatitis A spread?

Hepatitis A is spread primarily through food or water contaminated by feces from an infected person. Rarely, it spreads through contact with infected blood.

Who is at risk for hepatitis A?

People most likely to get hepatitis A are the following:

- International travelers, particularly those traveling to developing countries
- People who live with or have sex with an infected person
- People living in areas where children are not routinely vaccinated against hepatitis A, where outbreaks are more likely
- Day care children and employees, during outbreaks
- Men who have sex with men
- Users of illicit drugs

How can hepatitis A be prevented?

The hepatitis A vaccine offers immunity to adults and children older than age one. The Centers for Disease Control and Prevention recommends routine hepatitis A vaccination for children aged 12 to 23 months and for adults who are at high risk for infection. Treatment with immune globulin can provide short-term immunity to hepatitis A when given before exposure or within two weeks of exposure to the virus. Avoiding tap water when traveling internationally and practicing good hygiene and sanitation also help prevent hepatitis A.

What is the treatment for hepatitis A?

Hepatitis A usually resolves on its own over several weeks.

Hepatitis B

How is hepatitis B spread?

Hepatitis B is spread through contact with infected blood, through sex with an infected person, and from mother to child during childbirth, whether the delivery is vaginal or via cesarean section.

Who is at risk for hepatitis B?

People most likely to get hepatitis B are the following:

- People who live with or have sexual contact with an infected person
- Men who have sex with men
- People who have multiple sex partners
- Injection drug users
- Immigrants and children of immigrants from areas with high rates of hepatitis B
- Infants born to infected mothers
- Health care workers
- Hemodialysis patients
- People who received a transfusion of blood or blood products before 1987, when better tests to screen blood donors were developed
- International travelers

How can hepatitis B be prevented?

The hepatitis B vaccine offers the best protection. All infants and unvaccinated children, adolescents, and at-risk adults should be vaccinated. For people who have not been vaccinated, reducing exposure to the virus can help prevent hepatitis B. Reducing exposure means using latex condoms, which may lower the risk of transmission; not sharing drug needles; and not sharing personal items such as toothbrushes, razors, and nail clippers with an infected person.

What is the treatment for hepatitis B?

Drugs approved for the treatment of chronic hepatitis B include alpha interferon and peginterferon, which slow the replication of the virus in the body and also boost the immune system, and the antiviral drugs lamivudine, adefovir dipivoxil, entecavir, and telbivudine. Other drugs are also being evaluated. Infants born to infected mothers should receive hepatitis B immune globulin and the hepatitis B vaccine within 12 hours of birth to help prevent infection.

People who develop acute hepatitis B are generally not treated with antiviral drugs because, depending on their age at infection, the disease often resolves on its own. Infected newborns are most likely to progress to chronic hepatitis B, but by young adulthood, most people with acute infection recover spontaneously. Severe acute hepatitis B can be treated with an antiviral drug such as lamivudine.

Hepatitis C

How is hepatitis C spread?

Hepatitis C is spread primarily through contact with infected blood. Less commonly, it can spread through sexual contact and childbirth.

Who is at risk for hepatitis C?

People most likely to be exposed to the hepatitis C virus are the following:

- Injection drug users
- People who have sex with an infected person
- People who have multiple sex partners
- Health care workers
- Infants born to infected women
- Hemodialysis patients
- People who received a transfusion of blood or blood products before July 1992, when sensitive tests to screen blood donors for hepatitis C were introduced
- People who received clotting factors made before 1987, when methods to manufacture these products were improved

How can hepatitis C be prevented?

There is no vaccine for hepatitis C. The only way to prevent the disease is to reduce the risk of exposure to the virus. Reducing exposure means avoiding behaviors like sharing drug needles or personal items such as toothbrushes, razors, and nail clippers with an infected person.

What is the treatment for hepatitis C?

Chronic hepatitis C is treated with peginterferon together with the antiviral drug ribavirin.

If acute hepatitis C does not resolve on its own within two to three months, drug treatment is recommended.

Hepatitis D

How is hepatitis D spread?

Hepatitis D is spread through contact with infected blood. This disease only occurs at the same time as infection with hepatitis B or in people who are already infected with hepatitis B.

Who is at risk for hepatitis D?

Anyone infected with hepatitis B is at risk for hepatitis D. Injection drug users have the highest risk. Others at risk include the following:

- People who live with or have sex with a person infected with hepatitis D
- People who received a transfusion of blood or blood products before 1987

How can hepatitis D be prevented?

People not already infected with hepatitis B should receive the hepatitis B vaccine. Other preventive measures include avoiding exposure to infected blood, contaminated needles, and an infected person's personal items such as toothbrushes, razors, and nail clippers.

What is the treatment for hepatitis D?

Chronic hepatitis D is usually treated with pegylated interferon, although other potential treatments are under study.

Hepatitis E

How is hepatitis E spread?

Hepatitis E is spread through food or water contaminated by feces from an infected person. This disease is uncommon in the United States.

Who is at risk for hepatitis E?

People most likely to be exposed to the hepatitis E virus are the following:

- International travelers, particularly those traveling to developing countries
- People living in areas where hepatitis E outbreaks are common
- People who live with or have sex with an infected person

How can hepatitis E be prevented?

There is no U.S. Food and Drug Administration (FDA)–approved vaccine for hepatitis E. The only way to prevent the disease is to reduce the risk of exposure to the virus. Reducing risk of exposure means avoiding tap water when traveling internationally and practicing good hygiene and sanitation.

What is the treatment for hepatitis E?

Hepatitis E usually resolves on its own over several weeks to months.

Points to Remember

- Viral hepatitis is inflammation of the liver caused by the hepatitis A, B, C, D, or E viruses.
- Depending on the type of virus, viral hepatitis is spread through contaminated food or water, contact with infected blood, sexual contact with an infected person, or from mother to child during childbirth.
- Vaccines offer protection from hepatitis A and hepatitis B.
- No vaccines are available for hepatitis C, D, and E. Reducing exposure to the viruses offers the best protection.
- Hepatitis A and E usually resolve on their own. Hepatitis B, C, and D can be chronic and serious. Drugs are available to treat chronic hepatitis.

What else causes viral hepatitis?

Some cases of viral hepatitis cannot be attributed to the hepatitis A, B, C, D, or E viruses, or even the less common viruses that can infect the liver, such as cytomegalovirus, Epstein-Barr virus, herpesvirus, parvovirus, and adenovirus. These cases are called non-A–E hepatitis. Scientists continue to study the causes of non-A–E hepatitis.

Hope through Research

The National Institute of Diabetes and Digestive and Kidney Diseases, through its Division of Digestive Diseases and Nutrition, supports basic and clinical research into the nature and transmission of the hepatitis viruses, and the activation and mechanisms of the immune system. Results from these basic and clinical studies are used in developing new treatments and methods of prevention.

The U.S. Government does not endorse or favor any specific commercial product or company. Trade, proprietary, or company names appearing in this document are used only because they are considered necessary in the context of the information provided. If a product is not mentioned, the omission does not mean or imply that the product is unsatisfactory.

Section 20.2

Rates and Risks of HIV and Hepatitis Co-Infection

"HBV Less Likely than HCV to Cause Liver Disease Progression and Death in People with HIV," © 2007 HIVandHepatitis.com. Reprinted with permission.

It is well known that both hepatitis B virus (HBV) and hepatitis C virus (HCV) can cause advanced liver disease, including cirrhosis and hepatocellular carcinoma (HCC), and this appears to occur more rapidly among people with HIV. However, less is known about the comparative outcomes of hepatitis B and C in HIV positive individuals—an issue explored in two studies reported at the 14th Conference on Retroviruses and Opportunistic Infections in February 2007.

Study 1

In the first study, researchers analyzed all HIV positive patients co-infected with HBV (positive for HBV surface antigen) or HCV (detectable HCV antibodies or HCV RNA) in the Netherlands ATHENA observational HIV cohort. Data on liver disease were systematically collected from January 2001 onward.

Results

- Of 12,257 HIV-infected patients in the cohort, 1,129 (9%) were HCV co-infected and 815 (7%) were HBV co-infected.
- 31 patients (0.3%) triply infected with HIV, HBV, and HCV were excluded from the analysis.
- Among the co-infected patients, 31 (2%) developed liver fibrosis, 71 (4%) developed liver cirrhoses, and 5 (0.3%) developed HCC between 2001 and 2006.
- 246 co-infected patients (13%) died during follow-up.
- The risk of liver disease was nearly twice as high in HCV-HIV co-infected patients compared with HBV-HIV co-infected individuals (adjusted risk ratio 1.93).
- HIV-HCV co-infected patients also had significantly shorter survival than HIV-HBV co-infected individuals.
- Time to death did not differ between patients with and without HBV.

The researchers concluded that, "HCV co-infected HAART-treated patients have a faster progression to hepatitis-related liver disease and to death than HBV-HIV co-infected patients, suggesting that progression to liver-related disease may be faster in HCV co-infected patients."

HIV Monitoring Fndn, Academic Med Ctr, Univ of Amsterdam, Netherlands; Ctr for Immunity and Infection, Academic Med Ctr, Univ of Amsterdam, Netherlands; Imperial Coll Sch of Med, London, UK.

Study 2

In the second study, researchers in Texas analyzed serum samples from 129 co-infected patients seen at an inner city HIV clinic; about half had both baseline and follow-up samples.

- Forty-five patients had HIV-HBV coinfection, 43 had HIV-HCV confection, and 41 had HIV-HBV-HCV triple infection.
- Triply infected patients had significantly lower HBV viral loads compared with HIV-HBV co-infected patients.

- The triply infected group was more likely to also have hepatitis delta virus (HDV).
- Triply infected patients were more likely to have cirrhosis (31%) than those with HIV-HBV coinfection (9%) or HIV-HCV coinfection (10%).
- A higher proportion of deaths were seen in HIV-HCV co-infected patients (33%) compared with HIV-HBV co-infected (20%) and triply infected (23%) patients.

"The presence of HCV in those with triple infection appears to diminish HBV DNA levels as compared with the HIV/HBV setting but the reverse is not true," the researchers concluded. "Triply infected persons appear to have more severe disease and are more likely to have delta virus, possibly due to injection drug use and should be evaluated for these features."

Univ of Texas Southwestern Med Ctr, Dallas, TX.

References

C Smit, L Gras, A van Sighem, and others. Increased Progression to Liver Disease and Death in HIV/HCV than in HBV-co-infected Patients. 14th Conference on Retroviruses and Opportunistic Infections; February 25–28, 2007; Los Angeles, California. Abstract 932 (poster).

M Jain, R Joshi, N Attar, and others. Comparison of Triple Infection with HIV/HBV/HCV to HIV/HCV and HIV/HBV. 14th Conference on Retroviruses and Opportunistic Infections; February 25–28, 2007; Los Angeles, California. Abstract 933 (poster).

Chapter 21

Hepatitis B (HBV)

Chapter Contents

Section 21.1

Frequently Asked Questions about HBV

"Questions Frequently Asked about Hepatitis B," © 2007 Immunization Action Coalition (www.immunize.org). Reprinted with permission.

What is hepatitis B?

Hepatitis B is a serious public health problem that affects people of all ages in the U.S. and around the world. In 2006, an estimated 46,000 people contracted hepatitis B virus (HBV) infection in the U.S. Hepatitis B is caused by a highly infectious virus that attacks the liver and can lead to severe illness, liver damage, and in some cases, death.

The best way to be protected from hepatitis B is to be vaccinated with hepatitis B vaccine, a vaccine used in the U.S. for more than two decades and proved safe and effective.

Who is at risk for HBV infection?

About 5% of people in the U.S. will get infected with HBV sometime during their lives if they are not vaccinated. You might be infected with HBV and not even know it. If you engage in certain activities, your risk might be much higher. You might be at risk if you:

- have a job that exposes you to human blood;
- share a household with someone who has chronic (lifelong) HBV infection;
- inject drugs;
- have sex with a person infected with HBV;
- are sexually active but not in a long-term, mutually monogamous relationship;
- are a man who has sex with men;
- received a blood transfusion before 1975, when excellent blood testing became available;

- are a person who was born, or who has a parent born, in Asia, Africa, the Amazon River Basin in South America, the Pacific Islands, Eastern Europe, or the Middle East;
- were adopted from Asia, Africa, the Amazon River Basin in South America, the Pacific Islands, Eastern Europe, or the Middle East;
- have hemophilia;
- are a patient or worker in an institution for developmentally challenged people;
- are an inmate of a correctional facility; or
- travel internationally to areas with moderate or high rates of HBV infection.

How is HBV spread?

HBV is found in the blood of people infected with the virus and certain of their body fluids, such as serum, semen, and vaginal secretions. HBV is not found in sweat, tears, urine, or respiratory secretions. Contact with microscopic amounts of infected blood can cause infection.

Hepatitis B virus can be spread by:

- unprotected sex;
- injection drug use;
- an HBV-infected mother to her child during birth;
- contact with blood or open sores of an HBV-infected person;
- human bites from an HBV-infected person;
- sharing a household with a person with chronic (lifelong) HBV infection;
- sharing items such as razors, toothbrushes, or washcloths;
- pre-chewing food for babies or sharing chewing gum;
- using unsterilized needles in ear- or body-piercing, tattooing, or acupuncture; or
- using the same immunization needle on more than one person.

Hepatitis B virus IS NOT spread by:

- casual contact, like holding hands;
- eating food prepared by an infected person;

- kissing or hugging;
- sharing silverware, plates, or cups;
- visiting an infected person's home;
- sneezing or coughing; or
- breastfeeding.

What are the symptoms of hepatitis B?

Most babies and young children who get HBV infection don't look or feel sick at all. About half of adults who get infected don't have any symptoms or signs of the disease. If people do have signs or symptoms, they might experience any or all of the following:

- loss of appetite;
- nausea, vomiting;
- fever;
- weakness, fatigue, inability to work for weeks or months;
- abdominal pain;
- yellowing of skin and eyes (jaundice);
- joint pain;
- cola-colored urine; and
- clay-colored stools.

I'm not in a risk group. How did I get HBV infection?

Many people don't know when or how they got the infection. When they get the results of a blood test indicating they've been infected with HBV, they are taken by surprise. Studies have demonstrated that about 15% of people who acquire hepatitis B are unable to identify a risk factor that explains why they have the disease.

Do people usually recover from HBV infection?

About 95% of adults recover after several months. They clear the infection from their bodies and become immune. This means they won't get infected with HBV again. They are no longer contagious and cannot pass HBV to others.

Unfortunately, about 5% of adults and up to 90% of children under age five years are unable to clear the infection from their bodies and develop chronic HBV infection.

How do I know if I have or have had HBV infection?

The only way to know if you are currently infected with HBV, have recovered, are chronically infected, or could become infected, is by having blood tests. The three standard blood tests are the following:

- **HBsAg (hepatitis B surface antigen):** When this is "positive" or "reactive," it means the person is currently infected with HBV and is able to pass the infection on to others.
- **Anti-HBs [sometimes written as HBs-Ab] (antibody to hepatitis B surface antigen):** When this is "positive" or "reactive," it means the person is immune to HBV infection, either from vaccination or from past infection. (This test is not done routinely by most blood banks on donated blood.)
- **Anti-HBc [sometimes written as HBc-Ab] (antibody to hepatitis B core antigen):** When this is "positive" or "reactive," it might mean the person has had contact with HBV. This is a very complicated test to explain because the "anti-HBc" can possibly be a "false-positive" test result. Blood banks routinely run an "anti-HBc" on donated blood. The interpretation of this test result, if it is positive, depends on the results of the other two blood tests previously described.

A fourth blood test that is sometimes done is IgM anti-HBc (IgM class antibody to hepatitis B core antigen). When this is positive or "reactive," it means that the person has had HBV infection in the past six months, indicating acute (recently acquired) HBV infection.

What does it mean if my blood bank said I tested positive for hepatitis B and can no longer donate blood?

If the blood bank told you your test was "positive," it is important to find out which test was positive. If the "HBsAg" was positive, this means that you are either chronically infected with HBV or were recently infected. If only the "anti-HBc" was positive, it is most likely that you either had a "false-positive" test or are immune to HBV infection (had HBV infection sometime in the past). It is important that you understand the full meaning of your test results. If you are not sure how to interpret these test results, call your blood bank for an explanation or have the blood bank send the test results to your health care provider. You may need to provide written permission for the blood bank to release these results to your health care provider. Your health care provider may want to repeat the blood tests or perform additional tests such as an "anti-HBs." Bring this information along with you on your visit to your health care provider. The blood bank does not usually test for anti-HBs or IgM anti-HBc.

And remember, you cannot get HBV from donating blood because the equipment used during blood donation is sterile.

Chronic Hepatitis B Virus Infection

What does it mean to be chronically infected with HBV?

People who do not recover from HBV infection are chronically infected, usually for life. There are over one million chronically infected people in the U.S. today. A chronically infected person is someone who has had HBV in her/his blood for more than six months. While approximately 5% of adults who acquire HBV infection become chronically infected, children younger than age five years have a greater risk (up to 90%). The younger the child is at the time of infection, the greater the risk that the child will develop chronic infection. Many babies born to chronically infected mothers will also become chronically infected with HBV unless the babies are given two shots in the hospital immediately after birth—the first dose of hepatitis B vaccine and a dose of hepatitis B immune globulin (HBIG)—and at least two doses of hepatitis B vaccine during the six months after birth to protect them from the infection. The final dose should not be given before 24 weeks of age.

A chronically infected person might have no signs or symptoms of HBV infection but usually remains infected for years or for a lifetime and is capable of passing HBV on to others. Sometimes chronically infected people will spontaneously clear the infection from their bodies, but most will not. Although most chronically infected people have no serious problems with hepatitis B and lead normal, healthy lives, some develop liver problems later. Chronically infected people are at significantly higher risk than the general population for liver failure or liver cancer.

How can I take care of myself if I am chronically infected with HBV?

A person with HBV infection should see a physician knowledgeable about the management of liver disease every 6–12 months. The physician will do blood tests to check the health of the liver, as well as test for evidence of liver cancer. It is best for chronically infected people to avoid alcohol because alcohol can injure the liver. Additionally, your physician should know about all the medicines you are taking, even over-the-counter drugs, because some medicines can hurt the liver. If the result of any liver test is abnormal, it's important that you consult a liver specialist.

If your liver disease has progressed...

If your physician tells you your liver disease has progressed, read the following for some extra precautions you should take.

- Avoid alcohol and medicine that has not been prescribed by your doctor—even over-the-counter medicines.
- Get vaccinated against hepatitis A. Hepatitis A virus infection can further damage your liver.
- Get a yearly influenza (flu) vaccination. Patients with severe liver disease (cirrhosis) should also receive pneumococcal vaccine.
- Don't eat raw oysters. They may carry the bacteria *Vibrio vulnificus*, which can cause serious blood infections in people with liver disease. Approximately 50% of people with this blood infection die from it.

What can I do to protect others from HBV infection?

People with HBV infection might feel healthy but are still capable of passing the infection on to other people. To protect others from getting HBV infection, it is important to protect them from contact with your infected blood and other infectious body fluids, including semen and vaginal secretions. Sweat, tears, urine, and respiratory secretions do not contain HBV. Transmission of HBV by saliva has only been documented through biting.

Important DOs and DON'Ts for people with chronic HBV infection

DO

- Cover all cuts and open sores with a bandage.
- Discard used items such as Band-Aids and menstrual pads carefully so no one is accidentally exposed to your blood.
- Wash your hands well after touching your blood or infectious body fluids.

- Clean up blood spills. Then reclean the area with a bleach solution (one part household chlorine bleach to 10 parts water).
- Tell your sex partner(s) you have hepatitis B so they can be tested and vaccinated (if not already infected). Sex partners should be tested for anti-HBs 1–2 months after the three doses are completed to be sure the vaccine worked.
- Use condoms (rubbers) during sex unless your sex partner has had hepatitis B or has been vaccinated and has had the anti-HBs blood test demonstrating immunity. (Condoms may also protect you from other sexually transmitted diseases.)
- Tell household members to see their health care providers for testing and vaccination for hepatitis B.
- Tell your health care providers that you are chronically infected with HBV.
- See your health care provider every 6–12 months to check the health of your liver with blood tests and liver scanning.
- If you are pregnant, tell your health care provider that you have HBV infection. It is critical that your baby is started on the hepatitis B shots (both vaccine and HBIG) within 12 hours of birth.

DON'T

- Don't share chewing gum, toothbrushes, razors, washcloths, needles for ear or body piercing, or anything that might have come in contact with your blood or infectious body fluids.
- Don't pre-chew food for babies.
- Don't share syringes and needles.
- Don't donate blood, plasma, body organs, tissue, or sperm.
- Don't take any medicines not prescribed by your doctor, even over-the-counter medicines.

What are the long-term effects of HBV infection?

Each year, approximately 3,000–5,000 people in the U.S. die of HBV-related chronic liver disease. HBV infection is the most common cause of liver cancer worldwide and ranks second only to tobacco as the world's leading cause of cancer.

Is there a cure for hepatitis B?

As of this writing, there are several drugs used for the treatment of people with chronic hepatitis B. These drugs usually don't get rid of the virus completely, but may reduce your risk for serious liver disease such as cirrhosis and liver cancer. Check with your doctor to find out if treatment with medication is the right choice for you. Researchers continue to find additional treatments and look for cures for hepatitis B.

Why is hepatitis B so serious in pregnant women?

Pregnant women who are infected with HBV can transmit the disease to their babies. If babies aren't protected with vaccinations, many of them develop lifelong HBV infections, and up to 25% of those who become infected will develop liver failure or liver cancer later in life. All pregnant women should be tested early in every pregnancy to determine if they are infected with HBV. If the blood test is positive, the baby should be vaccinated within 12 hours of birth with two shots, one of HBIG and the other the first dose of hepatitis B vaccine. The infant will need at least two more doses of hepatitis B vaccine by age six months. The final dose should not be given before age 24 weeks.

How can hepatitis B be prevented?

Hepatitis B vaccine can provide protection in 90%–95% of healthy young adults. The vaccine can safely be given to infants, children, and adults, including pregnant women. Usually, three doses of vaccine are given over a six-month period. Hepatitis B vaccine is very safe, and side effects are rare. Since 1982, more than 100 million children, teens, and adults in the U.S. have been vaccinated. Hepatitis B vaccine is our first vaccine that prevents cancer—liver cancer.

At what age are hepatitis B vaccines given routinely?

The hepatitis B vaccine series can begin at any age. For newborns, it's recommended that the first dose be given in the hospital at birth. Hepatitis B vaccine is recommended routinely for all children age 0–18 years living in the U.S. Older children and teens should be vaccinated at the earliest opportunity. Any adult who is at risk for HBV infection or who simply wants to be protected from HBV infection should start the vaccine series right away.

Where can I get hepatitis B vaccine?

Check with your health care provider's office first. Children's health insurance usually covers the cost of this vaccine since it is routinely recommended for all children in the U.S. If your child is uninsured, ask your local health department for assistance. The federal Vaccines For Children (VFC) program helps families by providing free vaccines to health care providers who serve eligible children. VFC is administered at the national level by the Centers for Disease Control and Prevention (CDC), which contracts with vaccine manufacturers to buy vaccines at reduced rates. For adults, contact your health care provider to find out if the vaccine is available and how much it costs. If you are uninsured or don't have a health care provider, call your local health department for advice.

How many doses of vaccine are needed?

Three doses are needed usually for the best protection against HBV infection, but protection is sometimes provided from receiving as little as one dose. Hepatitis B vaccine is usually given on a schedule of zero, one, and six months, but there is flexibility in the timing of these injections. As with all other vaccines, if you fall behind on the schedule, you just continue from where you left off. Hepatitis B vaccine will not help or cure a person who is already infected with HBV.

What should I do if I'm in a risk group and am not infected with HBV?

If you are in a risk group for hepatitis B, be sure to get vaccinated. All people in risk groups (risk groups are listed in the second question on this question-and-answer series) should protect themselves from HBV infection. You don't have to "admit" that you have a risk factor to be vaccinated. You simply need to ask to be vaccinated. Every day you delay getting vaccinated increases your chances of being in contact with this highly contagious liver disease. The problems caused by hepatitis B—liver cancer and liver failure—are too great to take a chance. See your health care provider or visit your health department.

How does hepatitis B differ from hepatitis A and C?

Hepatitis A, B, and C are all different viruses that attack and injure the liver, and all can cause similar symptoms. Usually, people get hepatitis A virus (HAV) infection from household or sexual contact with a person who has the infection. Hepatitis C is caused by the hepatitis C virus (HCV) and is spread through HCV-infected blood. Both HCV and HBV infections are spread by blood through some of the same activities (e.g., injection drug use). Both HBV and HCV infections can cause lifelong liver problems. HAV infection does not. Vaccines to prevent HAV infection are also available. Hepatitis A vaccine won't protect you from HBV or HCV infection, nor will hepatitis B vaccine protect you from HAV or HCV infection. There is no vaccine yet for hepatitis C. If you've been infected with HAV or HCV in the past, it is still possible to get infected with HBV.

Section 21.2

Pregnancy, Children, and HBV

Should I be tested for hepatitis B if I am pregnant?

Yes. ALL pregnant women should be tested for hepatitis B. Testing is especially important for women who fall into high-risk groups such as health care workers, women from ethnic communities where hepatitis B is common, spouses or partners living with an infected person, etc. If you are pregnant, be sure your doctor tests you for hepatitis B before your baby is born.

Why are these tests so important for pregnant women?

If you test positive for hepatitis B and are pregnant, the virus can be passed on to your newborn baby during delivery. If your doctor is aware that you have hepatitis B, he or she can make arrangements to have the proper medications in the delivery room to prevent your baby from being infected. If the proper procedures are not followed, your baby has a 95% chance of developing chronic hepatitis B.

Will a hepatitis B infection affect my pregnancy?

A hepatitis B infection should not cause any problems for you or your unborn baby during your pregnancy. It is important for your doctor to be aware of your hepatitis B infection so that he or she can monitor your health and so your baby can be protected from an infection after it is born.

If I am pregnant and have hepatitis B, how can I protect my baby?

If you test positive for hepatitis B, then your newborn must be given two shots immediately in the delivery room:

- first dose of the **hepatitis B vaccine**; and
- one dose of the **hepatitis B immune globulin (HBIG).**

If these two medications are given correctly within the first 12 hours of life, a newborn has more than a 90% chance of being protected against a lifelong hepatitis B infection. You must make sure your baby receives the second and third dose of the hepatitis B vaccine at one and six months of age to ensure complete protection.

There is no second chance to protect your newborn baby.

Can I breastfeed my baby if I have hepatitis B?

The Centers for Disease Control recommends that all women with hepatitis B should be encouraged to breastfeed their newborns. The benefits of breastfeeding outweigh the potential risk of infection, which is minimal. In addition, since it is recommended that all infants be vaccinated against hepatitis B at birth, any potential risk is further reduced.

How will being diagnosed with chronic hepatitis B affect my child?

Hepatitis B does not usually affect a child's normal growth and development. Most children with chronic hepatitis B infections will enjoy long and healthy lives. Unlike other chronic medical conditions, there are generally no physical disabilities associated with hepatitis B, nor are there usually any physical restrictions for these children.

I am planning to adopt a child, should I request that he or she be tested?

Your adoption agency should be able to tell you if a child has been tested for hepatitis B. With an international adoption, it is advised that you do not request that your child be tested in the originating country since the blood test itself could be a source of infection.

What if the child I am planning to adopt tests positive for hepatitis B?

Finding out that the child you wish to adopt has chronic hepatitis B can be upsetting, but should not be cause for alarm or stopping an adoption. We hope that a hepatitis B diagnosis will not change your decision to adopt a child. You can be reassured that most children will enjoy a long and healthy life. Hepatitis B does not usually affect a child's normal growth and development, and there are generally no physical disabilities or restrictions associated with this diagnosis.

How can I protect other family members if my child tests positive for hepatitis B?

All parents, siblings, and other household members should be vaccinated. Extended family members, child care providers, family, friends, and others should consider vaccination if they have frequent and close contact with your child.

Is there treatment available for a child with hepatitis B?

There are currently two approved treatment options available in the United States for children with chronic hepatitis B: (1) Intron A (interferon alpha) and (2) Epivir-HBV (lamivudine). However, not every child (or adult) with hepatitis B needs to be treated. You should see a pediatric liver specialist to determine if your child would benefit from one of these approved treatments. Whether you decide to start treatment or not, your child should see a liver specialist or doctor skilled in hepatitis B on a regular basis.

Section 21.3

HBV Treatment

Will I recover?

The first question most people ask is whether or not they will recover from a hepatitis B infection. The answer is directly related to that age at which a person is infected. Most infected adults will recover without any problems, but unfortunately, most infected babies and children will develop chronic hepatitis B infections.

Acute vs. chronic?

A hepatitis B infection is considered to be "acute" during the first six months after being exposed. This is the average period of time it takes to recover from a hepatitis B infection. If you still test positive for the hepatitis B virus (HBsAg+) after six months, you are considered to have a "chronic" hepatitis B infection, which can last a lifetime.

What should I do if I am diagnosed with chronic hepatitis B?

Make an appointment with a hepatologist (liver specialist) or gastroenterologist familiar with hepatitis B. This specialist will order blood tests and possibly a liver ultrasound to evaluate your hepatitis B status and the health of your liver. Your doctor will probably want to see you at least once or twice a year to monitor you and determine if you would benefit from treatment.

Most people with chronic hepatitis B can expect to live long, healthy lives. It is important to know that you can pass the virus along to others, even if you don't feel sick. This is why it's so important that you make sure that all close household contacts and sex partners are vaccinated against hepatitis B.

Consider following these helpful tips:

- Avoid alcohol and smoking as they can be extremely harmful to a liver already infected with the hepatitis B virus.
- Talk to your doctor before taking any prescription, over-the-counter medication, or herbal remedies.
- Although there is no special diet for people who have chronic hepatitis B, a healthy, well-balanced diet that is low fat and includes plenty of vegetables is recommended.
- Avoid eating raw shellfish, since they can contain bacteria that are harmful to your liver.

Is there a cure for chronic hepatitis B?

Right now, there is no cure for chronic hepatitis B, but the good news is there are treatments that can help slow the progression of liver disease by slowing down the virus. If there is less hepatitis B virus being produced, then there is less damage being done to the liver. Sometimes these drugs can even get rid of the virus, although this is not common. With all of the new exciting research, there is great hope that a complete cure will be found for chronic hepatitis B in the near future.

Should I be on medication?

It is important to understand that not every person with chronic hepatitis B needs to be on medication. You should talk to your doctor about whether you are a good candidate for drug therapy or a clinical trial. Be sure that you understand the pros and cons of each treatment option. Whether you decide to start treatment or not, you should be seen regularly by a liver specialist or a doctor knowledgeable about hepatitis B.

Section 21.4

HBV and Liver Cancer

"Hepatitis B and Primary Liver Cancer," © 2008 Hepatitis B Foundation (www.hepb.org). All rights reserved. Reprinted with permission.

Chronic hepatitis B infections cause 80% of all primary liver cancer worldwide.

Patients with chronic hepatitis B infections are at increased risk for progressing to liver cancer or hepatocellular carcinoma (HCC), whether they develop cirrhosis or not.

In the U.S. the overall incidence of cancer is decreasing, except for primary liver cancer (as reported by the National Cancer Institute in 2005). This is due in large part to the increased number of Americans who are chronically infected with hepatitis B and hepatitis C. Although survival rates for most types of common cancers have improved over the years, the five-year survival rate for liver cancer is still below 10%.

In the world, primary liver cancer is the third leading cause of death. According to the World Health Organization, at least 550,000 people die each year from primary liver cancer.

The hepatitis B vaccine was named the first "Anti-Cancer Vaccine" vaccine by the U.S. Food and Drug Administration since it prevents hepatitis B infections, the leading cause of primary liver cancer.

Who should be screened for liver cancer?

Early detection improves the chances of survival after treatment. Since liver cancer develops quietly, usually without symptoms, patients with chronic hepatitis B should undergo regular liver cancer screening. A reasonable approach is to begin regular liver cancer screening at 30 years of age (although experts are recommending starting at an even earlier age since liver cancer can strike children, though rare).

It is important to stress that Asians and Asian Americans, who generally develop chronic hepatitis B infections soon after birth, have a high risk of developing liver cancer at an early age whether they have cirrhosis or not. The risk is greater in men and those with a positive family history for liver cancer.

What is liver cancer screening?

This generally consists of a simple blood test for alpha-fetoprotein (AFP) levels every six months and an ultrasound of the liver at least once a year. Either test alone can miss the diagnosis. Some doctors prefer CT scans to ultrasounds. Once the patient develops cirrhosis, or has a family history of liver cancer, more frequent screening is generally recommended.

What are the symptoms of liver cancer?

Liver cancer is a silent killer because the majority of patients appear to be perfectly healthy and have no early signs or symptoms. Both small and large tumors may be undetected due to the shielded location of the liver underneath the ribs.

Pain is uncommon until the tumor is quite large, and some large tumors don't even cause pain or any symptoms. Later stages of liver cancer, when the cancer is very large or when it impairs the functions of the liver, can produce more obvious symptoms such as abdominal pain, weight loss, lack of appetite, and finally the development of jaundice and abdominal swelling.

How is liver cancer treated?

Treatment of HCC is particularly challenging when compared with other types of cancer because in addition to the cancer itself, many patients have livers that have been damaged by chronic hepatitis B infections. For each individual patient, the potential benefits of the various treatment options must be balanced with the risk of liver failure and how it affects the patient's quality of life.

Surgical treatment: When the tumor is small and the patient's liver condition is stable, surgical removal offers the best chance for long-term survival. Despite complete removal of the tumor, however, patients are still at risk for recurrent disease. They will need to be followed closely long-term, especially during the first year when the risk of recurrence is greatest.

Nonsurgical treatment: For patients who cannot undergo surgery, a number of treatment options, though limited in effectiveness, are available or being investigated in an attempt to control the disease long-term and with the aim of maintaining normal quality of life. Traditional chemotherapy is generally ineffective, causes many side effects that may severely impair the patient's quality of life, and often does not prolong survival.

TACE (or TAC): Since HCC are hypervascular tumors often fed by one or more blood vessels from the hepatic arteries, they present the unique opportunity to target the therapy directly into the tumor. Intrahepatic arterial chemoembolization or chemoinfusion (TACE or TAC) is used in the treatment of selected patients with tumors that cannot be surgically removed.

Long-term treatments with TACE or TAC have been associated with prolonged patient survival, and those who have good control or shrinkage of the tumor may even become suitable candidates for surgical resection or transplantation.

What about a liver transplant?

Liver transplant is the only treatment option for patients with liver cancer tumors that cannot be surgically or medically removed. The tumor must be small (less than five centimeters or fewer than four lesions), confined to the liver, and without invasion into the blood vessels. Larger or more extensive tumors have a high risk for early recurrence after liver transplantation.

What does the future hold?

Early diagnosis of small tumors is the only effective way of improving the outcome of liver cancer treatment, and that is only possible through screening of the high-risk population. Universal hepatitis B vaccination is ultimately the only hope for reducing the incidence of this frequently fatal cancer worldwide.

Chapter 22

Hepatitis C (HCV)

Chapter Contents

Section 22.1

Facts about HCV Infection

"Hepatitis C: A Simple FactSheet," © 2006 AIDS Treatment Data Network – The Network (www.atdn.org). Reprinted with permission.

What Is Hepatitis C?

Hepatitis C is caused by a virus. The hepatitis C virus (HCV) can cause damage to the liver. HCV testing is recommended for anyone who is HIV-positive. About 33% of all people with HIV also have HCV. Keeping an HIV-positive person's liver healthy increases their ability to tolerate HIV medication. Keeping a person's HIV under control may also help to slow HCV disease progression. HCV disease appears to progress more quickly in people with HIV disease. HCV can cause serious liver disease, including liver failure, in people with or without HIV.

HCV Transmission

HCV is transmitted mainly by blood-to-blood contact, although it may be transmitted through unsafe sex. Most people have no idea that they have been infected with HCV, although millions of people worldwide are HCV-positive. Many people do not know how they became infected with HCV when they find out. Some people became infected with HCV through blood products or blood transfusions. The blood supply in the United States has been screened for HCV since 1992.

A person can become infected with HCV by using needles and other contaminated injection equipment. HCV infection is an ongoing risk for health care providers, police and firefighters, and correctional officers. It is also possible, but rare, for a mother to transmit HCV to her unborn child during delivery. HCV is also sometimes transmitted during sex, especially those acts that involve contact with blood. HCV is more likely to be transmitted through sex if the other person's HCV viral load is high. Sharing razors, manicure equipment, toothbrushes, and any other personal care items with blood on them are another possible route of transmission. Body piercing or tattooing with unsterilized equipment or shared inkwells and needles can spread HCV.

About one out of six people infected with HCV will clear the infection. No virus can be found in their blood. For most people, however, HCV becomes a chronic disease. Some people will never have any symptoms, and won't develop serious liver damage from HCV. Other people will slowly develop liver damage 10 to 30 years after infection. About half the people infected with HCV won't develop serious liver damage during their lifetime. Some people will develop fibrosis (mild to moderate scarring of liver tissue). One in five people with chronic HCV will develop cirrhosis (serious scarring of the liver, which interferes with the liver's ability to do its job). A small group of people (about 1% to 4%) with HCV will develop liver cancer and/or liver failure as a result of HCV. A liver transplant is the only treatment for liver failure.

It is recommended that people who are HIV positive get tested for HCV. People who are co-infected with HIV and HCV are more likely to develop cirrhosis and/or fibrosis. People with HIV sometimes falsely test negative for HCV, so routine screening is suggested on a regular basis.

Symptoms of HCV

Three out of four people don't have any symptoms when first infected with HCV. Initial symptoms can include: fatigue, nausea, loss of appetite, low fever, stiff and aching joints, jaundice (yellowing of the eyes and skin), dark brown urine, pale feces, and liver pain (on the right side of the body, under the ribcage). Later symptoms of liver damage caused by HCV can include jaundice, fatigue, itchiness, mood alterations, depression, forgetfulness, and liver pain.

Diagnostic Testing

HCV antibodies will appear by 12 weeks after infection. Follow-up testing such as a RIBA or qualitative viral load test is recommended to confirm HCV infection. HCV viral load results are usually much higher than HIV viral load test results. HCV viral load results range from undetectable to millions of copies. The HCV viral load is usually used to monitor the success of treatment. In people who are HIV infected, antibodies my take longer to develop, sometimes months.

Monitoring Disease Progression

Ultrasound/sonogram testing is a non-invasive test that uses sound waves to identify liver abnormalities. Usually, a total abdomen scan is done to see if liver damage is affecting other organs such as the pancreas, gall bladder, or the spleen. Blood tests, including measurements of liver enzyme levels, as well as HCV viral load testing are also used to determine how well your liver is working. These tests, however, can't predict if, or when, serious liver disease will develop. A liver biopsy, a procedure where a thin needle is inserted between the ribs into the liver to remove a small tissue sample, is the only way to determine the actual condition of the liver itself. When done properly, a liver biopsy takes a few minutes to perform, and leaves only a pencil point scar.

The liver is responsible for many things, including processing drugs, herbs, and body chemicals, clearing toxic substances from the bloodstream, and turning food into energy. The liver has to stay in good working order for the body to function. Some HIV treatments are harder for the liver to tolerate than others. Certain HIV medications, as well as drugs used for other purposes, should be avoided by people with hepatitis.

There are at least six different types, or genotypes, of HCV. The most common genotypes in the U.S. are 1a and 1b. Some people have type 2, 3, or 4. It appears that the hardest types of HCV to treat are types 1 and 4. Types 2 and 3 are easier to treat, although the same treatments are used for all genotypes. Regardless of your genotype, treatment must be used for at least six months before it can really said to be effective. Most people will take treatment for a year, especially people co-infected with HIV, as well as people with genotypes 1 and 4. Some researchers believe that 18 months of treatment is needed for people who are HIV/HCV co-infected.

HCV Treatment Decisions

The results of blood tests, and other procedures you may have had done (liver biopsy or ultrasound, for example), can help you decide whether you need to start HCV treatment. Deciding when to start treatment is a difficult choice. HCV treatment may be easier to tolerate for people with higher CD4 counts, and people who are in better general health. There are things that people with HCV can do to stay healthy regardless of whether they decide to start treatment.

Many people experience fatigue, depression and, occasionally, more severe side effects when they start HCV treatment. The symptoms of untreated HCV disease can sometimes be severe as well. Symptoms of HCV disease may also improve with treatment.

HCV Treatments

A combination of ribavirin and a Pegylated interferon is now the standard treatment for HCV. There are two FDA approved pegylated interferons, Peg-Intron and Pegasys. Pegylated interferon is taken as an injection under the skin once a week. Ribavirin is a nucleoside analog like AZT or ddI. It is a pill. The pills are taken twice a day. Studies have shown that after 48 weeks of combination treatment, some people can get rid of HCV (undetectable HCV viral load). Successful treatment is called a Sustained Virologic Response (SVR), meaning that the HCV is no longer detectable in blood tests for at least five months after the 48-week treatment. SVR depends on many different factors, including HIV co-infection, HCV genotype, and the person's age, gender, race, and the condition of his/her liver. The treatment outcome ranges from 89% SVR for someone mono-infected (no HIV infection), relatively healthy with genotypes 2 or 3, to a disappointing 30% SVR for someone co-infected (with HIV), with advanced liver fibrosis, or with HCV genotype 1. However, even if the treatment doesn't wipe out the virus, it can sometimes help improve the condition of the liver.

Studies have shown that people who do not respond to treatment in the first 12-week period, by showing a reduction in liver enzymes or at least a 2_{log} drop in HCV viral load, are unlikely to benefit from continued treatment. It is very important to be fully aware of what side effects might occur and how they can be managed, before you begin treatment. This reduces the chance you will stop treatment before completing the very crucial 12-week starting period.

The Side Effects

The most common side effects of pegylated interferon include: a decrease in white blood cells and platelets, anemia, nausea, diarrhea, fever, chills, muscle and joint pain, difficulty in concentrating, thyroid dysfunction, hair loss, sleeplessness, irritability, mild to serious depression, and rarely, suicidal thoughts. Other serious adverse events include bone marrow toxicity, cardiovascular disorders, hypersensitivity, endocrine disorders, pulmonary disorders, colitis, pancreatitis, and ophthalmologic disorders (eye and vision problems).

Pegylated interferon may also cause or make worse fatal or life-threatening neuropsychiatric, autoimmune, ischemic, and infectious disorders. If you decide to go on treatment, your doctor should monitor you closely with periodic clinical and laboratory tests. Patients with persistently severe or worsening signs or symptoms of these conditions should stop therapy. In many, but not all cases, these disorders resolve after stopping therapy.

Side effects of ribavirin include nausea and anemia. Anemia caused by ribavirin is usually easily treatable. Ribavirin can also cause birth defects (see warning below). Ribavirin should not be taken with the HIV drug ddI (didanosine, Videx, Videx EC), as lactic acidosis with fatal hepatic steatosis (fatty liver) has occurred. This may be more prevalent in people who are co-infected. It is very important to inform your doctor and liver specialist of any symptoms you experience.

Ribavirin/pregnancy warning

Ribavirin can cause severe birth defects. Women and men who that take ribavirin should not plan a pregnancy for six months after stopping, because ribavirin stays in the body for a long time.

Paying for Treatment

The drugs used to treat HCV are expensive. Make sure to discuss how you will be able to pay for your HCV and HIV treatments and the associated care with your case manager before starting. A case manager can also help you throughout the treatment process. The Network can also provide you with information on what treatments and services are covered by your state ADAP or Medicaid Program. Contact The Network at 212-260-8868 or 800-734-7104.

Schering-Plough, the maker of Peg-Intron, Rebetol, and Rebetron, has a "COMMITMENT TO CARE" reimbursement assistance program. Call 800-521-7157 to enroll.

Hoffmann-La Roche, the maker of Pegasys, also has a patient assistance program. Call 877-PEGASYS to enroll.

Section 22.2

Risks of Sexual Transmission of HCV

"Sexual Transmission of Hepatitis C," reprinted with permission of the Hepatitis C Support Project, http://www.hcvadvocate.org, © 2009.

The hepatitis C virus often causes liver inflammation. In up to 75% of people initially infected with HCV, the disease becomes chronic, potentially leading to long-term liver damage. A small percentage (about 10–25%) of those who are HCV positive will progress to liver cirrhosis, and approximately 3–5% of those with chronic HCV infection will develop liver cancer. Experts estimate that at least four million Americans are currently chronically infected with HCV; the number of new cases of HCV in the U.S. is decreasing. Fortunately, there are several measures people can take to protect themselves from this potentially life threatening disease.

How Is HCV Spread?

HCV is a blood-borne disease, that is, it is transmitted by blood-to-blood contact. Any activity that lets one person's blood or body fluids come into contact with another person's blood or mucous membranes can potentially transmit HCV. However, some activities are much more likely than others to spread the virus. HCV can be transmitted by sharing equipment (including water) for injection and non-injection drugs (for example, needles, cottons, cookers, cocaine/crank straws, and crack pipes).

Sharing tattoo ink and needles as well as needles used for body piercing and acupuncture may also spread HCV if safety precautions are not followed carefully. Sharing personal items like razors, toothbrushes, or nail files is a less likely—but still possible—transmission route. In the past, many people contracted HCV through blood transfusions, but since 1992 there has been a reliable HCV blood test and now donated blood is considered safe. Today, transfusion-associated cases of HCV occur in less than one per two million transfused units of blood.

Sex and HCV

We know that blood-borne viruses can be transmitted through certain types of sexual activity. HCV has rarely been detected in semen and vaginal fluids. Most studies suggest that the virus is not often found in these body fluids, or that it is present in very small amounts and that the virus particles may be non-infectious.

Most experts believe that the risk of sexual transmission of HCV is low. Most studies show that only a small percentage of people—usually ranging from 0–3%—contract HCV through unprotected heterosexual intercourse with a long term, monogamous HCV-positive partner.

Some studies indicate that sexual transmission from men to women is more efficient than transmission from women to men. Since HCV is spread through blood, the risk of sexual transmission may be higher when a woman is having her menstrual period.

According to the most recent (2002) National Institutes of Health Consensus Statement, people who have multiple sex partners should practice safer sex. Those in stable, monogamous relationships do not need to change their current sexual practices, although they should discuss safer sex options if either partner is concerned about sexual transmission.

Among people in so-called "high risk" groups (gay men, prostitutes, people with multiple sex partners, people seen at STD clinics), sexual transmission of HCV appears to be more common. The fact that people with more sex partners and other sexual risk factors have higher rates of HCV indicates that the disease can be sexually transmitted. On the other hand, if sexual transmission of HCV were common, we would expect to see many more new cases of the disease among people whose partners are HCV positive.

Sexual transmission of HCV between men who have sex with men and women who have sex with women has not been well studied. Many recent studies show higher rates of HCV infection in gay men, but it is not known whether this is related to the type of sexual activity, such as fisting or multiple sexual partners, or to concomitant drug use. Anal sex may be a more efficient route of transmission than vaginal sex because the delicate lining of the rectum is more prone to damage that allows contact with blood. There are no known cases of HCV being transmitted through oral sex on a man (fellatio) or a woman (cunnilingus). However, it is theoretically possible that the virus could be transmitted this way if a person has mouth sores, bleeding gums, or a throat infection.

There are no known cases of HCV being spread through kissing, including deep, open mouth, or "French" kissing. It is theoretically possible that HCV could be transmitted this way if one partner has mouth sores, bleeding gums, or any other condition that could permit blood-to-blood contact. But this mode of transmission is believed to be very rare.

Special Considerations

Experts believe that HCV (like HIV) is more likely to be transmitted if either the positive or the negative partner has a sexually transmitted disease (STD), especially one that causes sores or lesions (for example, herpes or syphilis). Always have any suspicious symptoms checked by a doctor, and get prompt treatment for curable STDs such as Chlamydia, gonorrhea, and syphilis. Some studies suggest that people who are co-infected with both HCV and HIV are more likely to transmit HCV; the same may also be true for people co-infected with both HCV and hepatitis B virus (HBV). In addition, a person with HIV whose immune system is compromised may be at higher risk for contracting HCV.

Other sexual transmission routes that are not well-documented, but may pose a higher risk are rough or traumatic sex, dry sex, use of sex toys, cutting, whipping, or any practice where there is a potential for blood exposure.

Safer Sex

Some people feel more secure knowing that they are doing everything they can to prevent sexual transmission of HCV. Safer sex practices can also help prevent the spread of hepatitis A and B, HIV, and other STDs.

Using condoms is the surest way to prevent transmission of HCV and STDs. Latex condoms are best for disease prevention; natural skin condoms have small pores that can let viruses through. Polyurethane (plastic) condoms are also a good choice, especially for people who are sensitive to latex. Internal or "female" condoms (brand name "Reality") are polyurethane sheaths worn inside the vagina rather than on the penis.

Learn how to use condoms correctly. Most "condom failure" is caused by incorrect use. Pinch the tip as the condom is rolled on in order to create an air pocket that will leave room for the semen. Hold onto the base of a regular condom or hold an internal condom in place when withdrawing after sex to keep the semen from spilling. Tie the condom to prevent spills, and dispose of it properly. Condoms (both regular condoms and internal condoms) should be used only once. Some people choose to use condoms for oral sex on a man. For oral sex on a woman, barriers can be used to reduce the risk of disease transmission. Commonly used barriers include latex dental dams, sheets of plastic wrap, and latex sheets sold specifically for sex.

To prevent disease transmission through broken skin, some people use latex or nitrile (plastic) gloves or "finger cots" for manual sex. It is a good idea to cover any cuts or sores with a bandage that will not allow fluids to seep through.

Use only water-based lubricants with latex condoms or barriers. KY jelly and most commercial lubricants sold specifically for sex are water-based. Avoid oil-based lubricants (such as Vaseline, coconut oil, or moisturizing lotion) since these damage latex and can cause a condom or barrier to break. Avoid lubricants or pre-lubricated condoms that contain nonoxynol-9. Most manufacturers have recently stopped including this ingredient after it was shown that nonoxynol-9 caused irritation and damage to mucous membranes of the vagina, rectum, and penis that may actually increase the risk of disease transmission.

To reduce the risk of HCV transmission during oral sex or deep kissing, practice regular good oral hygiene—healthy teeth and gums may be the best defense against the spread of diseases through the mouth. Many experts recommend that people avoid brushing or flossing their teeth right before or after oral sex or deep kissing, since these can cause bleeding gums and tiny abrasions.

Conclusion

While sexual transmission of HCV remains somewhat controversial, most studies indicate that transmission through sexual activity is uncommon, and most experts believe the risk of sexual transmission is low. According to the National Institutes of Health, people in stable, monogamous relationships do not need to change their current sexual practices, although they should discuss safer sex options if either partner is concerned about sexual transmission. People with multiple sex partners should practice safer sex, in particular the use of latex condoms.

Section 22.3

Dispelling Myths about HCV

As the saying goes, "knowledge is power." This is particularly true when it comes to living with a chronic illness such as hepatitis C. In this day and age of managed health care, it is extremely important that people learn as much as possible about any healthcare issue so that they can advocate for themselves in order to get the best medical care possible. Conversely, misinformation about a condition like hepatitis C can be especially dangerous, and could potentially lead to living in fear and isolation, making life with HCV even more difficult.

Considering that the hepatitis C virus was only identified in 1989, it is incredible how far we have come in our understanding of hepatitis C, and remarkable that we have medications that can eradicate the virus in up to 50% of people infected with HCV genotype 1 and up to 80–90% in HCV genotypes 2 and 3. However, we have a long way to go before we can completely understand hepatitis C and discover medications that can eliminate the virus in everyone with hepatitis C.

This section will focus on some of the most common myths.

Myth: New drugs to treat hepatitis C will be on the market in the very near future.

There are many new drugs under investigation to treat hepatitis C, but the reality is that it will most likely not be until 2010–2011 before more effective medications are approved by the FDA to treat hepatitis C. It is also important to remember that pegylated interferon and ribavirin will be part of the "drug cocktail" for many years to come. Newer treatments offer the promise of higher effectiveness and perhaps shorter duration of treatment. This is important to know because some people who should be treated are waiting for the magic bullet.

People with hepatitis C should consult with their medical provider to decide if and when they should be treated. For some, waiting until new therapies are available is a wise decision, but for others HCV treatment is more urgent.

Myth: Hepatitis C is a death sentence.

After an initial diagnosis of hepatitis C, one must confront his or her mortality. Many people believe that every HCV-infected person will die of hepatitis C, and that it will happen very soon. This is one of the biggest fears that people with HCV face, especially those who are newly diagnosed. In recent years we have studied many different populations that have acquired hepatitis C within the last 10, 20, or 30 years or more, and it has been well-documented that only 10–25% of people chronically infected with HCV will experience serious liver disease progression that may result in death. The remaining 75–90% of people with chronic hepatitis C will live long and productive lives. However, we can not predict who will and who will not have serious disease progression. That is why it is so important that people with chronic hepatitis C are seen regularly by their medical providers to monitor their HCV health and status. There are also many strategies to staying healthy with hepatitis C that include good nutrition, daily exercise, stress management, avoiding alcohol, and HCV treatment.

The percentage of people progressing to serious liver disease would drop even lower if expanded testing and care were available to everyone at risk for hepatitis C. But this is not to say that people with hepatitis C do not suffer and die. Conservatively, it is estimated that there are approximately four million people in the United States and 170 million people worldwide who are infected with hepatitis C; so even though a minority of people who are infected with hepatitis C develop serious complications, the large number of people who are infected with hepatitis C means that the future disease burden is going to challenge our medical system in ways we haven't seen before.

Myth: Everyone with hepatitis C should be treated with current HCV medications.

The vast majority of people with chronic HCV will not experience serious disease progression and may never need to be treated. Hepatitis C behaves differently in different people, and as a result everyone with HCV should be evaluated on an individual basis. Currently, the major goals of HCV therapy are viral eradication, improvement in quality of life, and stopping or slowing disease progression. Treatment decisions should be made in partnership with a medical provider based on several considerations, including current health status, existing disease progression, likelihood of responding to current therapies, and quality of life. For example, people with minimal disease progression (little or no scarring of the liver) may want to wait until more effective medications are available that do not have as many undesired side effects. Conversely, someone with a decreased quality of life or serious disease progression (moderate to severe scarring of the liver) should be more aggressive in seeking medical treatment. But it is important to remember that people with minimal liver disease respond better to HCV medications, so this needs to be factored into the decision making process.

The wait and see exception is people with HCV genotypes 2 and 3 since they have such a high treatment response rate (up to 80–90% sustained virological response in some studies). Most experts believe that people who are infected with genotypes 2 or 3 should be treated.

It is also important to remember that everyone who would like to be treated should have access to care, management and HCV medications and that no one should be excluded from HCV treatment. The 2002 National Institutes of Health Consensus Conference Statement states that "All patients with chronic hepatitis C are potential candidates for antiviral therapy." In addition, from a public health standpoint, successful treatment of hepatitis C will lower the future disease burden and help to stop the spread of hepatitis C.

Myth: There are no effective medical treatments for hepatitis C.

Treatments for hepatitis C have improved dramatically since the early days of interferon monotherapy, when sustained virological response rates (SVR, remaining virus-free during and six months after the end of treatment) were measured in the single digits. Today we have two FDA-approved regimens of pegylated interferon plus ribavirin: Peg-Intron plus Rebetol (ribavirin), and Pegasys plus Copegus (ribavirin) which produce SVR rates up to ~50% for people with genotype 1 and up to 80–90% in people with genotypes 2 and 3. Furthermore, clinical studies have shown that, of people who have achieved an SVR, 98–99% continue to be HCV RNA (viral load) negative for five years post-treatment.

Myth: Most people can not tolerate the side effects from current HCV medications

This common myth prevents many people from seeking treatment because they have heard horror stories or worst-case scenarios experienced by some people taking the current HCV medications. Just as we have come a long way in improving treatment response rates since the early interferon monotherapy days, there have also been dramatic improvements in the way that side effects are managed. The truth is that therapy can be difficult, but most people can complete the treatment regimen if they receive appropriate support from medical providers, family, friends, and others. The key to successfully managing side effects is a team approach that treats physical and psychological side effects as soon as they surface and well before they become unmanageable. Unfortunately, some people do not have access to the supportive care that is such a critical part of the treatment process. Of course, there are people who cannot tolerate HCV therapy for a variety of reasons, but they are the exception rather than the rule.

Myth: Hepatitis C is a sexually transmitted disease.

HCV is transmitted in the vast majority of cases by blood-to-blood exposure. However, like many myths, this one is grounded in some truth. Hepatitis C can be transmitted sexually, but the risk is very low. It is difficult to study sexual transmission of HCV, but the majority of studies conducted to date have shown a 0–3% prevalence of HCV in people in stable monogamous heterosexual relationships. In fact, the Centers for Disease Control and Prevention do not recommend barrier protection to prevent HCV transmission for heterosexual couples in exclusive relationships. However, this recommendation must be considered carefully, since there is still a 1-in-1,000 to 1-in-10,000 chance of transmitting HCV to one's sexual partner even in this setting. Safer sex is recommended for people in so-called "high-risk" groups, usually defined as people with multiple sexual partners, men who have sex with men, women who have sex with women, prostitutes, and people seen at STD clinics. In these populations the risk of contracting HCV through unsafe sex is believed to be higher, but more studies are needed to clearly define the rate of sexual transmission.

Myth: HCV viral load correlates with disease progression.

It is logical to assume that if a person has more virus or a high HCV RNA (viral load), this it would mean a faster disease progression, but study after study has not shown a correlation between the amount of virus and the stage or degree of liver damage. In fact, the only reasons for measuring HCV viral load are to confirm active infection (to make sure that there is replicating HCV), to predict treatment response (the lower the viral load, the better chance one has of eradicating the virus), to make sure HCV medications are working, and after treatment is completed to make sure the virus is still undetectable.

Myth: HCV viral load correlates with the symptoms of HCV.

There have been no studies that have shown that someone with a higher viral load has more symptoms compared to someone with a lower viral load. In other words, people with a low viral load can experience as many symptoms as people with a high viral load and vice-versa.

Myth: People with "normal" levels have minimal disease progression.

ALT (alanine aminotransferase) is an enzyme that is produced in liver cells when there is damage taking place in the liver. Most people with hepatitis C and "normal" ALT levels have minimal liver disease progression, but some people (about 20%) with "normal" ALT levels have moderate to severe HCV disease progression. For this reason, many experts believe that the only way to really tell if an HCV positive person has liver damage is by a liver biopsy rather than through the measurement of ALT levels. Studies have found that people with "normal" ALT levels can be successfully treated with current HCV medications.

Myth: People with HCV should not take Tylenol.

This myth grows out of the liver-related problems that people have when taking large amounts of acetaminophen (brand name Tylenol) or paracetamol especially when consuming alcohol. Medical providers often recommend acetaminophen to relieve symptoms associated with hepatitis C infection and treatment-related side effects. But it is very important that people follow the recommended acetaminophen dose and duration of use prescribed by their healthcare provider and read the product label of any medications they are taking since acetaminophen is often a common ingredient in many over-the-counter and prescribed medications. It should also be noted that people with advanced liver disease should avoid acetaminophen.

Myth: Genotype 1 is the "worst" genotype.

This myth is the result of earlier studies that reported a faster rate of disease progression in people infected with HCV genotype 1. Like many reports in the early years of HCV research, this has been debunked by more recent research which has not shown a correlation between genotype 1 and more rapid disease progression. In regards to the other genotypes, genotype 3 causes steatosis which could potentially increase the rate of HCV disease progression and lower treatment response, but more studies are needed of steatosis in people with genotype 3 to completely understand this. The exact way that hepatitis C causes steatosis is unknown.

Genotype information is important, though, for people seeking treatment, since genotypes 2 and 3 have been shown to respond more favorably to current HCV medications. People with genotypes 2 or 3 have the added benefits of a lower dose of ribavirin and a shorter duration of treatment compared to people with genotype 1.

Myth: HCV is an asymptomatic disease.

This is another myth that is grounded in some truth, but has led to a misunderstanding of the symptoms from which people with HCV suffer. It is well-documented that people with decompensated cirrhosis may have severe or even life-threatening conditions such as itching, ascites (accumulation of fluid in the abdomen), uncontrolled bleeding, and encephalopathy (brain disease). However, people with HCV may experience many debilitating symptoms even if they have mild disease. This is because HCV is not only a liver disease but affects other parts of the body through various mechanisms—most notably those involving autoimmune processes. The more common symptoms reported by people with HCV include fatigue (mild to severe), muscle pain, joint pain, headaches, depression, anxiety, "brain fog," abdominal pain, and other extrahepatic manifestations (diseases outside of the liver). Many patients report that their symptoms are not acknowledged or taken seriously by their medical providers, especially if the providers are not well versed in hepatitis C.

Myth: There is a vaccine to protect against hepatitis C.

This myth results from people confusing hepatitis A or hepatitis B—both preventable with vaccines—with hepatitis C. At this time there is NO vaccine to protect against getting hepatitis C. Unfortunately, developing an effective HCV vaccine will be very difficult because the virus constantly mutates. Research is underway, but an effective vaccine is not expected for at least 10 years.

Myth: Sharing household items such as razors and toothbrushes poses a very high risk for transmitting HCV.

There is a potential risk of transmitting HCV by sharing personal items, but experts believe that the risk is very low. Here's what would have to happen to transmit hepatitis C in a household setting: the blood of an HCV-infected person would have to get into the blood of another household member. To prevent HCV transmission in a household setting, do not share personal items, such as toothbrushes or razor blades, and cover items that could infect another person. And it is a good idea to keep any personal items (razors, toothbrushes, etc.) in a separate area so that people will not mistakenly use them. The good news is that we know hepatitis C is not spread by sneezing, hugging, sharing eating utensils or drinking glasses, preparing food, or any other kind of casual contact.

Myth: I am feeling worse than usual so my liver is becoming more damaged.

The general mild flu-like symptoms that people experience from hepatitis C are believed to be the result of the immune system fighting the virus and not necessarily the virus damaging the liver. People also report that the symptoms come in cycles. Sometimes they feel ok or mildly sick and other times feel like they can't get out of bed. Since some of these flu-like symptoms are from the immune system fighting the virus it does not necessarily mean that the liver is becoming more damaged. Of course, anyone who feels that they are getting more symptoms or that their symptoms are getting worse should be evaluated by a medical provider, but it does not necessarily mean that the liver disease progression is getting worse.

Chapter 23

Herpes Infections

Chapter Contents

Section 23.1

Genital Herpes Overview

"Genital Herpes," National Institute of Allergy and Infectious Diseases (www3.niaid.nih.gov), June 24, 2007. Reprinted with permission.

Genital herpes is a sexually transmitted infection (STI). According to the Centers for Disease Control and Prevention, one out of five American teenagers and adults is infected with genital herpes. Women are more commonly infected than men. In the United States, one out of four women has herpes.

Although at least 45 million people in the United States have genital herpes infection, there has been a substantial decrease in cases from 21% to 17%, according to a 1999 to 2004 CDC survey. Much of the decrease was in the 14- to 19-year age group, and continued through the young adult group.

Cause

Genital herpes is caused by herpes simplex virus (HSV). There are two types of HSV.

- HSV type 1 most commonly infects the mouth and lips, causing sores known as fever blisters or cold sores.
- HSV type 2 is the usual cause of genital herpes, but it also can infect the mouth.

Transmission

If you have genital herpes infection, you can easily pass or transmit the virus to an uninfected partner during sex.

Most people get genital herpes by having sex with someone who is shedding the herpes virus either during an outbreak or an asymptomatic (without symptoms) period. People who do not know they have herpes play an important role in transmission because they are unaware they can infect a sexual partner.

You can transmit herpes through close contact other than sexual intercourse, through oral sex or close skin-to-skin contact, for example.

The virus is spread rarely, if at all, by objects such as a toilet seat or hot tub.

Reduce Your Risk of Spreading Herpes

People with herpes should follow a few simple steps to avoid spreading the infection to other places on their body or other people.

- Avoid touching the infected area during an outbreak, and wash your hands after contact with that area.
- Do not have sexual contact (vaginal, oral, or anal) from the time of your first genital symptoms until your symptoms are completely gone.

Symptoms

Symptoms of herpes are called outbreaks. The first outbreak appears within two weeks after you become infected and can last for several weeks. These symptoms might include tingling or sores (lesions) near the area where the virus has entered your body, such as on your genital or rectal area, on your buttocks or thighs. Occasionally, these sores may appear on other parts of your body where the virus has entered through broken skin. Sores also can appear inside the vagina and on the cervix (opening to the womb) in women, or in the urinary passage of women and men. Small red bumps appear first, develop into small blisters, and then become itchy, painful sores that might develop a crust and will heal without leaving a scar.

Sometimes, there is a crack or raw area or some redness without pain, itching, or tingling. Other symptoms that may accompany the first (and less often future) outbreak of genital herpes are fever, headache, muscle aches, painful or difficult urination, vaginal discharge, and swollen glands in the groin area.

Often, though, people don't recognize their first or subsequent outbreaks. People who have mild or no symptoms at all may not think they are infected with herpes. They can still transmit the virus to others, however.

Recurrence of Herpes Outbreaks

In most people, the virus can become active and cause outbreaks several times a year. This is called a recurrence, and infected people can have symptoms. HSV remains in certain nerve cells of your body for life. When the virus is triggered to be active, it travels along the nerves to your skin. There, it makes more virus and sometimes new sores near the site of the first outbreak. Recurrences are generally much milder than the first outbreak of genital herpes. HSV-2 genital infection is more likely to result in recurrences than HSV-1 genital infection. Recurrences become less common over time.

Symptoms from recurrences might include itching, tingling, vaginal discharge, and a burning feeling or pain in the genital or anal area. Sores may be present during a recurrence, but sometimes they are small and easily overlooked.

Sometimes, the virus can become active but not cause any visible sores or any symptoms. During these times, small amounts of the virus may be shed at or near places of the first infection, in fluids from the mouth, penis, or vagina, or from barely noticeable sores. This is called asymptomatic shedding. Even though you are not aware of the shedding, you can infect a sexual partner during this time. Asymptomatic shedding is an important factor in the spread of herpes.

Diagnosis

Your health care provider can diagnose typical genital herpes by looking at the sores. Some cases, however, are more difficult to diagnose.

The virus sometimes, but not always, can be detected by a laboratory test called a culture. A culture is done when your health care provider uses a swab to get and study material from a suspected herpes sore. You may still have genital herpes, however, even if your culture is negative (which means it does not show HSV).

A blood test called type-specific test can tell whether you are infected with HSV-1 or HSV-2. The type-specific test results plus the location of the sores will help your health care provider to find out whether you have genital infection.

Coping with Herpes

A diagnosis of genital herpes can have substantial emotional effects on you and your sexual partner, whether or not you have symptoms. Proper counseling and treatment can help you and your partner learn to cope with the disease, recurrent episodes, personal relationships, and fertility issues.

Treatment

Although there is no cure for genital herpes, your health care provider might prescribe an antiviral medicine to treat your symptoms and to help prevent future outbreaks. This can decrease the risk of passing herpes to sexual partners. Medicines to treat genital herpes are the following:

- Acyclovir (Zovirax)
- Famciclovir (Famvir)
- Valacyclovir (Valtrex)

For updated information on treatment for genital herpes, read the CDC STD Treatment Guidelines at www.cdc.gov/std/treatment/.

Prevention

Because herpes can be transmitted from someone who has no symptoms, using the precautions listed below is not enough to prevent transmission. Recently, the Food and Drug Administration approved Valtrex for use in preventing transmission of genital herpes. It has to be taken continuously by the infected person, and while it significantly decreases the risk of the transmission of herpes, transmission can still occur.

Do not have oral-genital contact if you or your sexual partner has any symptoms or findings of oral herpes.

Using barriers such as latex condoms during sexual activity may decrease transmission when you use them consistently and correctly, but transmission can still occur since condoms may not cover all infected areas.

You can get tested to find out if you are infected with the herpes virus.

Complications

Genital herpes infections usually do not cause serious health problems in healthy adults. In some people whose immune systems do not work properly, however, genital herpes outbreaks can be unusually severe and long lasting.

Occasionally, people with normal immune systems can get herpes infection of the eye, called ocular herpes. Ocular herpes is usually caused by HSV-1 but sometimes by HSV-2. It can occasionally result in serious eye disease, including blindness.

A woman with herpes who is pregnant can pass the infection to her baby. A baby born with herpes might die or have serious brain, skin, or eye problems. A pregnant woman who has herpes, or whose sex partner has herpes, should discuss the situation with her health care provider. Together they can make a plan to reduce her or her baby's risk of getting infected. Babies who are born with herpes do better if the disease is recognized and treated early.

Genital herpes, like other genital diseases that cause sores, is important in the spread of HIV infection. A person infected with herpes may have a greater risk of getting HIV. This may be due to the open sores caused by the herpes infection or by other factors in the immune system. In addition, HIV-positive people may be more contagious for herpes.

Research

The National Institute of Allergy and Infectious Diseases (NIAID) supports research on genital herpes and HSV. Studies are currently underway to develop better treatments for the millions of people who suffer from genital herpes. While some scientists are carrying out clinical trials to determine the best way to use existing medicines, others are studying the biology of HSV. NIAID scientists have identified certain genes and enzymes (proteins) that the virus needs to survive. They are hopeful that drugs aimed at disrupting these viral targets might lead to the design of more effective treatments.

Meanwhile, other researchers are devising methods to control the virus' spread. Two important means of preventing HSV infection are vaccines and topical microbicides.

Several different vaccines are in various stages of development. These include vaccines made from proteins on the HSV cell surface, peptides or chains of amino acids, and the DNA of the virus itself. NIAID and GlaxoSmithKline are supporting a large clinical trial in women of an experimental vaccine that may help prevent transmission of genital herpes. The Herpevac Trial is being conducted at more than 50 sites in the U.S. and Canada.

Topical microbicides, preparations containing microbe-killing compounds, are also in various stages of development and testing. These include gels, creams, or lotions that a woman could insert into the vagina prior to intercourse to prevent infection. The NIAID Sexually Transmitted Infections Clinical Trials Group is conducting a Phase

1 study to evaluate the safety of a microbicide gel to prevent genital herpes.

A NIAID-supported clinical trial demonstrated that once-daily suppressive therapy using valacyclovir significantly reduces risk of transmission of genital herpes to an uninfected partner. This is the first time an antiviral medication had been shown to reduce the risk of transmission of an STI. This strategy may contribute to preventing the spread of genital herpes.

Section 23.2

Oral Herpes Overview

"Fact Sheet: Oral Herpes," © 2007 Washtenaw County Public Health (http://publichealth.ewashtenaw.org). Reprinted with permission.

What is Herpes?

Herpes is a viral infection caused by the herpes simplex virus. There are two types of herpes, herpes simplex I (oral) and herpes simplex II (genital). The first infection with HSV I usually occurs before five years of age. Antibodies to HSV I are found in 50–90% of adults. Cold sores (HSV I) are typically found on the lips and in the mouth, but can be passed to the genital area during oral sex.

What are the symptoms?

HSV I will usually start with sores or blisters in or around the mouth ("cold sores"). These crust and heal within a few days. Some people find that stress, illness, injuries, certain foods, or eating poorly may cause the sores to return.

How is it spread?

HSV I is primarily spread through skin to skin contact with the infected person; however, it can be transmitted occasionally through sharing of drinks, lip products (i.e.: Chapstick, lipstick) and moist washcloths and towels. Wash your hands after touching the sores. HSV

I can be transmitted to any area of the body, including the genitals and the eyes.

How is it treated?

Herpes is a virus and cannot be treated with antibiotics. Your health care provider can prescribe anti-viral medications that may decrease the severity of the outbreaks.

How is it prevented?

- Avoid skin-to-skin contact of the infected area with another person until the skin is completely healed.
- Wash hands thoroughly after touching the affected area.
- Learn to know your own symptoms if you have herpes and consider treatment if you have more than 6–9 outbreaks per year.
- Learn what kinds of things trigger your symptoms and avoid them when possible.
- Don't share washcloths, towels, or other personal items during a recurrence.

Section 23.3

Herpes Complications

This section excerpted from "Herpes Simplex,"

Complications

The severity of symptoms depends on where and how the virus enters the body. Except in very rare instances and in special circumstances, the disease is not life threatening, although it can be very debilitating and cause great emotional distress.

Herpes and Pregnancy

Pregnant women who are infected with either herpes simplex virus 2 (HSV-2) or herpes simplex virus 1 (HSV-1) genital herpes have a higher risk for miscarriage, premature labor, retarded fetal growth, or transmission of the herpes infection to the infant while in the uterus or at the time of delivery. Herpes in newborn babies (neonatals) can be a very serious condition.

Fortunately, neonatal herpes is rare. Although about 25–30% of pregnant women have genital herpes, less than 0.1% of babies are born with neonatal herpes. The baby is at greatest risk from an asymptomatic infection during a vaginal delivery in women who acquired the virus for the first time late in the pregnancy. In such cases, 30–50% of newborns become infected. Recurring herpes and a first infection that is acquired early in the pregnancy pose a much lower risk to the infant.

The reasons for the higher risk with a late primary infection are:

- during a first infection, the virus is shed for longer periods, and more viral particles are excreted;
- an infection that first occurs in the late term does not allow the mother to develop antibodies that would help her baby fight off the infection at the time of delivery.

The risk for transmission also increases if infants with infected mothers are born prematurely, if there is invasive monitoring, or if instruments are required during vaginal delivery. Transmission can occur if the amniotic membrane of an infected woman ruptures prematurely, or as the infant passes through an infected birth canal. This increased risk is present if the woman is having or has recently had an active herpes outbreak in the genital area.

Very rarely, the virus is transmitted across the placenta, a form of the infection known as congenital herpes. Also rarely, newborns may contract herpes during the first weeks of life from being kissed by someone with a herpes cold sore.

Infants may acquire congenital herpes from a mother with an active herpes infection at the time of birth. Aggressive treatment with antiviral medication is required, but may not help systemic herpes.

Unfortunately, only 5% of infected pregnant women have a history of symptoms, so in many cases herpes infection is not suspected, or symptoms are missed, at the time of delivery. If there is evidence of an active outbreak, doctors usually advise a Cesarean section to prevent the baby contacting the virus in the birth canal during delivery.

Approach to the Pregnant Herpes Patient

The approach to a pregnant woman who has been infected by either HSV-1 or HSV-2 in the genital area is usually determined by when the infection was acquired and the mother's condition around the time of delivery.

- Obtaining routine herpes cultures on all women during the prenatal period is not recommended.
- Performing chorionic villus sampling, amniocentesis, and percutaneous fetal blood draws can safely be performed during pregnancy.
- Using fetal scalp techniques if considered necessary is considered reasonable if there has been no recent genital herpes outbreaks
- If lesions in the genital area are present at the time of birth, Cesarean section is usually recommended. (Even a Cesarean section is no guarantee that the child will be virus-free, and the newborn must still be tested.)
- If lesions erupt shortly before the baby is due then samples must be taken and sent to the laboratory. Samples are cultured to detect the virus at three- to five-day intervals prior to delivery

to determine whether viral shedding is occurring. If no lesions are present and cultures indicate no viral shedding, a vaginal delivery can be performed and the newborn is examined and cultured after delivery.

- Some doctors recommend anti-viral medication for pregnant women who are infected with HSV-2. Recent studies indicate that acyclovir (Zovirax) or valacyclovir (Valtrex) or famciclovir (Famvir) can help reduce the recurrence of genital herpes and the need for Cesarean sections. Women begin to take the drug on a daily basis beginning in the 36th week of pregnancy (last trimester).
- Breast-feeding after delivery is safe unless there is a herpes lesion on the breast.

Potential Effects of Herpes in the Newborn

Herpes infection in a newborn causes vague symptoms, such as skin rash, fevers, mouth sores, and eye infections. If left untreated, neonatal herpes is a very serious and even life-threatening condition. Neonatal herpes can spread to the brain and central nervous system causing encephalitis and meningitis and leading to mental retardation, cerebral palsy, and death. Herpes can also spread to internal organs, such as the liver and lungs.

Infants infected with herpes are treated with acyclovir. It is important to treat babies quickly, before the infection spreads to the brain and other organs.

Effects on the Brain and Central Nervous System

Herpes encephalitis: Each year in the U.S., herpes accounts for about 2,100 cases of encephalitis, a rare but extremely serious brain disease. Herpes simplex virus 1 (HSV-1) is usually the cause, except in newborns. In about 70% of cases of infant herpes encephalitis, the disease occurs when a latent herpes simplex virus 2 (HSV-2) is activated. Untreated, herpes encephalitis is fatal over 70% of the time. Respiratory arrest can occur within the first 24–72 hours. Fortunately, rapid diagnostic tests and treatment with acyclovir have both significantly improved survival rates and reduced complication rates. For those who recover, nearly all suffer some impairment, ranging from very mild neurological changes to paralysis. Recovery from herpes encephalitis depends on the patient's age, the level of consciousness, duration of the disease, and the promptness of treatment. The best chances for a favorable outcome occur in patients who are treated with acyclovir within two days of becoming ill.

Herpes meningitis: Herpes meningitis, an inflammation of the membranes that line the brain and spinal cord, occurs in up to 10% of cases of primary genital HSV-2. Women are at higher risk than men for herpes meningitis. Symptoms include headache, fever, stiff neck, vomiting, and sensitivity to light. Fortunately, herpes meningitis usually resolves without complications, lasting for up to a week, although recurrences have been reported.

Eczema Herpeticum

A form of herpes infection called eczema herpeticum, also known as Kaposi's varicellum eruption, can affect patients with skin disorders and immunocompromised patients. The disease tends to develop into widespread skin infection that resembles impetigo. Symptoms appear abruptly and can include fever, chills, and malaise. Clusters of dimpled blisters emerge over 7–10 days and spread widely. They can become secondarily infected with staphylococcal or streptococcal organisms. When treated, lesions heal in 2–6 weeks. Untreated, this condition can be extremely serious and possibly fatal.

Ocular Herpes and Vision Loss

Herpetic infections of the eye (ocular herpes) occur in about 50,000 Americans each year. In most cases it causes inflammation and sores on the lids or outside of the cornea that go away in a few days.

Stromal keratitis: Stromal keratitis occurs in up to 25% of cases of ocular herpes. In this condition, deeper layers of the cornea are involved, possibly as an abnormal immune response to the original infection. In these rare cases, scarring and corneal thinning develop, which may cause the eye's globe to rupture, resulting in blindness. Although rare, it is the major cause of corneal blindness in the U.S.

Iridocyclitis: Iridocyclitis is another serious complication of ocular herpes, in which the iris and the area around it become inflamed.

Gingivostomatitis

Herpes can cause multiple painful ulcers on the gums and mucous membranes of the mouth, a condition called gingivostomatitis. This condition usually affects children one to five years of age. It nearly always subsides within two weeks. Rarely, it can lead to a viral infection. Children with gingivostomatitis commonly develop herpetic whitlow (herpes of the fingers).

A herpetic whitlow is an infection of the herpes virus around the fingernail. In children, this is often caused by thumb-sucking or finger sucking while they have a cold sore. It is seen in adult health care workers, such as dentists, because of increased exposure to the herpes virus. The use of rubber gloves prevents herpes whitlow in health care workers.

Herpes in Patients with Compromised Immune Systems

Herpes simplex is particularly devastating when it occurs in immunocompromised patients and, unfortunately, co-infection is common. People infected with herpes have a three-fold increased risk for contracting HIV. Furthermore, studies have reported that 68–81% of patients with HIV are also infected with herpes simplex virus 2 (HSV-2).

Patients with HIV are particularly vulnerable to complications. When a person has both viruses, there appears to be a synergy between them, with each virus increasing the severity of the other. HSV-2 infection increases HIV levels in the genital tract, which makes it easier for the HIV virus to be transmitted to sexual partners. In addition, episodes of herpes recurrence increase, at least temporarily, HIV viral load. Researchers are investigating whether treatment of HSV-2 may help reduce the risk of HIV transmission.

Herpes simplex in any patient with a seriously compromised immune system can cause serious and even life-threatening complications, including:

- pneumonia;
- inflammation of the esophagus;
- encephalitis (inflammation of the brain);
- destruction of the adrenal glands;
- disseminated herpes (spread of infection throughout the body);
- liver damage, including hepatitis.

Section 23.4

Herpes Treatment Options and Vaccine Trials

Treatment for Genital Herpes

No drug can cure herpes simplex virus. The infection may recur after treatment has been stopped, and, even during therapy, a patient can still transmit the virus to another person. Drugs can, however, reduce symptoms and improve healing times.

Acyclovir and Related Drugs

Antiviral drugs called nucleosides or nucleotide analogues are the main drugs used to treat genital herpes. They are taken by mouth. (Acyclovir is also available as an ointment, but the oral form is much more effective.) These drugs limit herpes viral replication and its spread to other cells. They are not cures, however.

Three drugs are approved to treat genital herpes:

- Acyclovir (Zovirax or generic)
- Valacyclovir (Valtrex)
- Famciclovir (Famvir)

When a patient has herpes for the first time, the drug is taken several times a day for 7–10 days. Then the drugs are used either to suppress the virus or to treat outbreaks.

To treat outbreaks, drug regimens depend on whether it is the first episode or a recurrence and on the medication and dosage prescribed. Most medications need to be taken several times a day. For a first episode, treatment usually lasts 7–10 days. For a recurrent episode, treatment takes one to five days depending on the type of medication and dosage.

To suppress outbreaks, treatment requires taking pills daily on a long-term basis. (Acyclovir and famciclovir are taken twice a day, valacyclovir once a day.) Suppressive treatment can reduce outbreaks by 70–80%. It is generally recommended for patients who have frequent recurrences (six or more outbreaks per year). Valacyclovir may work especially well for preventing herpes transmission among heterosexual patients when one partner has herpes simplex virus 2 (HSV-2) and the other partner does not. However, valacyclovir may not be as effective as acyclovir or famciclovir for patients who have very frequent recurrences of herpes (more than 10 outbreaks per year).

Because the frequency of herpes recurrences often diminishes over time, patients should discuss annually with their doctors whether they should stay with drug therapy or discontinue it. Studies suggest that daily drug therapy is safe and effective for up to six years with acyclovir, and up to one year with valacyclovir or famciclovir.

Side effects: Nausea and headache are the most common side effects, but in general these drugs are safe. Although there is some evidence these drugs may reduce shedding, they probably do not prevent it entirely. The use of condoms during asymptomatic periods is still essential, even when patients are taking these medications.

Risk for resistant viruses: As with antibiotics, doctors are concerned about signs of increasing viral resistance to acyclovir and similar drugs, particularly in immunocompromised patients (such as those with AIDS). Most patients on long-term suppressive drug therapy show few signs of drug resistance. However, patients who do not respond to standard regimens should be monitored for emergence of drug resistance.

Investigational Vaccine for Herpes

In 2002, the U.S. National Institute of Allergy and Infectious Diseases (NIAID) launched the Herpevac Trial for Women to investigate a vaccine for preventing herpes in women who are not infected with HSV-1 or HSV-2. (Previous studies found that the vaccine is not effective for men.) The study of over 7,000 women is currently in its final phases at 40 sites in the U.S. and Canada.

Treatment for Oral Herpes

Oral Treatments

Acyclovir (Zovirax), valacyclovir (Valtrex), and famciclovir (Famvir)—the anti-viral pills used to treat genital herpes—can also treat the cold sores associated with oral herpes. In addition, acyclovir is available in topical form, as is penciclovir (a related drug).

Topical Treatments

These ointments or creams help shorten healing time and duration of symptoms. However, none are truly effective in eliminating outbreaks.

- Penciclovir (Denavir) heals herpes simplex virus 1 (HSV-1) sores on average about half a day faster than without treatment, stops viral shedding, and reduces the duration of pain. Ideally, the patient should apply the cream within the first hour of symptoms, although benefits have also been noted with later application. It is continued for four consecutive days, and should be reapplied every two hours while awake.
- Acyclovir cream (Zovirax) works best when applied early on (at the first sign of pain or tingling).
- Docosanol cream (Abreva) is the only FDA-approved nonprescription ointment for oral herpes. The patient applies the cream five times a day, beginning at the first sign of tingling or pain. Studies have been mixed on the cream's benefits.
- Over-the-counter topical anesthetics may provide modest relief. They include Anbesol gel, Blistex lip ointment, Campho-Phenique, Herpecin-L, Viractin, and Zilactin.

Home Remedies

Patients can manage most herpes simplex infections that develop on the skin at home with over-the-counter painkillers and measures to relieve symptoms.

Symptomatic Relief

Several simple steps can produce some relief.

- Hygiene is important. Avoid touching the sores. Wash hands frequently during the day. Fingernails should be scrubbed daily. Keep the body clean.
- Drink plenty of water.
- Keep blisters or sores clean and dry with cornstarch or similar product. (Women should not use talcum powder because it may increase their risk for ovarian cancer.)

- Some people report that drying the genital area with a blow dryer on the cool setting offers relief.
- Avoid tight-fitting clothing, which restricts air circulation and slows healing of the sores.
- Choose cotton underwear, rather than synthetic materials.
- Local application of ice packs may alleviate the pain and help reduce recurrences by suppressing the virus.
- Lukewarm baths may be helpful.
- Wearing sun block helps prevent sun-triggered recurrence of herpes simplex virus 1 (HSV-1).
- Avoid sex during both outbreaks and prodromes (the early symptoms of herpes), which include tingling, itching, or tenderness in the infected areas.
- Over-the-counter medications such as aspirin, acetaminophen (Datril, Panadol, Tylenol), or ibuprofen (Advil, Medipren, Motrin, Nuprin), can be used to reduce fever and local tenderness.

Herbs and Supplements

Generally, manufacturers of herbal remedies and dietary supplements do not need FDA approval to sell their products. Just like a drug, herbs and supplements can affect the body's chemistry, and therefore have the potential to produce side effects that may be harmful. There have been several reported cases of serious and even lethal side effects from herbal products. Always check with your doctor before using any herbal remedies or dietary supplements.

Many herbal and dietary supplement products claim to help fight herpes infection by boosting the immune system. There has been little research on these products, and little evidence to show that they really work. Some are capsules taken by mouth. Others come in the form of ointment that is applied to the skin. Popular herbal and supplement remedies for herpes simplex include:

- echinacea (*Echinacea purpurea*);
- Siberian ginseng (*Eleutherococcus senticosus*);
- aloe (*Aloe vera*);
- bee products that contain propolis, a tree resin collected by bees;

- lysine;
- zinc.

The following are special concerns for people taking natural remedies for herpes simplex:

- Echinacea can lower white blood cell levels when taken for long periods of time. This herb can also interfere with drugs that are used to treat immune system disorders.
- Siberian ginseng can raise blood pressure levels.
- Bee products (like propolis) can cause allergic reactions in people who are allergic to bee stings.
- Lysine should not be taken with certain types of antibiotics.
- Taking zinc in large amounts (more than 200 mg/day) can cause stomach upset.

Chapter 24

HIV and AIDS

Chapter Contents

Section 24.1

HIV and AIDS Overview

"HIV Infection and AIDS: An Overview," National Institute of Allergy and Infectious Diseases (www3.niaid.nih.gov), October 2007.

AIDS was first reported in the United States in 1981 and has since become a major worldwide epidemic. AIDS is caused by the human immunodeficiency virus, or HIV. By killing or damaging cells of the body's immune system, HIV progressively destroys the body's ability to fight infections and certain cancers. People diagnosed with AIDS may get life-threatening diseases called opportunistic infections. These infections are caused by microbes such as viruses or bacteria that usually do not make healthy people sick.

Since 1981, more than 980,000 cases of AIDS have been reported in the United States to the Centers for Disease Control and Prevention (CDC). According to CDC, more than 1,000,000 Americans may be infected with HIV, one-quarter of whom are unaware of their infection. The epidemic is growing most rapidly among minority populations and is a leading killer of African American males ages 25 to 44. According, AIDS affects nearly seven times more African Americans and three times more Hispanics than whites. In recent years, an increasing number of African American women and children are being affected by HIV/AIDS.

Transmission

HIV is spread most often through unprotected sex with an infected partner. The virus can enter the body through the lining of the vagina, vulva, penis, rectum, or mouth during sex.

Risky Behavior

HIV can infect anyone who practices risky behaviors such as the following:

- Sharing drug needles or syringes
- Having sexual contact, including oral sexual contact, with an infected person without using a condom

- Having sexual contact with someone whose HIV status is unknown

Infected Blood

HIV also is spread through contact with infected blood. Before donated blood was screened for evidence of HIV infection and before heat-treating techniques to destroy HIV in blood products were introduced, HIV was transmitted through transfusions of contaminated blood or blood components. Today, because of blood screening and heat treatment, the risk of getting HIV from blood transfusions is extremely small.

Contaminated Needles

HIV is often spread among injection drug users when they share needles or syringes contaminated with very small quantities of blood from someone infected with the virus.

It is rare for a patient to be the source of HIV transmitted to a health care provider or vice versa by accidental sticks with contaminated needles or other medical instruments.

Mother-to-Child

Women can transmit HIV to their babies during pregnancy or birth. Approximately one-quarter to one-third of all untreated pregnant women infected with HIV will pass the infection to their babies. HIV also can be spread to babies through the breast milk of mothers infected with the virus. If the mother takes certain drugs during pregnancy, she can significantly reduce the chances that her baby will get infected with HIV. If health care providers treat HIV-infected pregnant women and deliver their babies by cesarean section, the chances of the baby being infected can be reduced to a rate of 1%. HIV infection of newborns has been almost eradicated in the United States because of appropriate treatment.

A study sponsored by the National Institute of Allergy and Infectious Diseases (NIAID) in Uganda found a highly effective and safe drug for preventing transmission of HIV from an infected mother to her newborn. Independent studies have also confirmed this finding. This regimen is more affordable and practical than any other examined to date. Results from the study show that a single oral dose of the antiretroviral drug nevirapine (NVP) given to an HIV-infected woman in labor and another to her baby within three days of birth reduces the transmission rate of HIV by half compared with a similar short course of AZT (azidothymidine).

Saliva

Although researchers have found HIV in the saliva of infected people, there is no evidence that the virus is spread by contact with saliva. Laboratory studies reveal that saliva has natural properties that limit the power of HIV to infect, and the amount of virus in saliva appears to be very low. Research studies of people infected with HIV have found no evidence that the virus is spread to others through saliva by kissing. The lining of the mouth, however, can be infected by HIV, and instances of HIV transmission through oral intercourse have been reported.

Scientists have found no evidence that HIV is spread through sweat, tears, urine, or feces.

Casual Contact

Studies of families of HIV-infected people have shown clearly that HIV is not spread through casual contact such as the sharing of food utensils, towels and bedding, swimming pools, telephones, or toilet seats.

HIV is not spread by biting insects such as mosquitoes or bedbugs.

Sexually Transmitted Infections

People with a sexually transmitted infection, such as syphilis, genital herpes, chlamydia, gonorrhea, or bacterial vaginosis, may be more susceptible to getting HIV infection during sex with infected partners.

Symptoms

Early Symptoms

Many people will not have any symptoms when they first become infected with HIV. They may, however, have a flu-like illness within a month or two after exposure to the virus. This illness may include the following symptoms:

- Fever
- Headache
- Tiredness

- Enlarged lymph nodes (glands of the immune system easily felt in the neck and groin)

These symptoms usually disappear within a week to a month and are often mistaken for those of another viral infection. During this period, people are very infectious, and HIV is present in large quantities in genital fluids.

Later Symptoms

More persistent or severe symptoms may not appear for 10 years or more after HIV first enters the body in adults, or within two years in children born with HIV infection. This period of asymptomatic infection varies greatly in each person. Some people may begin to have symptoms within a few months, while others may be symptom-free for more than 10 years.

Even during the asymptomatic period, the virus is actively multiplying, infecting, and killing cells of the immune system. The virus can also hide within infected cells and be inactive. The most obvious effect of HIV infection is a decline in the number of CD4 positive T (CD4+) cells found in the blood—the immune system's key infection fighters. The virus slowly disables or destroys these cells without causing symptoms.

As the immune system becomes more debilitated, a variety of complications start to take over. For many people, the first signs of infection are large lymph nodes, or swollen glands that may be enlarged for more than three months. Other symptoms often experienced months to years before the onset of AIDS include the following:

- Lack of energy
- Weight loss
- Frequent fevers and sweats
- Persistent or frequent yeast infections (oral or vaginal)
- Persistent skin rashes or flaky skin
- Pelvic inflammatory disease in women that does not respond to treatment
- Short-term memory loss

Some people develop frequent and severe herpes infections that cause mouth, genital, or anal sores, or a painful nerve disease called shingles. Children may grow slowly or get sick frequently.

What Is AIDS?

Symptoms of opportunistic infections common in people with AIDS include the following:

- Coughing and shortness of breath
- Seizures and lack of coordination
- Difficult or painful swallowing
- Mental symptoms such as confusion and forgetfulness
- Severe and persistent diarrhea
- Fever
- Vision loss
- Nausea, abdominal cramps, and vomiting
- Weight loss and extreme fatigue
- Severe headaches
- Coma

Children with AIDS may get the same opportunistic infections as do adults with the disease. In addition, they also may have severe forms of the typically common childhood bacterial infections, such as conjunctivitis (pink eye), ear infections, and tonsillitis.

People with AIDS are also particularly prone to developing various cancers, especially those caused by viruses such as Kaposi's sarcoma and cervical cancer, or cancers of the immune system known as lymphomas. These cancers are usually more aggressive and difficult to treat in people with AIDS. Signs of Kaposi's sarcoma in light-skinned people are round brown, reddish, or purple spots that develop in the skin or in the mouth. In dark-skinned people, the spots are more pigmented.

During the course of HIV infection, most people experience a gradual decline in the number of CD4+ T cells, although some may have abrupt and dramatic drops in their CD4+ T-cell counts. A person with CD4+ T cells above 200 may experience some of the early symptoms of HIV disease. Others may have no symptoms even though their CD4+ T-cell count is below 200.

Many people are so debilitated by the symptoms of AIDS that they cannot hold a steady job or do household chores. Other people with AIDS may experience phases of intense life-threatening illness followed by phases in which they function normally.

A small number of people first infected with HIV 10 or more years ago have not developed symptoms of AIDS. Scientists are trying to determine what factors may account for the lack of progression to AIDS in some people, such as the following:

- Whether their immune systems have particular characteristics
- Whether they were infected with a less aggressive strain of the virus
- If their genes may protect them from the effects of HIV

Scientists hope that understanding the body's natural method of controlling infection may lead to ideas for protective HIV vaccines and use of vaccines to prevent the disease from progressing.

Diagnosis

Because early HIV infection often causes no symptoms, a health care provider usually can diagnose it by testing blood for the presence of antibodies (disease-fighting proteins) to HIV. HIV antibodies generally do not reach noticeable levels in the blood for one to three months after infection. It may take the antibodies as long as six months to be produced in quantities large enough to show up in standard blood tests. Hence, to determine whether a person has been recently infected (acute infection), a health care provider can screen blood for the presence of HIV genetic material. Direct screening of HIV is extremely critical in order to prevent transmission of HIV from recently infected individuals.

Anyone who has been exposed to the virus should get an HIV test as soon as the immune system is likely to develop antibodies to the virus—within 6 weeks to 12 months after possible exposure to the virus. By getting tested early, a health care provider can give advice to an infected person about when to start treatment to help the immune system combat HIV and help prevent the emergence of certain opportunistic infections (see section on treatment). Early testing also alerts an infected person to avoid high-risk behaviors that could spread the virus to others.

Most health care providers can do HIV testing and will usually offer counseling at the same time. Of course, testing can be done anonymously at many sites if a person is concerned about confidentiality.

Health care providers diagnose HIV infection by using two different types of antibody tests: ELISA (enzyme-linked immunosorbent assay) and Western blot. If a person is highly likely to be infected with

HIV but has tested negative for both tests, a health care provider may request additional tests. A person also may be told to repeat antibody testing at a later date, when antibodies to HIV are more likely to have developed.

Babies born to mothers infected with HIV may or may not be infected with the virus, but all carry their mothers' antibodies to HIV for several months. If these babies lack symptoms, health care providers cannot make a definitive diagnosis of HIV infection using standard antibody tests. Instead, they are using new technologies to detect HIV and more accurately determine HIV infection in infants between ages 3 months and 15 months. Researchers are evaluating a number of blood tests to determine which ones are best for diagnosing HIV infection in babies younger than three months.

Treatment

When AIDS first surfaced in the United States, there were no drugs to combat the underlying immune deficiency and few treatments existed for the opportunistic diseases that resulted. Researchers, however, have developed drugs to fight both HIV infection and its associated infections and cancers.

HIV Infection

The Food and Drug Administration (FDA) has approved a number of drugs for treating HIV infection. The first group of drugs, called reverse transcriptase (RT) inhibitors, interrupts an early stage of the virus making copies of itself. Nucleoside/nucleotide RT inhibitors are faulty DNA building blocks. When these faulty pieces are incorporated into the HIV DNA (during the process when the HIV RNA is converted to HIV DNA), the DNA chain cannot be completed, thereby blocking HIV from replicating in a cell. Non-nucleoside RT inhibitors bind to reverse transcriptase, interfering with its ability to convert the HIV RNA into HIV DNA. This class of drugs may slow the spread of HIV in the body and delay the start of opportunistic infections.

FDA has approved a second class of drugs for treating HIV infection. These drugs, called protease inhibitors, interrupt the virus from making copies of itself at a later step in its life cycle.

FDA also has introduced a third new class of drugs, known as fusion inhibitors, to treat HIV infection. Fuzeon (enfuvirtide or T-20), the first approved fusion inhibitor, works by interfering with the ability of HIV-1 to enter into cells by blocking the merging of the virus with the cell membranes. This inhibition blocks HIV's ability to enter and infect the human immune cells. Fuzeon is designed for use in combination with other anti-HIV treatments. It reduces the level of HIV infection in the blood and may be effective against HIV that has become resistant to current antiviral treatment schedules.

Because HIV can become resistant to any of these drugs, health care providers must use a combination treatment to effectively suppress the virus. When multiple drugs (three or more) are used in combination, it is referred to as highly active antiretroviral therapy, or HAART, and can be used by people who are newly infected with HIV as well as people with AIDS. Recently, FDA approved the first one-a-day three drug–combination pill called Atripla.

Researchers have credited HAART as being a major factor in significantly reducing the number of deaths from AIDS in this country. While HAART is not a cure for AIDS, it has greatly improved the health of many people with AIDS and it reduces the amount of virus circulating in the blood to nearly undetectable levels. Researchers, however, have shown that HIV remains present in hiding places, such as the lymph nodes, brain, testes, and retina of the eye, even in people who have been treated.

Side Effects

Despite the beneficial effects of HAART, there are side effects associated with the use of antiviral drugs that can be severe. Some of the nucleoside RT inhibitors may cause a decrease of red or white blood cells, especially when taken in the later stages of the disease. Some may also cause inflammation of the pancreas and painful nerve damage. There have been reports of complications and other severe reactions, including death, to some of the antiretroviral nucleoside analogs when used alone or in combination. Therefore, health experts recommend that anyone on antiretroviral therapy be routinely seen and followed by their health care provider.

The most common side effects associated with protease inhibitors include nausea, diarrhea, and other gastrointestinal symptoms. In addition, protease inhibitors can interact with other drugs resulting in serious side effects. Fuzeon may also cause severe allergic reactions such as pneumonia, trouble breathing, chills and fever, skin rash, blood in urine, vomiting, and low blood pressure. Local skin reactions are also possible since it is given as an injection underneath the skin. People taking HIV drugs should contact their health care providers immediately if they have any of these symptoms.

Opportunistic Infections

A number of available drugs help treat opportunistic infections. These drugs include the following:

- Foscarnet and ganciclovir to treat CMV (cytomegalovirus) eye infections
- Fluconazole to treat yeast and other fungal infections
- TMP/SMX (trimethoprim/sulfamethoxazole) or pentamidine to treat PCP (Pneumocystis carinii pneumonia)

Cancers

Health care providers use radiation, chemotherapy, or injections of alpha interferon-a genetically engineered protein that occurs naturally in the human body to treat Kaposi's sarcoma or other cancers associated with HIV infection.

Prevention

Because there is no vaccine for HIV, the only way people can prevent infection with the virus is to avoid behaviors putting them at risk of infection, such as sharing needles and having unprotected sex.

Many people infected with HIV have no symptoms. Therefore, there is no way of knowing with certainty whether a sexual partner is infected unless he or she has repeatedly tested negative for the virus and has not engaged in any risky behavior. Abstaining from having sex or use male latex condoms or female polyurethane condoms may offer partial protection during oral, anal, or vaginal sex. Only water-based lubricants should be used with male latex condoms.

Although some laboratory evidence shows that spermicides can kill HIV, researchers have not found that these products can prevent a person from getting HIV.

Recently, NIAID supported two studies that found adult male medical circumcision reduces a man's risk of acquiring HIV infection by approximately 50%. The studies, conducted in Uganda and Kenya, pertain only to heterosexual transmission. As with most prevention strategies, adult male medical circumcision is not completely effective at preventing HIV transmission. Circumcision will be most effective when it is part of a more complete prevention strategy including the ABCs (Abstinence, Be Faithful, Use Condoms) of HIV prevention.

Research

NIAID-supported investigators are conducting an abundance of research on all areas of HIV infection, including developing and testing preventive HIV vaccines, prevention strategies, and new treatments for HIV infection and AIDS-associated opportunistic infections. Researchers also are investigating exactly how HIV damages the immune system. This research is identifying new and more effective targets for drugs and vaccines. NIAID-supported investigators also continue to trace how the disease progresses in different people.

Scientists are investigating and testing chemical barriers, such as topical microbicides, that people can use in the vagina or in the rectum during sex to prevent HIV transmission. They also are looking at other ways to prevent transmission, such as controlling STIs, modifying personal behavior, and pre-exposure prophylaxis (PrEP), as well as ways to prevent transmission from mother to child.

Section 24.2

The Link between STDs and HIV Infection

"The Role of STD Detection and Treatment in HIV Prevention—CDC Fact Sheet," Centers for Disease Control and Prevention (www.cdc.gov), April 10, 2008.

Testing and treatment of sexually transmitted diseases (STDs) can be an effective tool in preventing the spread of HIV, the virus that causes AIDS. An understanding of the relationship between STDs and HIV infection can help in the development of effective HIV prevention programs for persons with high-risk sexual behaviors.

What is the link between STDs and HIV infection?

Individuals who are infected with STDs are at least two to five times more likely than uninfected individuals to acquire HIV infection if they are exposed to the virus through sexual contact. In addition, if an HIV-infected individual is also infected with another STD, that person is more likely to transmit HIV through sexual contact than other HIV-infected persons.

There is substantial biological evidence demonstrating that the presence of other STDs increases the likelihood of both transmitting and acquiring HIV.

- **Increased susceptibility:** STDs appear to increase susceptibility to HIV infection by two mechanisms. Genital ulcers (e.g., syphilis, herpes, or chancroid) result in breaks in the genital tract lining or skin. These breaks create a portal of entry for HIV. Additionally, inflammation resulting from genital ulcers or non-ulcerative STDs (e.g., chlamydia, gonorrhea, and trichomoniasis) increase the concentration of cells in genital secretions that can serve as targets for HIV (e.g., CD4+ cells).
- **Increased infectiousness:** STDs also appear to increase the risk of an HIV-infected person transmitting the virus to his or her sex partners. Studies have shown that HIV-infected individuals who are also infected with other STDs are particularly likely to shed HIV in their genital secretions. For example, men who are infected with both gonorrhea and HIV are more than twice as likely to have HIV in their genital secretions than are those who are infected only with HIV. Moreover, the median concentration of HIV in semen is as much as 10 times higher in men who are infected with both gonorrhea and HIV than in men infected only with HIV. The higher the concentration of HIV in semen or genital fluids, the more likely it is that HIV will be transmitted to a sex partner.

How can STD treatment slow the spread of HIV infection?

Evidence from intervention studies indicates that detecting and treating STDs may reduce HIV transmission.

- STD treatment reduces an individual's ability to transmit HIV. Studies have shown that treating STDs in HIV-infected individuals decreases both the amount of HIV in genital secretions and how frequently HIV is found in those secretions.
- Herpes can make people more susceptible to HIV infection, and it can make HIV-infected individuals more infectious. It is critical that all individuals, especially those with herpes, know whether

they are infected with HIV and, if uninfected with HIV, take measures to protect themselves from infection with HIV.

- Among individuals with both herpes and HIV, trials are underway studying if treatment of the genital herpes helps prevent HIV transmission to partners.

What are the implications for HIV prevention?

Strong STD prevention, testing, and treatment can play a vital role in comprehensive programs to prevent sexual transmission of HIV. Furthermore, STD trends can offer important insights into where the HIV epidemic may grow, making STD surveillance data helpful in forecasting where HIV rates are likely to increase. Better linkages are needed between HIV and STD prevention efforts nationwide in order to control both epidemics.

In the context of persistently high prevalence of STDs in many parts of the United States and with emerging evidence that the U.S. HIV epidemic increasingly is affecting populations with the highest rates of curable STDs, the CDC/HRSA Advisory Committee on HIV/AIDS and STD Prevention (CHAC) recommended the following:

- Early detection and treatment of curable STDs should become a major, explicit component of comprehensive HIV prevention programs at national, state, and local levels.
- In areas where STDs that facilitate HIV transmission are prevalent, screening and treatment programs should be expanded.
- HIV testing should always be recommended for individuals who are diagnosed with or suspected to have an STD.
- HIV and STD prevention programs in the United States, together with private and public sector partners, should take joint responsibility for implementing these strategies.

CHAC also notes that early detection and treatment of STDs should be only one component of a comprehensive HIV prevention program, which also must include a range of social, behavioral, and biomedical interventions.

Section 24.3

Understanding Your HIV Diagnosis

Finding out that you have HIV can be scary and overwhelming. If you feel overwhelmed, try to remember that you can get help and that these feelings will get better with time.

There are some things that you should know about HIV that may ease some of the stress or confusion you are feeling.

Remember:

- You are not alone. Many people are living with HIV, even if you don't know that they are.
- HIV does not equal death: Having HIV does not mean that you are going to die of it.
- A diagnosis of HIV does not automatically mean that you have AIDS.
- Don't freeze: Learning how to live with HIV and getting in touch with a health care team that knows how to manage HIV will help you to feel better and get on with your life.
- Testing positive for HIV is a serious matter. This section will take you through the steps you need to take to protect your health.

Understand Your Diagnosis

When your doctor tells you that you are HIV positive, it means that you have been infected with the virus. The HIV test does not tell you if you have AIDS or how long you have been infected or how sick you might be.

Soon after your diagnosis, your doctor will run other tests to determine your overall health condition, and the condition of your immune system. For descriptions of these tests, see Section 24.2, "Medical Tests If You Have HIV."

Learn about HIV and AIDS

The more you know about HIV and how to treat it, the less confused and anxious you will be about your diagnosis. The more you learn, the better you will be at making decisions about your health.

There are many ways to learn about HIV and AIDS:

1. Start with the Basics section at HIV InSite (http://hivinsite.ucsf.edu/insite?page=basics-00-00) and read through all the sections.
2. Check out government or nonprofit educational organizations that deal with HIV and AIDS issues.
3. Use your local library: The most current information will be in the library's collection of newspapers and magazines (books about HIV and AIDS may be out of date by the time they are published).
4. Talk with others who have been diagnosed with HIV and AIDS. Ask your doctors if they know of any support groups. Or you can go online, where you can find message boards and chat rooms. Always discuss what you learn from these sources with your doctor. The information may not be accurate; and even if it is, it may not be right for your particular situation.

Find Support

Finding support means finding people who are willing to help you through the emotional and physical issues you are going to face. If you let the right people in your life know that you are HIV positive, they can:

- offer you support and understanding;
- provide you with assistance, such as running errands and helping with child care, doctor visits, and work;
- learn from you how HIV is spread and work with you to prevent the virus from spreading.

Telling Others

Deciding to tell others that you are HIV positive is an important personal choice. It can make a big difference in how you cope with the disease. It can also affect your relationships with people.

If you decide to share information about your diagnosis, it is best to tell people you trust or people who are directly affected. These include:

- family members;
- people you spend a lot of time with, such as good friends;
- all your health care providers, such as doctors, nurses, and dentists.

You don't have to tell everyone about your HIV status right away. You might want to talk with a counselor or social worker first.

Join a Support Group

Joining a group of people who are facing the same challenges you are facing can have important benefits. These include feeling better about yourself, finding a new life focus, making new friendships, improving your mood, and better understanding your needs and those of your family. People in support groups often help each other deal with common experiences associated with being HIV positive.

Support groups are especially helpful if you live alone or don't have family and friends nearby.

There are different types of support groups, from hotlines to face-to-face encounter groups. Here are descriptions of some of the most popular types, and suggestions about how to find them.

Hotlines

Find a hotline in your area by talking to a social worker or other health care professional. Or look in the telephone book, in the yellow pages under "Social Service Organizations." Ask the hotline to "match" you with another person with a history like yours. He or she can give you practical advice and emotional support over the telephone.

Professional Help

Ask your doctor for referrals to mental health professionals, such as psychologists, nurse therapists, clinical social workers, or psychiatrists. You also will likely have a social worker who is part of the HIV clinic where you will receive care. You can also get help for drug abuse.

Self-Help Organizations

Self-help groups enable people to share experiences and pool their knowledge to help each other and themselves. They are run by members, not by professionals (though professionals are involved). Because members face similar challenges, they feel an instant sense of community. These groups are volunteer, nonprofit organizations, with no fees (though sometimes there are small dues).

Work with Your Doctor

HIV is the virus that causes AIDS. If left untreated, it can lead to illness and death. This is why it is so important to get medical care if you find out you have HIV. Do not be afraid to seek a doctor with experience in treating HIV-infected patients—he or she can help you to stay well.

Treatments for HIV are not perfect, but can be very effective for many people. A doctor or other health care provider can explain the best options for you.

If you work with your health care provider in planning your care, you can deal with the disease in a way that is best for you.

Before Appointments

Start with a list or notebook. Prepare for your appointment with your doctor by writing down:

1. any questions that you have (print out questions to ask your doctor and take it to your appointment);
2. any symptoms or problems you want to tell the doctor about (include symptoms such as poor sleep, trouble concentrating, feeling tired);
3. a list of the medications that you are taking (include herbs and vitamins);
4. upcoming tests or new information you've heard about;
5. changes in your living situation, such as a job change.

That way you won't forget anything during the appointment.

You may want to ask a friend or family member to come with you and take notes. It can be difficult for you to take notes and pay attention to what your doctor is saying at the same time.

During Appointments

Go over your lab work, and keep track of your results. If your doctor wants you to have some medical tests, make sure you understand what the test is for and what your doctor will do with the results. If you don't understand what your doctor is saying, ask the doctor to explain it in everyday terms.

If you feel your doctor has forgotten something during the appointment, it is better to ask about it than to leave wondering whether something was supposed to happen that didn't. It's your right to ask questions of your doctor. You also have a legal right to see your medical records. After all, it's your body.

Be honest. Your doctor isn't there to judge you, but to make decisions based on your particular circumstances. Tell your doctor about your sexual or drug use history. These behaviors can put you at risk of getting other sexually transmitted diseases as well as hepatitis. If your body is fighting off these other diseases, it will not be able to fight off HIV as effectively. You may get sicker, faster.

Monitor Your Health

Once you have been diagnosed with HIV, you need to pay closer attention to your health than you did before.

You can keep track of your immune system in two ways. First, have regular lab tests done. Lab tests often can show signs of illness before you have any noticeable symptoms.

Second, listen to what your body is telling you, and be on the alert for signs that something isn't right. Note any change in your health—good or bad. And don't be afraid to call a doctor.

Have Regular Lab Tests

Your doctor will use laboratory tests to check your health. Some of these tests will be done soon after you learn you are HIV positive.

The lab tests look at several things:

- How well your immune system is functioning
- How rapidly HIV is progressing
- Certain basic body functions (tests look at your kidneys, liver, cholesterol, and blood cells)
- Whether you have other diseases that are associated with HIV

For your first few doctor visits, be prepared to have a lot of blood drawn. Don't worry. You are not going to have so much blood drawn at every appointment.

For information on specific tests, see Section 24.2, "Medical Tests If You Have HIV."

Be Aware of Possible Complications

Certain changes can happen to HIV-positive people who are living longer and taking HIV medicines. Some people have experienced visible changes in body shape and appearance. Sometimes these changes can raise the risk of heart disease and diabetes.

Also, by weakening your immune system, HIV can leave you vulnerable to certain cancers and infections. These infections are called "opportunistic" because they take the opportunity to attack you when your immune system is weak.

Know When to Call a Doctor

You don't need to panic every time you have a headache or get a runny nose. But if a symptom is concerning you or is not going away, it is always best to have a doctor check it out even if it doesn't feel like a big deal. The earlier you see a doctor when you have unusual symptoms, the better off you are likely to be.

The following symptoms may or may not be serious, but don't wait until your next appointment before calling a doctor if you are experiencing them.

Breathing Problems

- Persistent cough
- Wheezing or noisy breathing
- Sharp pain when breathing
- Difficulty catching your breath

Skin Problems

- Appearance of brownish, purple or pink blotches on the skin
- Onset of rash—especially important if you are taking medication

Eye or Vision Problems

- Blurring, wavy lines, sudden blind spots
- Eye pain
- Sensitivity to light

Aches and Pains

- Numbness, tingling, or pain in hands and feet
- Headache, especially when accompanied by a fever
- Stiffness in neck
- Severe or persistent cough
- Persistent cramps
- Pain in lower abdomen, often during sex (women in particular)

Other Symptoms

- Mental changes—confusion, disorientation, loss of memory or balance
- Appearance of swollen lymph nodes, especially when larger on one side of the body
- Diarrhea—when severe, accompanied by fever, or lasting more than three days
- Weight loss
- High or persistent fever
- Fatigue
- Frequent urination

Protect Others

Once you have HIV, you can give the virus to others by having unprotected sex or by sharing needles (or, if you have a child, by breastfeeding). This is true even if you are feeling perfectly fine. Using condoms and clean needles can prevent infecting other people. It can also protect you from getting other sexually transmitted diseases.

Sometimes it can be difficult to explain that you have HIV to people you have had sex with or shared needles with in the past. However, it is important that they know so that they can decide whether to get tested. If you need help telling people that you may have exposed them to HIV, most city or county health departments will tell them for you, without using your name. Ask your doctor about this service.

Before telling your partner that you have HIV, take some time alone to think about how you want to bring up the subject.

- Decide when and where would be the best time and place to have a conversation. Choose a time when you expect that you will both be comfortable, rested, and as relaxed as possible.

- Think about how your partner may react to stressful situations. If there is a history of violence in your relationship, consider your safety first and plan the situation with a case manager or counselor.

Know When to Consider Treatment

Whether or not to start treatment for HIV is a decision that each person must make with his or her doctor. While anti-HIV drugs (also known as antiretrovirals) can be lifesavers, there are good reasons to delay taking them right away.

In general, you and your doctor will need to consider:

- how well you feel;
- how healthy your immune system is;
- whether or not you have AIDS;
- whether you can stick to a treatment plan.

Move Forward with Your Life

Life does not end with a diagnosis of HIV. In fact, with proper treatment, people with HIV can live fairly healthy lives. Taking care of your overall health can help you deal with HIV:

- Get regular medical and dental checkups.
- Eat a healthy diet.
- Exercise regularly.
- Avoid smoking and recreational drug use.
- Go easy on alcohol.
- Practice safer sex (it can protect others from getting HIV, and can protect you from other sexually transmitted diseases).

Section 24.4

HIV Treatment

"Treatment of HIV Infection," National Institute for Allergy and Infectious Diseases (www3.niaid.nih.gov), November 2007.

In the early 1980s when the HIV/AIDS epidemic began, people with AIDS were not likely to live longer than a few years. With the development of safe and effective drugs, however, people infected with HIV now have longer and healthier lives.

The discovery and development of new therapeutic strategies against HIV is a high priority for the National Institute of Allergy and Infectious Diseases (NIAID). Research supported by NIAID has already greatly advanced our understanding of HIV and how it causes disease. This knowledge provides the foundation for NIAID's HIV/AIDS research effort and continues to support studies designed to further extend and improve the quality of life of those infected with HIV.

Drugs for HIV/AIDS

Currently, there are 30 antiretroviral drugs approved by the Food and Drug Administration to treat people infected with HIV. These drugs fall into four major classes.

1. Reverse transcriptase (RT) inhibitors interfere with the critical step during the HIV life cycle known as reverse transcription. During this step, RT, an HIV enzyme, converts HIV RNA to HIV DNA. There are two main types of RT inhibitors.
    - Nucleoside/nucleotide RT inhibitors are faulty DNA building blocks. When these faulty pieces are incorporated into the HIV DNA (during the process when the HIV RNA is converted to HIV DNA), the DNA chain cannot be completed, thereby blocking HIV from replicating in a cell.

- Non-nucleoside RT inhibitors bind to RT, interfering with its ability to convert the HIV RNA into HIV DNA.

2. Protease inhibitors interfere with the protease enzyme that HIV uses to produce infectious viral particles.
3. Entry and fusion inhibitors interfere with the virus' ability to fuse with the cellular membrane, thereby blocking entry into the host cell.
4. Integrase inhibitors block integrase, the enzyme HIV uses to integrate genetic material of the virus into its target host cell.
5. Multidrug combination products combine drugs from more than one class into a single product.

Currently available drugs do not cure HIV infection or AIDS. They can suppress the virus, even to undetectable levels, but they cannot eliminate HIV from the body. Hence, people with HIV need to continuously take antiretroviral drugs.

Highly Active Antiretroviral Therapy (HAART) Counters Drug Resistance

As HIV reproduces itself, variants of the virus emerge, including some that are resistant to antiretroviral drugs. Therefore, doctors recommend that people infected with HIV take a combination of antiretroviral drugs known as highly active antiretroviral therapy, or HAART. This strategy, which typically combines drugs from at least two different classes of antiretroviral drugs, has been shown to effectively suppress the virus when used properly. Developed by NIAID-supported researchers, HAART has revolutionized how people infected with HIV are treated. HAART works by suppressing the virus and decreasing the rate of opportunistic infections.

HIV Transmission and Antiretroviral Drugs

Although the use of HAART has greatly reduced the number of deaths due to HIV/AIDS, and possibly the transmission of HIV/AIDS as well, this powerful combination of drugs cannot suppress the virus completely. Therefore, people infected with HIV who take antiretroviral drugs can still transmit HIV to others through unprotected sex and needle-sharing.

Antiretroviral Drug Effects on Opportunistic Infections and AIDS-Associated Co-Infections

People infected with HIV have impaired immune systems that can leave them susceptible to opportunistic infections (OIs) and AIDS-associated co-infections, caused by a wide range of microorganisms such as protozoa, viruses, fungi, and bacteria. One example of an associated co-infection is hepatitis C virus infection, which can lead to liver cancer.

Potent HIV therapies such as HAART, however, have produced dramatic responses in patients. These therapies often allow the immune system to recover, sustain, and protect the body from other infections. Hence, antiretroviral drugs provide a way for the immune system to remain effective, thereby improving the quality and length of life for people with HIV.

Side Effects of Antiretroviral Drugs

People taking antiretroviral drugs may have low adherence to complicated drug regimens. Current recommended regimens involve taking several antiretroviral drugs each day from at least two different classes, some of which may cause unpleasant side effects such as nausea and vomiting. In addition, antiretroviral drugs may cause more serious medical problems, including metabolic changes such as abnormal fat distribution, abnormal lipid and glucose metabolism, and bone loss. Therefore, NIAID is investigating simpler, less toxic, and more effective drug regimens.

Development of New Safe and Effective Antiretroviral Drugs

NIAID supports the development and testing of new therapeutic agents, classes, and combinations of antiretroviral drugs that can continuously suppress the virus with few side effects. Through human clinical trials, NIAID-supported studies provide accurate and extensive information about the safety and efficacy of drug candidates and combinations, and identify potential uncommon but important toxicities of newly approved agents. Studies are also under way to assess rare toxicities of older approved agents, especially as a result of long-term use.

Through the Multicenter AIDS Cohort Study and Women's Interagency HIV Study, NIAID supports long-term studies of HIV disease and its treatment in both men and women. Since their inception, these cohort studies have enrolled and collected data from more than 10,000 people. In addition, NIAID supports treatment studies conducted through three HIV/AIDS clinical trials networks: the AIDS Clinical Trials Group, the International Maternal Pediatric Adolescent AIDS Clinical Trials Group, and the International Network for Strategic Initiatives in Global HIV Trials. For more information about HIV/AIDS drugs and treatment trials, please visit the AIDSinfo website at www.aidsinfo.nih.gov.

NIAID Research on the Complications of Antiretroviral Drugs

NIAID supports studies aimed at understanding the side effects of antiretroviral drugs as well as strategies to reduce exposure to potentially toxic drug regimens, such as the following:

- Structured treatment interruption (STI) protocols
- Use of immune-based therapies with HAART
- Studies to compare different drug dosing schedules or combinations
- Studies to compare early versus delayed treatment

NIAID also supports projects evaluating regimens containing agents associated with toxicities. For example, NIAID-funded researchers are conducting studies to evaluate treatments for several drug-associated metabolic complications, including fat redistribution, lipid and glucose abnormalities, and bone loss. In addition, researchers are studying the long-term metabolic effects of various antiretroviral regimens in pregnant women and their infants and in HIV-infected children and adolescents.

Down the Road: New Drugs in the Pipeline

The Pharmaceutical Research and Manufacturers Association of America maintains a database of new drugs in development to treat HIV infection. They include new protease inhibitors and more potent, less toxic RT inhibitors, as well as other drugs that interfere with entirely different steps in the virus' lifecycle. These new categories of drugs include the following types:

- Entry inhibitors that interfere with HIV's ability to enter cells

- Integrase inhibitors that interfere with HIV's ability to insert its genes into a cell's normal DNA
- Assembly and budding inhibitors that interfere with the final stage of the HIV life cycle, when new virus particles are released into the bloodstream
- Cellular metabolism modulators that interfere with the cellular processes needed for HIV replication
- Gene therapy that uses modified genes inserted directly into cells to suppress HIV replication (These cells are designed to produce T cells that are genetically resistant to HIV infection.)

In addition, scientists are exploring whether immune modulators help boost the immune response to the virus and may make existing anti-HIV drugs more effective. Therapeutic vaccines also are being evaluated for this purpose and could help reduce the number of anti-HIV drugs needed or the duration of treatment.

Section 24.5

Medical Tests If You Have HIV

Laboratory tests can help keep tabs on your health. Some of these tests will be done soon after you learn you are HIV positive. Then depending on your immune status, whether you are on medication or not, and a variety of other factors, your provider will set up a schedule for you.

The lab tests look at:

- how well your immune system is functioning;
- how rapidly HIV is progressing;

- how well your body is functioning (tests look at your kidneys, liver, cholesterol, and blood cells); and
- whether you have other diseases that are associated with HIV.

When done shortly after you find out you have HIV, these tests establish a starting point or "baseline." Future tests will let you know how far from this baseline you have moved. This can help you tell how fast or slow the disease is moving and indicate whether treatments are working.

Most labs include a "normal" range (high and low values) when they report test results. The most important results are the ones that fall outside these normal ranges. Test results often go up and down over time so don't worry about small changes. Instead look for overall trends.

What follows are descriptions of the most common tests.

CD4 count (or T-cell test)

The CD4 count is like a snapshot of how well your immune system is functioning. CD4 cells (also known as CD4+ T cells) are white blood cells that fight infection. The more you have, the better. These are the cells that HIV kills. As HIV infection progresses, the number of these cells declines. When the CD4 count drops below 200 due to advanced HIV disease, a person is diagnosed with AIDS. A normal range for CD4 cells is between 600 and 1,500. The *higher* your CD4 count, the better.

The same test that measures your CD4 count usually includes a CD8 cell count, too. CD8 cells (also known as CD8+ T cells) are another type of white blood cell that seek out and destroy cells infected with viruses, including HIV-infected cells.

Viral Load (or "HIV RNA")

Viral load tests measure the amount of HIV in the blood. Lower levels are better than higher levels. The main goal of HIV drugs is to reduce viral load as much as possible for as long as possible. Some viral load tests measure down to 400 or 500 copies of HIV per unit of blood; others go as low as 200 or even 50 copies. High levels—from 30,000 (in women) to 60,000 (in men) and above—are linked to faster disease progression. Levels below 50 offer the best outcome for your health. The *lower* your viral load, the better.

CD4 counts and viral load tests are usually done every three months. Results can help you and your doctor decide when it's time to start taking anti-HIV drugs.

Resistance Test

This test determines whether the particular virus in your body is resistant to anti-HIV medications. This test used to be done later in the course of HIV disease, but now doctors are doing the test when HIV treatment is started.

HIV reproduces rapidly and, as the virus makes copies of itself, little changes (or mutations) sometimes result. These changes can lead to different HIV strains. A person can have many strains in his or her body.

If a strain that is resistant to your HIV drugs develops, the virus will be able to grow even though you are on medication. Your viral load will start to rise. The resistant virus soon will become the most common strain in your body.

Complete Blood Count (CBC)

This test looks at the different cells in your blood, including red blood cells, platelets, and white blood cells.

- Red blood cells carry oxygen to other cells in your body. If the level of your red blood cells is too low, you have anemia. Anemia can lead to fatigue. Tests looking at your red blood cells include red blood cell count, hemoglobin, and hematocrit.
- Platelets help with clotting, so if your platelets fall too low, your blood may not clot well. You may bleed more than usual, for example, when you brush your teeth or shave your skin. As the platelet count falls, the chance of internal bleeding rises.
- White blood cells come in many types, and all are involved in your immune system's effort to keep you healthy. High white blood cell counts may indicate that you are fighting an infection. Low counts may put you at risk of getting an infection.

These tests are usually done every 6 to 12 months, unless your lab values are fluctuating a lot, or you have symptoms of infections associated with HIV disease. Then the tests are done more often, every three to six months.

Blood Chemistry Tests

Chemistry tests examine the levels of different elements and waste products in the blood and help determine how well different organs are functioning. Usually, the tests are divided into two panels:

- Electrolyte tests (sometimes called "lytes"): These tests help measure how well your kidneys are working, and measure the balance of fluids, acids, and sugar in your body. They include tests for sodium, potassium, chloride, magnesium, blood urea nitrogen (BUN), creatinine, and glucose.
- Liver function tests (LFTs): These tests measure whether your liver is being damaged. (Things that can damage the liver are viral hepatitis, alcohol, medications, and street drugs.) These tests measure alkaline phosphatase, ALT, AST, albumin, and bilirubin. It is important to have a baseline measure of your liver health, because you may need to take HIV medications in the future, and some of these medications can cause liver damage.

Blood chemistry tests are usually done a couple of times a year.

Fasting Lipid Profile

The level of certain fatty substances in the blood can give clues to your risk of heart disease. Triglycerides and cholesterol are important for health, but too much of them in the blood can cause fatty deposits to form in the arteries. This increases the chances of a heart attack. Too much triglyceride can also lead to pancreatitis, a serious inflammation of the pancreas. High cholesterol and high triglycerides can occur in people living with HIV for many years. They can also be a side effect of HIV medications.

Cholesterol is measured by three different tests:

- Total cholesterol
- HDL (high-density lipoprotein), often referred to as "good" cholesterol because high levels lower your risk of heart disease
- LDL (low-density lipoprotein), often referred to as "bad" cholesterol because high levels raise your risk of heart disease

These tests are usually done at least once a year, and more often if you require medication to control triglyceride and cholesterol levels.

TB Test (or "PPD")

TB is short for tuberculosis, a lung disease that people with HIV are at high risk for getting. A PPD test is a special skin test to see if you have been exposed to TB. In some people with HIV, the PPD test is not reliable and a chest X-ray or sputum culture is done instead.

STD Screening

If you got infected with HIV from unprotected sex, there is a chance you may have become infected with other sexually transmitted diseases, too. These include gonorrhea, syphilis, and chlamydia.

The bacteria that cause these diseases can be found in the throat, penis, vagina, and rectum. The bacteria that cause syphilis are also found in the blood. Having one of these other diseases can make your HIV advance faster. They can also make you two to five times more likely to pass HIV along to your sexual partner. Syphilis, for example, can cause open sores on your genitals, which allows easy passage of HIV from you to your partner.

Hepatitis A, B, and C

Your liver is an organ that processes almost everything you put into your body, including drugs. The three most common types of viral hepatitis (A, B, and C) can damage your liver.

Some of the same behaviors that put people at risk for HIV (unprotected sex, injection drug use) can put them at risk for hepatitis.

If you have both HIV and hepatitis B or C, your treatments for either disease can be affected. If you have HIV, your hepatitis may progress faster. If your liver is damaged from hepatitis, it may be harder for your body to process your HIV medications.

What's more, some HIV treatments can damage your liver, so if you have hepatitis, your doctor may want you to try other treatments.

Chapter 25

Human Papilloma Virus (HPV) and Genital Warts

Chapter Contents

Section 25.1

HPV Overview

"Genital HPV Infection—CDC Fact Sheet," Centers for Disease Control and Prevention (www.cdc.gov), April 10, 2008.

What is genital HPV infection?

Genital human papillomavirus (HPV) is the most common sexually transmitted infection (STI). The virus infects the skin and mucous membranes. There are more than 40 HPV types that can infect the genital areas of men and women, including the skin of the penis, vulva (area outside the vagina), and anus, and the linings of the vagina, cervix, and rectum. You cannot see HPV. Most people who become infected with HPV do not even know they have it.

What are the symptoms and potential health consequences of HPV?

Most people with HPV do not develop symptoms or health problems. But sometimes, certain types of HPV can cause genital warts in men and women. Other HPV types can cause cervical cancer and other less common cancers, such as cancers of the vulva, vagina, anus, and penis. The types of HPV that can cause genital warts are not the same as the types that can cause cancer.

HPV types are often referred to as "low-risk" (wart-causing) or "high-risk" (cancer-causing), based on whether they put a person at risk for cancer. In 90% of cases, the body's immune system clears the HPV infection naturally within two years. This is true of both high-risk and low-risk types.

Genital warts usually appear as small bumps or groups of bumps, usually in the genital area. They can be raised or flat, single or multiple, small or large, and sometimes cauliflower shaped. They can appear on the vulva, in or around the vagina or anus, on the cervix, and on the penis, scrotum, groin, or thigh. Warts may appear within weeks or months after sexual contact with an infected person. Or, they may not appear at all. If left untreated, genital warts may go away, remain unchanged, or increase in size or number. They will not turn into cancer.

Cervical cancer does not have symptoms until it is quite advanced. For this reason, it is important for women to get screened regularly for cervical cancer.

Other less common HPV-related cancers, such as cancers of the vulva, vagina, anus, and penis, also may not have signs or symptoms until they are advanced.

How do people get genital HPV infections?

Genital HPV is passed on through genital contact, most often during vaginal and anal sex. A person can have HPV even if years have passed since he or she had sex. Most infected persons do not realize they are infected or that they are passing the virus to a sex partner.

Very rarely, a pregnant woman with genital HPV can pass HPV to her baby during vaginal delivery. In these cases, the child may develop warts in the throat or voice box—a condition called recurrent respiratory papillomatosis (RRP).

How does HPV cause genital warts and cancer?

HPV can cause normal cells on infected skin or mucous membranes to turn abnormal. Most of the time, you cannot see or feel these cell changes. In most cases, the body fights off HPV naturally and the infected cells then go back to normal.

- Sometimes, low-risk types of HPV can cause visible changes that take the form of genital warts.
- If a high-risk HPV infection is not cleared by the immune system, it can linger for many years and turn abnormal cells into cancer over time. About 10% of women with high-risk HPV on their cervix will develop long-lasting HPV infections that put them at risk for cervical cancer. Similarly, when high-risk HPV lingers and infects the cells of the penis, anus, vulva, or vagina, it can cause cancer in those areas. But these cancers are much less common than cervical cancer.

How common are HPV and related diseases?

HPV infection: Approximately 20 million Americans are currently infected with HPV, and another 6.2 million people become newly infected each year. At least 50% of sexually active men and women acquire genital HPV infection at some point in their lives.

Genital warts: About 1% of sexually active adults in the U.S. have genital warts at any one time.

Cervical cancer: The American Cancer Society estimates that in 2008, 11,070 women will be diagnosed with cervical cancer in the U.S.

Other HPV-related cancers are much less common than cervical cancer. The American Cancer Society estimates that there will be the following number of cases in 2008:

- 3,460 women diagnosed with vulvar cancer
- 2,210 women diagnosed with vaginal and other female genital cancers
- 1,250 men diagnosed with penile and other male genital cancers
- 3,050 women and 2,020 men diagnosed with anal cancer

Certain populations may be at higher risk for HPV-related cancers, such as gay and bisexual men, and individuals with weak immune systems (including those who have HIV/AIDS).

RRP is very rare. It is estimated that less than 2,000 children get RRP every year.

How can people prevent HPV?

A vaccine can now protect females from the four types of HPV that cause most cervical cancers and genital warts. The vaccine is recommended for 11- and 12-year-old girls. It is also recommended for girls and women age 13 through 26 who have not yet been vaccinated or completed the vaccine series.

For those who choose to be sexually active, condoms may lower the risk of HPV, if used all the time and the right way. Condoms may also lower the risk of developing HPV-related diseases, such as genital warts and cervical cancer. But HPV can infect areas that are not covered by a condom—so condoms may not fully protect against HPV. So the only sure way to prevent HPV is to avoid all sexual activity.

Individuals can also lower their chances of getting HPV by being in a mutually faithful relationship with someone who has had no or few sex partners. However, even people with only one lifetime sex partner can get HPV, if their partner was infected with HPV. For those who are not in long-term mutually monogamous relationships, limiting the number of sex partners and choosing a partner less likely to be infected may lower the risk of HPV. Partners less likely to be infected include those who have had no or few prior sex partners. But it may not be possible to determine if a partner who has been sexually active in the past is currently infected.

How can people prevent HPV-related diseases?

There are important steps girls and women can take to prevent cervical cancer. The HPV vaccine can protect against most cervical cancers (see above). Cervical cancer can also be prevented with routine cervical cancer screening and follow-up of abnormal results. The Pap test can identify abnormal or pre-cancerous changes in the cervix so that they can be removed before cancer develops. An HPV DNA test, which can find high-risk HPV on a woman's cervix, may also be used with a Pap test in certain cases. The HPV test can help health care professionals decide if more tests or treatment are needed. Even women who got the vaccine when they were younger need regular cervical cancer screening because the vaccine does not protect against all cervical cancers.

There is currently no vaccine licensed to prevent HPV-related diseases in men. Studies are now being done to find out if the vaccine is also safe in men, and if it can protect them against HPV and related conditions. The FDA will consider licensing the vaccine for boys and men if there is proof that it is safe and effective for them. There is also no approved screening test to find early signs of penile or anal cancer. Some experts recommend yearly anal Pap tests for gay and bisexual men and for HIV-positive persons because anal cancer is more common in these populations. Scientists are still studying how best to screen for penile and anal cancers in those who may be at highest risk for those diseases.

Generally, cesarean delivery is not recommended for women with genital warts to prevent RRP in their babies. This is because it is unclear whether cesarean delivery actually prevents RRP in infants and children.

Is there a test for HPV?

The HPV test on the market is only used as part of cervical cancer screening. There is no general test for men or women to check one's overall "HPV status." HPV usually goes away on its own, without causing health problems. So an HPV infection that is found today will most likely not be there a year or two from now. For this reason, there is no need to be tested just to find out if you have HPV now. However, you should get tested for signs of disease that HPV can cause, such as cervical cancer.

- Genital warts are diagnosed by visual inspection. Some health care providers may use acetic acid, a vinegar solution, to help identify flat warts. But this is not a sensitive test so it may wrongly identify normal skin as a wart.
- Cervical cell changes (early signs of cervical cancer) can be identified by routine Pap tests. The HPV test can identify high-risk HPV types on a woman's cervix, which can cause cervical cell changes and cancer.
- As noted above, there is currently no approved test to find HPV or related cancers in men. But HPV is very common and HPV-related cancers are very rare in men.

Is there a treatment for HPV?

There is no treatment for the virus itself, but a healthy immune system can usually fight off HPV naturally. The following are treatments for the diseases that HPV can cause:

Visible genital warts can be removed by patient-applied medications, or by treatments performed by a health care provider. Some individuals choose to forego treatment to see if the warts will disappear on their own. No one treatment is better than another.

Cervical cancer is most treatable when it is diagnosed and treated early. There are new forms of surgery, radiation therapy, and chemotherapy available for patients (see http://www.cancer.org). But women who get routine Pap testing and follow-up as needed can identify problems before cancer develops. Prevention is always better than treatment.

Other HPV-related cancers are also more treatable when diagnosed and treated early. There are new forms of surgery, radiation therapy, and chemotherapy available for patients (see http://www.cancer.org).

Sources

American Cancer Society. Cancer Facts & Figures, 2008. Atlanta: American Cancer Society: 2008.

Centers for Disease Control and Prevention. Sexually Transmitted Diseases Treatment Guidelines 2006. *MMWR* 2006; 55 [No. RR-11].

Dunne EF, Unger ER, Sternberg M, McQuillan G, Swan DC, Patel SS, Markowitz LE. Prevalence of HPV infection among females in the United States. *JAMA*. 2007; 297(8):813–9.

FUTURE II Study Group. Prophylactic efficacy of a quadrivalent human papillomavirus (HPV) vaccine in women with virological evidence of HPV infection. *J Infect Dis*. 2007; 196:1438–1446.

FUTURE II Study Group. Quadrivalent vaccine against human papillomavirus to prevent high-grade cervical lesions. *N Engl J Med*. 2007; 356(19):1915–27.

Garland SM, Hernandez-Avila M, Wheeler CM, Perez G, Harper DM, Leodolter S, et al. Females United to Unilaterally Reduce Endo/Ectocervical Disease (FUTURE) I Investigators. Quadrivalent vaccine against human papillomavirus to prevent anogenital diseases. *N Engl J Med*. 2007; 356(19):1928–43.

Koutsky LA, Kiviat NB. Genital human papillomavirus. In: K. Holmes, P. Sparling, P. Mardh et al (eds). *Sexually Transmitted Diseases*, 3rd edition. New York: McGraw-Hill, 1999, p. 347–359.

Kiviat NB, Koutsky LA, Paavonen J. Cervical neoplasia and other STD-related genital tract neoplasias. In: K. Holmes, P. Sparling, P. Mardh et al (eds). *Sexually Transmitted Diseases*, 3rd edition. New York: McGraw-Hill, 1999, p. 811–831.

Markowitz LE, Dunne EF, Saraiya M, Lawson HW, Chesson H, Unger ER. Quadrivalent human papillomavirus vaccine: Recommendations of the Advisory Committee on Immunization Practices (ACIP). *MMWR*. 2007; 56: 1–24.

Myers ER, McCrory DC, Nanda K, Bastian L, Matchar DB. Mathematical model for the natural history of human papillomavirus infection and cervical carcinogenesis. *American Journal of Epidemiology*. 2000; 151(12):1158–1171.

Paavonen J, Jenkins D, Bosch FX, Naud P, Salmeron J, Wheeler CM et al. Efficacy of a prophylactic adjuvanted bivalent L1 virus-like-particle vaccine against infection with human papillomavirus types 16 and 18 in young women: an interim analysis of a phase III double-blind, randomised controlled trial. *Lancet*. 2007; 370(9596):1414.

Weinstock H, Berman S, Cates W. Sexually transmitted disease among American youth: Incidence and prevalence estimates, 2000. *Perspectives on Sexual and Reproductive Health.* 2004;36: 6–10.

Winer R, Hughes JP, Feng Q, et al. Consistent condom use from time of first vaginal intercourse and the risk of genital human papillomavirus infection in young women. *N Engl J Med.* 2006;354:2645–2654.

Section 25.2

Genital Warts

What Causes Genital Warts?

Genital warts, caused by some types of HPV, can appear on the skin anywhere in the genital area as white or flesh-colored, smooth, small bumps, or larger, fleshy, cauliflower-like lumps. There are more than 100 different subtypes of HPV, and around 30 of them specifically affect the genitals. Other HPV subtypes cause warts to grow on different parts of the body, such as the hands.

Not everyone infected with HPV will develop genital warts. Some will be infected with a strain that does not produce warts, or they will remain asymptomatic (i.e., no warts will appear) even though the virus is present in the skin or mucous membranes around the genital area or on the cervix in women.

Those who do go on to develop warts will usually notice them one to three months after initial infection.

What Do Genital Warts Look Like? What Are the Symptoms?

If symptoms do appear then the infected person may notice pinkish/white small lumps or larger cauliflower-shaped lumps on the genital area. Warts can appear on or around the penis, the scrotum, the thighs, or the anus. In women warts can develop around the vulva or inside the vagina and on the cervix. If a woman has warts on her cervix, this may cause slight bleeding or, very rarely, an unusual colored vaginal discharge.

Warts may occur singly or in groups. The warts may itch, but they are usually painless. Sometimes the warts can be difficult to spot. In severe cases, it is possible for warts to spread from the genitals to the area around the anus, even if anal intercourse has not occurred.

Occasionally, people can confuse skin problems caused by other STDs (such as genital herpes, syphilis, or molluscum) with genital warts. Others may become very worried because they mistake perfectly normal and non-infectious lumps and bumps for genital warts. Conditions that may be confused with genital warts include:

- Pearly penile papules—small white or skin-colored bumps that, when numerous, appear in a ring around the edge of the head of the penis. More rarely, similar papules may be found on the vulva.
- Angiokeratomas—bright red or purple spots that look a little like blood blisters.
- Sebaceous glands (also known as "Fordyce spots")—hard white, yellowish, or skin-colored little bumps that may be found all over the skin of the penis and scrotum in men, and the vulva in women. Sebaceous glands produce a substance called sebum, which keeps the skin healthy.
- Pimples or spots—caused by blocked sebaceous glands, pimples and spots can form just as easily around the genital area as they do on the face, and may become sore and inflamed in a similar way.

All of the above are common, non-infectious skin manifestations that are not sexually transmitted.

Any doubt about lumps and bumps on the genitals can usually be resolved by a quick visit to a doctor or sexual health clinic.

How Is HPV Passed On?

Genital HPV is transmitted by genital skin-to-skin contact, or through the transfer of infected genital fluids. This is usually during vaginal or anal sex, but it is also possible to pass it on through non-penetrative sexual activity.

In rare circumstances, a woman can pass HPV on to her baby during vaginal child birth.

How Do You Know If You Have Genital Warts?

A doctor or nurse can usually tell whether you have genital warts just by looking closely at the affected area. If warts are suspected but are not obvious, the doctor may apply a weak vinegar-like solution to the genital area; this turns any warts white and therefore makes them more visible.

To check for hidden warts, the doctor may carry out an internal examination of the vagina, cervix, and/or anus.

If a person suspects they have been exposed to HPV, but does not yet have symptoms, their doctor may be able to take a swab to test for high-risk strains of the virus (this isn't available in all countries). In women, this may be performed alongside a cervical Pap smear test (see below).

Not everyone diagnosed with HPV will develop warts, and patients may be asked to come back for another examination at a later date if nothing is yet visible.

Where to Go for Help

If you have any symptoms or you are worried you may have been infected with an STD, you should discuss your worries with a doctor. They may be able to run tests or offer you treatment themselves, or refer you on to someone who can.

Some countries have specific sexual health clinics that can help you directly. Check our help and advice page or your local telephone directory to see if you have a clinic near you.

Treatment for Genital Warts

There is no treatment that can completely eliminate genital warts once a person has been infected. Often outbreaks of genital warts will become less frequent over time, until the body naturally clears the virus and the warts disappear of their own accord. However, in some people the infection may linger.

A doctor can give patients various treatments to clear genital warts, but they may reappear even after treatment. Genital warts are caused by a virus, not a bacterium, so antibiotics will not get rid of them. Common treatments include:

- Podophyllin resin—a brown liquid which is painted on to the wart(s) by a doctor or nurse and must be washed off four hours later (or sooner, if the area is irritated). Podophyllin resin and podofilox lotion remove genital warts by stopping cell growth and may require several applications to work effectively. Podophyllin has to be applied by a medical professional as it must be applied carefully to avoid damaging the healthy tissue around the wart.
- Podofilox lotion/gel—can be applied to the wart(s) by the patient at home. The usual schedule is twice a day for three days, followed by four days without any lotion. This cycle is repeated for four weeks. It has few side effects and is well-suited for treatment at home.
- Cryocautery (also called cryotherapy)—uses liquid nitrogen to freeze more persistent warts every one to three weeks for a short period. It may cause some discomfort and is not recommended for young children.
- Laser treatments—this approach, which uses an intense beam of light, can be expensive and is usually reserved for very extensive and tough-to-treat warts.
- Electrocautery—an electrical current is used to super-heat a needle which burns the wart cells and cauterizes the blood vessels. A local anesthetic is used to prevent any pain and the procedure is usually carried out at a doctor's surgery. Electrocautery is used only after other treatments have failed.
- Surgical excision—the doctor will perform minor surgery to remove the wart under local anesthetic.

The doctor or nurse should give the patient advice about having sex whilst receiving treatment.

There are some non-prescription treatments available for genital HPV, but it is advisable to always seek medical advice. Never try to treat genital warts by yourself.

It is important that a woman who is pregnant, or trying to become pregnant, informs her doctor. Podophyllin treatment could harm the developing baby and an alternative treatment should be used.

Is There a Vaccine against Genital Warts?

In June 2006 the first vaccine to prevent four major subtypes of cervical genital HPV was licensed for use in the United States of America.

The vaccine is called Gardasil® and it protects women against HPV subtypes 6 and 11, which cause 90% of genital warts, and 16 and 18, which together cause 70% of cervical cancers in American women.

The vaccine is claimed to be between 95–100% effective. It is approved for use in the U.S. for girls and women aged 9–26 years old. The vaccine may be less effective in women who are already sexually active, as they may have already been infected with HPV.

Taking Care of Yourself and Your Partner

If you have genital warts, following these suggestions will make an outbreak easier to deal with, and will help protect your partner.

- Use condoms when having sex. But remember that condoms will only prevent the transmission of genital warts if they cover the affected areas. Talk to your doctor or nurse for more advice on safer sex.
- Make sure that your partner has a check-up too, as they may have warts that they haven't noticed.
- Keep your genitals clean and dry.
- Don't use scented soaps and bath oils or vaginal deodorants, as these may irritate the warts.

Follow-Up

It is important to return regularly for treatment until all of the genital warts have gone so that the doctor or nurse can check progress and make any necessary changes in your treatment. Sometimes treatment can take a long time.

The majority of people whose genital warts initially disappear will get a recurrence.

In the majority of cases, the immune system keeps the virus under control and eventually destroys it a few years after the initial infection.

HPV and the Cervix

Some types of the human papilloma virus (notably types 16 and 18) have been linked to changes in cervical cells that can lead to cancer. This is why it is important that all sexually active women have a regular cervical Pap smear test.

A smear test is performed by opening the vagina using a speculum (a metal instrument that gently stretches the entrance and the walls of the vagina) and taking a small sample of cells from the cervix with a special swab.

The cells will be looked at under a microscope. If any changes to the cells are noted, the woman may be asked to repeat the test or will be referred for treatment that can prevent the cells from developing into cervical cancer.

It is important to note that cell changes (also called cervical dysplasia) do not indicate that a woman already has cancer. They simply suggest that she is more likely to develop cancer in the future if she does not receive treatment.

A woman who has received an abnormal Pap smear result may sometimes be given a colposcopy to look at cells on the cervix. A colposcope is a kind of small microscope with a light which is used to view the cervix. The scope magnifies the cervix so the doctor can see any changes or problems. The doctor may take a small sample of cells (called a biopsy), which will be looked at in a laboratory.

The colposcopy may feel slightly uncomfortable. If the patient has a biopsy taken then they may have a dull ache like a mild period cramp, with slight bleeding.

Treatment to remove abnormal cells on the cervix will usually consist of cryocautery (freezing the cells using a special cold probe), electrocautery (heating the cells with electricity), or using laser treatment to "zap" the cells. None of these procedures should be painful, but they may lead to dull aching (like period pains) and watery vaginal discharge that may last several weeks.

A woman who has had visible genital warts in the past is not necessarily at any greater risk of cervical cancer, as genital warts tend to be linked to non-cancer causing subtypes of HPV.

HPV and the Anus and Rectum

The subtypes of HPV than can lead to cervical cancer may also pose a risk for men and women who have regular anal sex. Though few countries offer regular screening for anal and rectal cancer, many doctors recommend that people who have frequent anal sex (such as gay or bisexual men) should still receive a regular Pap smear test of the rectum and anus. As with cervical cell changes, early detection and treatment can help to prevent cancer from developing.

Section 25.3

HPV and Cervical Cancer

"Cervical Cancer," © National Cervical Cancer Coalition (www.nccc-online.org), undated. Reprinted with permission. Reviewed in January 2009 by Dr. David A. Cooke, M.D., Diplomate, American Board of Internal Medicine.

Cervical cancer affects approximately 10,000 women in the United States each year. Cervical cancer is the second most common type of cancer for women worldwide, but because it develops over time, it is also one of the most preventable types of cancer. Deaths from cervical cancer in the United States continue to decline by approximately 2% a year. This decline is primarily due to the widespread use of the Pap test to detect cervical abnormalities and allow for early treatment. Most women who have abnormal cervical cell changes that progress to cervical cancer have never had a Pap test or have not had one in the previous three to five years.

Cancer of the cervix tends to occur during midlife. Half of the women diagnosed with the disease are between 35 and 55 years of age. It rarely affects women under age 20, and approximately 20% of diagnoses are made in women older than 65. For this reason, it is important for women to continue cervical cancer screening until at least the age of 70.

Types of Cervical Cancer

The cervix is the narrow opening into the uterus from the vagina. The normal "ectocervix" (the portion of the uterus extending into the vagina) is a healthy pink color and is covered with flat, thin cells called squamous cells. The "endocervix" or cervical canal is made up of another kind of cell called columnar cells. The area where these cells meet is called the "transformation zone" (T-zone) and is the most likely location for abnormal or precancerous cells to develop.

Most cervical cancers (80 to 90%) are squamous cell cancers. Adenocarcinoma is the second most common type of cervical cancer, accounting for the remaining 10 to 20% of cases. Adenocarcinoma develops from the glands that produce mucus in the endocervix. While less common than squamous cell carcinoma, the incidence of adenocarcinoma is on the rise, particularly in younger women.

Causes of Cervical Cancer

Human papillomavirus (HPV) is found in about 99% of cervical cancers. There are over 100 different types of HPV, the majority of which are considered low risk and do not cause cervical cancer. High-risk HPV types may cause cervical cell abnormalities or cancer. More than 70% of cervical cancer cases can be attributed to two types of the virus, HPV-16 and HPV-18, often referred to as high-risk HPV types.

HPV is estimated to be the most common sexually transmitted infection in the United States. In fact, by age 50 approximately 80% of women have been infected with some type of HPV. The majority of women infected with the HPV virus do NOT develop cervical cancer. For most women the HPV infection is transient and 90% of infections resolve spontaneously within two years. A small proportion of women do not clear the HPV virus and are considered to have persistent infection. A woman with a persistent HPV infection is at greater risk of developing cervical cell abnormalities and cancer than a woman whose infection resolves on its own.

Signs and Symptoms of Cervical Cancer

Precancerous cervical cell changes and early cancers of the cervix generally do not cause symptoms. Abnormal or irregular vaginal bleeding, pain during sex, or vaginal discharge may be symptoms of more advanced disease.

Notify your health care provider if you experience:

- abnormal bleeding, such as:
  - bleeding between regular menstrual periods,
  - bleeding after sexual intercourse,
  - bleeding after douching,
  - bleeding after a pelvic exam;
- pelvic pain not related to your menstrual cycle;
- heavy or unusual discharge that may be watery, thick, and possibly have a foul odor;
- increased urinary frequency;
- pain during urination.

Detecting Cervical Cancer

The best way to determine if precancerous or cancerous cells are present is with a Pap test. The Pap test can determine if cell changes have taken place that may indicate precancerous or cancerous development. In addition to a Pap test, your doctor may recommend an HPV test. The HPV test does not indicate the presence of precancerous or cancerous cells. It determines whether or not a woman has an HPV infection with any of the 13 high-risk HPV types. The test cannot tell you whether your infection is new or if it is persistent. This information will assist you and your doctor to determine appropriate follow-up and intervals for cervical cancer screening.

Protecting Myself from Cervical Cancer

Cervical cancer is one of the most preventable cancers today. If caught early, the five-year survival rate is almost 100%. Regular Pap testing is the best method to protect against invasive cervical cancer. It is most important to remember that cervical cancer takes many years to develop. Regular Pap tests will help detect any precancerous or abnormal cells early enough so that cervical cancer can be prevented.

In addition to routine Pap testing, you may want to consider minimizing risk factors that could contribute to cervical cancer. Those factors include:

- multiple sexual partners;
- multiple full-term pregnancies;
- sexual intercourse at an early age;
- chlamydia infection;
- cigarette smoking;
- use of oral contraceptives;
- weakened immune system or HIV infection.

Section 25.4

HPV and Oral Cancer

"Mouth, throat cancers strongly linked to HPV; oral sex increases risk," by Keith Alcorn. © 2007 NAM (www.aidsmap.com). Reprinted with permission.

Oral sex with multiple partners and oral infection with human papilloma virus are the strongest risk factors for cancers of the mouth and throat, far outweighing the contribution of alcohol and tobacco, researchers from the Johns Hopkins University Kimmel Cancer Center report in the May 10, 2007 issue of the *New England Journal of Medicine*.

"It's the virus that drives the cancer," said lead researcher Dr. Maura Gillison, an assistant professor of oncology and epidemiology at Johns Hopkins. "Since HPV has already disrupted the cell enough to steer its change to cancer, then tobacco and alcohol use may have no further impact."

Oral cancers have in the past been blamed on heavy smoking and drinking, and an infectious cause has been debated.

Cervical and anal cancers, also caused by human papilloma virus, have been on the rise among HIV-positive people over the past 10 years despite the success of antiretroviral therapy, and the Johns Hopkins findings will alert physicians to the need to be more vigilant to the emergence of cancers of the mouth and throat in HIV-positive people. One large study showed a slightly elevated rate of certain mouth and throat cancers in HIV-positive people, particularly women, in New York state between 1981 and 1994.

The newly published study compared risk factors in 100 HIV-negative patients newly diagnosed with an oropharyngeal cancer (mainly of the tongue or tonsil) and 200 control patients who did not have cancer matched for sex and age. HPV antibody testing of blood took place, and tumors and oral fluid were also examined for the presence of HPV DNA.

Oral cancer was strongly associated with human papilloma virus type 16 infection (odds ratio 44.8, confidence interval 5.9–338.5) and with oral HPV-16 infection (OR 43.7, CI 4.2–452.7) in patients with no history of heavy tobacco or alcohol use, and a 19-fold increased risk among those who did drink or smoke heavily. HPV 16 is one of the two types of human papilloma virus to be associated with cervical, vaginal, and anal cancers, along with HPV 18.

The association dwarfs the connection between high cholesterol and heart attacks, say the researchers.

HPV 16 was present in the tumors of 72% of oropharyngeal cancer patients enrolled in the study, a figure that dwarfs the connection between high cholesterol and heart attacks. The researchers also were able to find higher risk in patients with traces of HPV in oral rinses, a first step to developing a "swish-and-spit" screening method for at-risk individuals.

However, HPV-16 was not the only type of human papilloma virus to be associated with an increased risk of oral and throat cancers. Any type of HPV was associated with an elevated risk (OR 12.3).

Study participants who reported having more than six oral sex partners in their lifetime were 8.6 times more likely to develop the HPV-linked cancer (confidence interval 2.2–34, $p<0.001$), while individuals with more than 26 lifetime vaginal sex partners were 4.2 times more likely to be diagnosed with an oral or throat cancer (CI 1.8–9.4, $p=0.001$). However there was no increased risk associated with sex with same-sex partners.

Dr. Gillison said that "people should be reassured that oropharyngeal cancer is relatively uncommon, and the overwhelming majority of people with an oral HPV infection probably will not get throat cancer."

"It is important for health care providers to know that people without the traditional risk factors of tobacco and alcohol use can nevertheless be at risk for oropharyngeal cancer," said Gypsyamber D'Souza, a co-author and assistant scientist at the Johns Hopkins Bloomberg School of Public Health.

Oral sex, including both fellatio and cunnilingus, is the main route of transmission for oral HPV infection, the investigators say, although mouth-to-mouth transmission remains possible and was not ruled out by the current study.

Human papilloma virus can also be transmitted by skin contact and is found in the mucous of the genital tract, and in saliva, urine, and semen. Both men and women contract the ubiquitous virus in equal numbers, which is believed to have infected a large proportion of people worldwide at some point in their lives. Most HPV infections clear with little or no symptoms, but a small percentage of men and women who acquire cancer-causing strains, such as HPV 16, may develop a cancer.

As for an oral rinse screening test, its feasibility still remains unproven. For this study, Gillison and her colleagues spent two years refining methods to detect HPV in oral samples. She also is working with manufacturers of the new FDA-approved vaccine for HPV to determine its potential in curbing oral cancers.

HPV-linked oral cancers have been on the rise since at least 1973, and Dr. Gillison expects the trend to continue to a point when HPV-associated cancers will far outpace those caused by tobacco and alcohol use. They currently account for 60% of oropharyngeal cancers and about a third of all oral cavity and pharynx cancers in the United States, totaling more than 11,000 individuals.

Reference

D'Souza G et al. Case-control study of human papillomavirus and oropharyngeal cancer. *N Engl J Med* 356: 1944–1956, 2007.

Chapter 26

Molluscum Contagiosum

What is molluscum contagiosum?

Molluscum contagiosum is caused by a virus and usually causes a mild skin disease. The virus affects only the outer (epithelial) layer of skin and does not circulate throughout the body in healthy people.

The virus causes small white, pink, or flesh-colored raised bumps or growths with a dimple or pit in the center. The bumps are usually smooth and firm. In most people, the growths range from about the size of a pinhead to as large as a pencil eraser (2 to 5 millimeters in diameter).

The bumps may appear anywhere on the body, alone or in groups. They are usually painless, although they may be itchy, red, swollen, and/or sore.

Molluscum usually disappears within 6 to 12 months without treatment and without leaving scars. Some growths may remain for up to 4 years.

Who gets molluscum contagiosum?

Molluscum infections occur worldwide but are more common in warm, humid climates and where living conditions are crowded. There is evidence that molluscum infections have been on the rise in the United States since 1966, but these infections are not routinely

---

"Molluscum (Molluscum Contagiosum)," Centers for Disease Control and Prevention (www.cdc.gov), August 15, 2006.

monitored because they are seldom serious and routinely disappear without treatment.

Molluscum is common enough that you should not be surprised if you see someone with it or if someone in your family becomes infected. Although not limited to children, it is most common in children 1 to 10 years of age. People with weakened immune systems (i.e., HIV-infected persons or persons being treated for cancer) are at higher risk for getting molluscum, and their growths may look different, be larger, and be more difficult to treat.

How do people become infected with the molluscum virus?

The virus that causes molluscum is spread from person to person by touching the affected skin. The virus may also be spread by touching a surface with the virus on it, such as a towel, clothing, or toys. Once someone has the virus, the bumps can spread to other parts of their body by touching or scratching a bump and then touching another part of the body. Molluscum can be spread from one person to another by sexual contact.

Although the virus might be spread by sharing swimming pools, baths, saunas, or other wet and warm environments, this has not been proven. Researchers who have investigated this idea think it is more likely the virus is spread by sharing towels and other items around a pool or sauna than through water.

How would I know if I had molluscum contagiosum?

Only a health care provider can diagnose molluscum infection. If you have any unusual skin irritation, rash, bump(s), or blister(s) that do not disappear in a few days, you should see a health care provider.

If you have molluscum, you will see small white, pink, or flesh-colored raised bumps or growths with a pit or dimple in the center. The bumps are usually smooth and firm. They can be as small as the head of a pin and as large as a pencil eraser (two to five millimeters in diameter). The growths are usually painless but may become itchy, sore, and red and/or swollen. They may occur anywhere on the body including the face, neck, arms, legs, abdomen, and genital area, alone or in groups. The bumps are rarely found on the palms of the hands or the soles of the feet.

What should I do if I think I have molluscum contagiosum?

If you have any unusual skin irritation, rash, bumps, or blisters that do not disappear in a few days, contact a health care provider.

Only a health care professional can diagnose molluscum. He or she will discuss treatment options and how to care for the affected skin.

How can I avoid becoming infected with molluscum?

The best way to avoid getting molluscum is by following good hygiene habits.

- Do not touch, pick, or scratch any skin with bumps or blisters (yours or someone else's).
- Good hand hygiene is the best way to avoid getting many infections including molluscum. For handwashing tips, see the Clean Hands Saves Lives website at http://www.cdc.gov/cleanhands. By washing your hands frequently you wash away germs picked up from other people or from contaminated surfaces.

What is the correct way to wash my hands?

- First wet your hands and apply soap.
- Next rub your hands vigorously together and scrub all surfaces.
- Continue for 10–15 seconds. Soap combined with scrubbing action helps dislodge and remove germs.
- Rinse well and dry your hands.

I have molluscum. How can I avoid spreading it to others?

It is important to keep the area with growths clean and covered with clothing or a bandage so that others do not touch the bumps and become infected with molluscum.

However, when there is no risk of others coming into contact with your skin, such as at night when you sleep, uncover the bumps to help keep your skin healthy.

Before participating in sports in which your body will come into contact with another person's body (i.e., wrestling) or shared equipment (swimming pools) cover all growths with clothing or a watertight bandage.

Do not share towels, clothing, or other personal items.

Do not shave or have electrolysis on areas with bumps.

If you have bumps in the genital area, avoid sexual activities until you see a health care provider.

How long does the molluscum contagiosum virus stay in my body?

The virus lives only in the skin and once the growths are gone, the virus is gone and you cannot spread the virus to others.

Molluscum contagiosum is not like herpes viruses, which can remain dormant ("sleeping") in your body for long periods and then reappear. So, assuming you do not come in contact with another infected person, once all the molluscum contagiosum bumps go away, you will not develop any new bumps.

How is molluscum treated?

You should discuss all treatment options with a health care provider. Usually no treatment is needed because the bumps disappear by themselves within 6–12 months, although this may take up to four years.

To prevent the spread of molluscum to other areas of your body or to other people, it is important to keep every blister or bump covered either with clothing or with a watertight bandage. However, to promote healthy skin, do remove the bandage at night and when there is no risk of others coming into contact with your skin.

A number of treatment options are available, but some (available from internet services) are not effective and may even be harmful. Therefore, always discuss any possible therapy with your health care provider. Treating the molluscum growths may prevent spread to other parts of the body and to other people. Not everyone agrees on how well treatments work.

Treatment is more difficult for persons with weakened immune systems (for example, people who are HIV positive or receiving cancer drugs). For people with weakened immune systems, the best treatment seems to be medications that help strengthen the immune system.

Treatment options in the health care setting: Cryotherapy (freezing the molluscum growth) is one treatment option. This is the same way that warts are removed from the skin. Another option is to remove the fluid inside the bumps (termed curettage). Lasers also can remove molluscum bumps.

All three options may be a little painful and should only be done by a health care professional. Both curettage and cryotherapy methods may leave scars. In a small percentage of cases, natural healing of molluscum contagiosum bumps lead to scars regardless of type of therapy.

Treatment options in the home setting: Check with a health care provider before using any of these treatments. Most of these creams and oral medicines are available by prescription.

Creams that include certain chemicals (i.e., salicylic acid, podophyllin, tretinoin, and cantharidin) may be used to remove the bumps. There is also a newer cream (imiquimod) that helps strengthen the skin's immune system. The creams are applied directly to each growth. Unfortunately these creams do not always remove the bumps and they may be harmful.

The oral medicine cimetidine has been used for treatment of molluscum in small children. This medicine is available only by prescription. As with all medications, cimetidine may cause unwanted side effects.

In general, medications should not be used by pregnant women, women who are breast feeding, or women who may become pregnant—without first asking a health care provider.

Once I am cured can I be reinfected with molluscum contagiosum?

Yes. Recovery from one infection with molluscum does not prevent future infections with molluscum so it is important not to pick at or scratch other people's skin.

However, molluscum contagiosum is not like herpes viruses, which can remain dormant ("sleeping") in your body for long periods of time and then reappear. If you get new molluscum contagiosum bumps after you are cured, it means you have come in contact with an infected person or object.

Should I try to remove the bumps caused by molluscum?

It is not a good idea to try to remove the molluscum growths or to get rid of the fluid inside them yourself.

Be aware that some treatments available through the internet are not effective and may even be harmful!

There are three important reasons not to treat the bumps without seeing a doctor first.

1. The treatment may be painful.
2. You might spread the bumps to another part of your body or to another person.
3. By scratching and scraping the skin you might cause a more serious bacterial infection. If you want to have the growths

removed or treated, talk to a health care provider. Molluscum bumps usually will disappear without treatment in 6 to 12 months and not leave scars, but it may not go away completely for up to four years.

Are there any complications of molluscum contagiosum infection?

The most common complication is a secondary infection caused by bacteria. Additionally, the removal of bumps by scratching, freezing (cryotherapy), or fluid removal (curettage) can leave scars on the skin.

Can my child go to day care or school if he or she has molluscum?

There should be no reason to keep a child with molluscum infection home from day care or school.

Growths not covered by clothing should be covered with a watertight bandage. Change the bandage daily or when obviously soiled.

If a child with bumps in the underwear/diaper area needs assistance going to the bathroom or needs diaper changes, then growths in this area should be bandaged too if possible.

Covering the bumps will protect other children and adults from getting molluscum and will also keep the child from touching and scratching the bumps, which could spread the bumps to other parts of his/her body or cause secondary (bacterial) infections.

Remind children to wash their hands frequently.

What do I need to know about swimming pools and molluscum?

Some investigations report that spread of molluscum contagiosum is increased in swimming pools. However, it has not been proved how or under what circumstances swimming pools might increase spread of the virus. Activities related to swimming might be the cause. For example, the virus might spread from one person to another if they share a towel or toys. More research is needed to understand if and for how long the molluscum virus can live in swimming pool water and if such water can infect swimmers.

Open sores and breaks in the skin can become infected by many different germs. Therefore, people with open sores or breaks from any cause should not go into swimming pools.

If a person has molluscum bumps, the following recommendations should be followed when swimming:

- Cover all visible bumps with watertight bandages
- Dispose of all used bandages at home
- Do not share towels, kick boards or other equipment, or toys

Is molluscum contagiosum a sexually transmitted disease?

Molluscum contagiosum can be spread by any contact between two people—this includes sexual contact. Many, but not all, cases of molluscum in adults are caused by sexual contact.

Treatment for molluscum is usually recommended if the growths are in the genital area (on or near the penis, vulva, vagina, or anus). If bumps are found in the genital area, it is a good idea to discuss with a health care provider the possibility that you might have another disease that is spread by sexual contact.

I am HIV positive. How could molluscum contagiosum affect me?

Persons with HIV disease are at increased risk for acquiring molluscum. The growths may be very large—the size of a dime or larger (at least 15 millimeters). Bumps may be anywhere on the body but are often on the face. These growths usually do not go away by themselves.

Treatment of molluscum among HIV-positive persons is more difficult than in people with normal immune systems. The best treatment for people with HIV seems to be helping to strengthen the immune system with antiretroviral (anti-HIV) medications.

The risk of a secondary infection caused by bacteria is always present. If you are HIV positive or think you might be, it is especially important that you see a health care provider. This person will discuss possible treatments for molluscum and ways to improve your overall health.

I have a weakened immune system. How could molluscum contagiosum affect me?

Persons with weakened immune systems (such as cancer, organ transplantation, HIV, etc.) are at increased risk for catching molluscum and may develop very large growths (the size of a dime or larger—

at least 15 millimeters in diameter). Bumps may be anywhere on the body but tend to occur on the face and not to go away by themselves.

Treatment of molluscum is more difficult among persons with weakened immune systems. The best treatment is to strengthen the immune system by treating the primary problem.

The risk of a secondary infection caused by bacteria is always present. Your health care provider will discuss possible treatments for molluscum and ways to improve your overall health.

Since molluscum contagiosum virus is a poxvirus, does the smallpox vaccination protect me from getting molluscum contagiosum?

No, the smallpox vaccination will not protect you from becoming infected with molluscum contagiosum virus. Although both molluscum contagiosum virus and smallpox (variola) virus are from the same group of viruses (poxviruses), they have significantly different genetic makeup and are easily distinguished by your immune system.

Chapter 27

Pelvic Inflammatory Disease

What is pelvic inflammatory disease (PID)?

PID is an infection of a woman's pelvic organs. The pelvic organs include the uterus (womb), fallopian tubes (tubes), ovaries, and other organs related to having babies.

What causes PID?

Bacteria (a type of germ) moves up from a woman's vagina, infecting her tubes, ovaries, and womb. Many different types of germs can cause PID. But, germs found in two common sexually transmitted diseases (STDs)—gonorrhea and chlamydia—are most often the cause of PID. After a person is infected, it can take from a few days to a few months to turn into PID.

It is rare, but you can get PID without having an STD. No one is sure why, but normal bacteria found in the vagina and on the cervix can sometimes cause PID.

Are some women more likely to get PID?

Yes. You are more likely to get PID if the following conditions apply to you:

- You have had an STD

"Pelvic Inflammatory Disease," National Women's Health Information Center, U.S. Department of Health and Human Services (www.womenshealth.gov), April 2007.

- You are under 25 and are having sex
- You have more than one sex partner
- You practice douching (Douching can push germs into the womb, ovaries, and tubes, causing infection. Douching can also hide the signs of an infection)
- You have an intrauterine device (IUD). You're less likely to get PID if you're tested and treated for any infections before getting an IUD.

How do I know if I have PID?

Many women have PID and don't know it. This is because sometimes women with PID don't have any symptoms. Still, some women do have symptoms, which can range from mild to severe. The most common symptom of PID is pain in your lower abdomen (stomach area). Other symptoms include the following:

- Fever (99.6° or higher)
- Vaginal discharge that may smell
- Painful sex
- Painful urination
- Irregular periods
- Pain in the upper right abdomen (stomach area)

PID can come on fast with extreme pain and fever, especially if it is caused by gonorrhea.

Are there any tests for PID?

It can be hard for your doctor to figure out if you have PID. Symptoms can be mild and are like symptoms of some other diseases. If you think that you may have PID, see a doctor right away. If you are treated right away, you'll be less likely to have long-term problems, such as infertility.

If you have pain in your lower abdomen (stomach area), your doctor will perform a physical exam. This will include a pelvic (internal) exam, which will help your doctor learn more about your pain. Your doctor will check for the following:

- Abnormal vaginal or cervical discharge

- Lumps near your ovaries and tubes
- Tenderness or pain of your pelvic organs

Your doctor will also give you tests for STDs, urinary tract infection, and if needed, pregnancy. Your doctor also might test you for HIV and syphilis.

If needed, your doctor may do other tests.

- **Ultrasound (sonogram):** A test that uses sound waves to take pictures of the pelvic area
- **Endometrial (uterine) biopsy:** A small piece of the endometrium (the inside lining of the womb) is removed and tested
- **Laparoscopy:** A small tube with a light inside is inserted through your abdomen (stomach area) to look at your pelvic organs

These tests will help your doctor find out if you have PID or if you have a different problem that looks like PID.

How is PID treated?

PID can be cured with antibiotics. Your doctor will work with you to find the best treatment for you. You must take all your medicine, even if your symptoms go away. The infection will not be fully cured if you do not take all of the medicine.

If PID is not treated, it can lead to severe problems like infertility, ectopic pregnancy, and constant pelvic pain.

Any damage done to your pelvic organs before you start treatment cannot be undone. Still, don't put off getting treatment. If you do, you may not be able to have children. If you think you may have PID, see a doctor right away.

Your doctor may suggest going into the hospital to treat your PID if you experience these conditions:

- Are very sick
- Are pregnant
- Do not respond to or cannot take medicine through your mouth—if this is the case, you will need intravenous (in the vein or IV) antibiotics
- Have a sore in a tube or ovary

If you still have symptoms or if the sore doesn't go away, you may need surgery. Problems of PID such as constant pelvic pain and scarring are often hard to treat, but sometimes they get better after surgery.

What if my partner is infected?

Even if your sex partner doesn't have any symptoms, she or he could still be infected with bacteria that can cause PID. Protect yourself from being re-infected with PID.

- Your sex partner(s) should be treated even if she or he doesn't have symptoms.
- Don't have sex with a partner who hasn't been treated.

My friend was told she can't get pregnant because she has PID. Is this true?

The more times you have PID, the more likely it is that you won't be able to have children. When you have PID, bacteria infect the tubes or cause inflammation of the tubes. This turns normal tissue into scar tissue, which can block your tubes and make it harder to get pregnant. Even having just a little scar tissue can keep you from getting pregnant.

How can I keep myself from getting PID?

PID is most often caused by an STD that hasn't been treated. You can keep from getting PID by not getting an STD.

- The best way to prevent an STD is to not have sex of any kind.
- Have sex with one partner who doesn't have any STDs.
- Use condoms every time you have vaginal, anal, or oral sex. Read and follow the directions on the package. If condoms are used correctly, they can lower your chances of getting an STD.
- Don't douche. Douching removes some of the normal bacteria in the vagina that protect you from infection. This makes it easier for you to get an STD.
- If you're having sex, ask your doctor to test you for STDs. STDs found early are easier to treat.

- Learn the common symptoms of STDs. If you think you might have an STD, see your doctor right away.

What should I do if I think I have an STD?

You may feel scared or shy about asking for information or help. Keep in mind, the sooner you seek treatment, the less likely the STD will cause you severe harm. And the sooner you tell your sex partner(s) that you have an STD, the less likely they are to re-infect you or spread the disease to others.

If you think you may have an STD, see a doctor right away. Doctors, local health departments, and STD and family planning clinics have information about STDs and many offer testing. The American Social Health Association (ASHA) keeps lists of clinics and doctors who provide treatment for STDs. Call ASHA at (800) 227-8922. You can get information from the phone line without leaving your name.

Chapter 28

Pubic Lice (Crabs)

Facts about Pubic Lice

What are pubic lice?

Also called crab lice or "crabs," pubic lice are parasitic insects found primarily in the pubic or genital area of humans. Pubic lice infestation is found worldwide and occurs in all races, ethnic groups, and levels of society.

What do pubic lice look like?

Pubic lice have forms: the egg (also called a nit), the nymph, and the adult.

Nit: Nits are lice eggs. They can be hard to see and are found firmly attached to the hair shaft. They are oval and usually yellow to white. Pubic lice nits take about 6–10 days to hatch.

Nymph: The nymph is an immature louse that hatches from the nit (egg). A nymph looks like an adult pubic louse but it is smaller. Pubic lice nymphs take about two to three weeks after hatching to mature into adults capable of reproducing. To live, a nymph must feed on blood.

This chapter includes "Pubic Lice Fact Sheet" and "Pubic Lice Treatment," Centers for Disease Control and Prevention (www.cdc.gov), May 16, 2008.

Adult: The adult pubic louse resembles a miniature crab when viewed through a strong magnifying glass. Pubic lice have six legs; their two front legs are very large and look like the pincher claws of a crab. This is how they got the nickname "crabs." Pubic lice are tan to grayish-white in color. Females lay nits and are usually larger than males. To live, lice must feed on blood. If the louse falls off a person, it dies within one to two days.

Where are pubic lice found?

Pubic lice usually are found in the genital area on pubic hair; but they may occasionally be found on other coarse body hair, such as hair on the legs, armpits, mustache, beard, eyebrows, or eyelashes. Pubic lice on the eyebrows or eyelashes of children may be a sign of sexual exposure or abuse. Lice found on the head are generally head lice, not pubic lice.

Animals do not get or spread pubic lice.

What are the signs and symptoms of pubic lice?

Signs and symptoms of pubic lice include the following:

- Itching in the genital area
- Visible nits (lice eggs) or crawling lice

How did I get pubic lice?

Pubic lice usually are spread through sexual contact and are most common in adults. Pubic lice found on children may be a sign of sexual exposure or abuse. Occasionally, pubic lice may be spread by close personal contact or contact with articles such as clothing, bed linens, or towels that have been used by an infested person. A common misunderstanding is that pubic lice are spread easily by sitting on a toilet seat. This would be extremely rare because lice cannot live long away from a warm human body and they do not have feet designed to hold onto or walk on smooth surfaces such as toilet seats.

Persons infested with pubic lice should be investigated for the presence of other sexually transmitted diseases.

How is a pubic lice infestation diagnosed?

A pubic lice infestation is diagnosed by finding a "crab" louse or egg (nit) on hair in the pubic region or, less commonly, elsewhere on the body (eyebrows, eyelashes, beard, mustache, armpit, perianal area, groin, trunk, scalp). Pubic lice may be difficult to find because there may be only a few. Pubic lice often attach themselves to more than one hair and generally do not crawl as quickly as head and body lice. If crawling lice are not seen, finding nits in the pubic area strongly suggests that a person is infested and should be treated. If you are unsure about infestation or if treatment is not successful, see a health care provider for a diagnosis. Persons infested with pubic lice should be investigated for the presence of other sexually transmitted diseases.

Although pubic lice and nits can be large enough to be seen with the naked eye, a magnifying lens may be necessary to find lice or eggs.

Pubic Lice Treatment

How is a pubic lice infestation treated?

A lice-killing lotion containing 1% permethrin or a mousse containing pyrethrins and piperonyl butoxide can be used to treat pubic lice. These products are available over-the-counter without a prescription at a local drug store or pharmacy. These medications are safe and effective when used exactly according to the instructions in the package or on the label.

Lindane shampoo is a prescription medication that can kill lice and lice eggs. However, lindane is not recommended as a first-line therapy. Lindane can be toxic to the brain and other parts of the nervous system; its use should be restricted to patients who have failed treatment with or cannot tolerate other medications that pose less risk. Lindane should not be used to treat premature infants, persons with a seizure disorder, women who are pregnant or breast-feeding, persons who have very irritated skin or sores where the lindane will be applied, infants, children, the elderly, and persons who weigh less than 110 pounds.

Malathion* lotion 0.5% (Ovide*) is a prescription medication that can kill lice and some lice eggs; however, malathion lotion (Ovide*) currently has not been approved by the U.S. Food and Drug Administration (FDA) for treatment of pubic lice.

Ivermectin has been used successfully to treat lice; however, ivermectin currently has not been approved by the FDA for treatment of lice.

How to treat pubic lice infestations: (Warning: See special instructions for treatment of lice and nits on eyebrows or eyelashes. The lice medications described in this section should not be used near the eyes.)

1. Wash the infested area; towel dry.

2. Carefully follow the instructions in the package or on the label. Thoroughly saturate the pubic hair and other infested areas with lice medication. Leave medication on hair for the time recommended in the instructions. After waiting the recommended time, remove the medication by following carefully the instructions on the label or in the box.
3. Following treatment, most nits will still be attached to hair shafts. Nits may be removed with fingernails or by using a fine-toothed comb.
4. Put on clean underwear and clothing after treatment.
5. To kill any lice or nits remaining on clothing, towels, or bedding, machine wash and machine dry those items that the infested person used during the two to three days before treatment. Use hot water (at least 130°F) and the hot dryer cycle.
6. Items that cannot be laundered can be dry cleaned or stored in a sealed plastic bag for two weeks.
7. All sex partners from within the previous month should be informed that they are at risk for infestation and should be treated.
8. Persons should avoid sexual contact with their sex partner(s) until both they and their partners have been successfully treated and reevaluated to rule out persistent infestation.
9. Repeat treatment in 9–10 days if live lice are still found.
10. Persons with pubic lice should be evaluated for other sexually transmitted diseases.

Special Instructions for Treatment of Lice and Nits Found on Eyebrows or Eyelashes

- If only a few live lice and nits are present, it may be possible to remove these with fingernails or a nit comb.
- If additional treatment is needed for lice or nits on the eyelashes, careful application of ophthalmic-grade petrolatum ointment (only available by prescription) to the eyelid margins two to four times a day for 10 days is effective. Regular Vaseline* should not be used because it can irritate the eyes if applied.

*Use of trade names is for identification purposes only and does not imply endorsement by the Public Health Service or by the U.S. Department of Health and Human Services.

Chapter 29

Scabies

What is scabies?

Scabies is an infestation of the skin with the microscopic mite *Sarcoptes scabei*. Infestation is common, found worldwide, and affects people of all races and social classes. Scabies spreads rapidly under crowded conditions where there is frequent skin-to-skin contact between people, such as in hospitals, institutions, child-care facilities, and nursing homes.

What are the signs and symptoms of scabies infestation?

- Pimple-like irritations, burrows, or rash of the skin, especially the webbing between the fingers; the skin folds on the wrist, elbow, or knee; the penis, the breast, or shoulder blades.
- Intense itching, especially at night and over most of the body.
- Sores on the body caused by scratching. These sores can sometimes become infected with bacteria.

How did I get scabies?

By direct, prolonged, skin-to-skin contact with a person already infested with scabies. Contact generally must be prolonged (a quick handshake or hug will usually not spread infestation). Infestation is

---

"Scabies Fact Sheet," Centers for Disease Control and Prevention (www.cdc.gov), February 4, 2008.

easily spread to sexual partners and household members. Infestation may also occur by sharing clothing, towels, and bedding.

Who is at risk for severe infestation?

People with weakened immune systems and the elderly are at risk for a more severe form of scabies, called Norwegian or crusted scabies. Scabies is spread more easily by persons who have Norwegian, or crusted, scabies than by persons with other types of scabies.

How long will mites live?

Once away from the human body, mites usually do not survive more than 48–72 hours. When living on a person, an adult female mite can live up to a month.

Did my pet spread scabies to me?

No. Pets become infested with a different kind of scabies mite. If your pet is infested with scabies (also called mange), and they have close contact with you, the mite can get under your skin and cause itching and skin irritation. However, the mite dies in a couple of days and does not reproduce. The mites may cause you to itch for several days, but you do not need to be treated with special medication to kill the mites. Until your pet is successfully treated, mites can continue to burrow into your skin and cause you to have symptoms.

How soon after infestation will symptoms begin?

For a person who has never been infested with scabies, symptoms may take four to six weeks to begin. For a person who has had scabies before, symptoms appear within several days.

How is scabies infestation diagnosed?

Diagnosis is most commonly made by looking at the burrows or rash. A skin scraping may be taken to look for mites, eggs, or mite fecal matter (scybala) to confirm the diagnosis. Even if a skin scraping or biopsy is taken and returns negative, it is still possible that you may be infested. Typically, there are fewer than 10 mites on the entire body of an infested person; this makes it easy for an infestation to be missed. However, persons with Norwegian, or crusted, scabies can be infested with thousands of mites and should be considered highly infectious.

Can scabies be treated?

Yes. Several creams or lotions that are available by prescription are U.S. Food and Drug Administration (FDA)-approved to treat scabies. Always follow the directions provided by your physician or the directions on the package label or insert. Apply the medication to a clean body from the neck down to the toes. After leaving the medication on the body for the recommended time, take a bath or shower to wash off the cream or lotion. Put on clean clothes. All clothes, bedding, and towels used by the infested person during the three days before treatment should be washed in hot water and dried in a hot dryer. A second treatment of the body with the same cream or lotion may be necessary. Pregnant women and children are often treated with milder scabies medications such as 5% permethrin cream.

Who should be treated for scabies?

Anyone who is diagnosed with scabies, as well as his or her sexual partners and persons who have close, prolonged contact to the infested person, should be treated. If your health care provider has instructed family members to be treated, everyone should receive treatment at the same time to prevent reinfestation.

How soon after treatment will I feel better?

Itching may continue for two to three weeks, and does not mean that you are still infested. Your health care provider may prescribe additional medication to relieve itching if it is severe.

Chapter 30

Syphilis

Chapter Contents

Section 30.1

What You Should Know about Syphilis

"Syphilis," National Institute for Allergy and Infectious Diseases (www3.niaid.nih.gov), November 14, 2006.

Syphilis is a sexually transmitted bacterial infection (STI) that initially causes genital ulcers (sores). If untreated, these ulcers can then lead to more serious symptoms of infection.

An ancient disease, syphilis is still of major importance today. Although syphilis rates in the United States declined by almost 90% from 1990 to 2000, the number of cases rose from 5,979 in 2000 to 7,980 in 2004. In a single year, from 2003 to 2004, the number of syphilis cases jumped 8%.

There also was a dramatic change in whom the disease affects. Between 2002 and 2003, the number of cases in men increased 13.5%, reflecting an increase in syphilis in men who have sex with men. During the same time the number of cases in women declined by 27.3%.

Syphilis also disproportionately affects African Americans, who represent 41% of all cases reported to the Centers for Disease Control and Prevention (CDC).

HIV infection and syphilis are linked. Syphilis increases the risk of transmitting as well as getting infected with HIV.

Cause

Syphilis is caused by a bacterium called *Treponema pallidum*.

Transmission

The most common way to get syphilis is by having sexual contact with an infected person. If you get infected, you can pass the bacteria from infected skin or mucous membranes (linings), usually your genital area, lips, mouth, or anus, to the mucous membranes or skin of your sexual partner.

Syphilis can be passed from mother to infant during pregnancy, causing a disease called congenital syphilis.

The bacteria are fragile; you can't get them from eating utensils or through using spas, pools, or toilets.

Symptoms

Syphilis is sometimes called "the great imitator" because it has so many possible symptoms, and its symptoms are similar to those of many other diseases. Having HIV infection at the same time can change the symptoms and course of syphilis. Syphilis (other than congenital syphilis) occurs in four stages that sometimes overlap.

Primary Syphilis

The first symptom of primary syphilis is often a small, round, firm ulcer called a chancre ("shanker") at the place where the bacteria entered your body. This place is usually the penis, vulva, or vagina, but chancres also can develop on the cervix, tongue, lips, or other parts of the body. Usually there is only one chancre, but sometimes there are many. Nearby lymph glands are often swollen. (Lymph glands, or nodes, are small bean-shaped organs of your immune system containing cells that help fight off germs. They are found throughout the body.) The chancre usually appears about three weeks after you're infected with the bacteria, but it can occur any time from 9 to 90 days after exposure.

Because a chancre is usually painless and can appear inside your body, you might not notice it. The chancre disappears in about three to six weeks whether or not you are treated. Therefore, you can have primary syphilis without symptoms or with only brief symptoms that could be overlooked. If primary syphilis is not treated, however, the infection moves to the secondary stage.

Secondary Syphilis

Most people with secondary syphilis have a non-itchy skin rash. Although the rash is usually on the palms of your hands and soles of your feet, it may cover your whole body or appear only in a few areas. The rash appears 2 to 10 weeks after the chancre, generally when the chancre is healing or already healed. Other common symptoms include the following:

- Sore throat
- Headache
- Tiredness
- Swollen lymph glands

Less frequent symptoms include fever, aches, weight loss, hair loss, aching joints, or lesions (sores) in the mouth or genital area.

Your symptoms may be mild. The sores of secondary syphilis contain many bacteria, and anyone who has contact with them can get syphilis. As with primary syphilis, secondary syphilis will disappear even without treatment. Without treatment, however, the infection will move to the next stages.

You may have recurrences of secondary syphilis.

Latent Syphilis

The latent (hidden) stage of syphilis begins when symptoms of secondary syphilis are over.

In early latent syphilis, you might notice signs and symptoms, but the infection remains in your body. When you are in this stage, you can still infect a sexual partner.

In late latent syphilis, the infection is quiet and the risk of infecting a sexual partner is low or absent. If you don't get treated for latent syphilis, you will progress to tertiary syphilis, the most serious stage of the disease.

Tertiary Syphilis

Even without treatment, only a small number of infected people develop the dreaded complications known as tertiary, or late, syphilis. In this stage, the bacteria will damage your heart, eyes, brain, nervous system, bones, joints, or almost any other part of your body. This damage can happen years or even decades after the primary stage.

Late syphilis can result in mental illness, blindness, deafness, memory loss or other neurological problems, heart disease, and death. Late neurosyphilis (brain or spinal cord damage) is one of the most severe signs of this stage.

Diagnosis

It can be very difficult for your health care provider to diagnose syphilis based on symptoms. This is because symptoms and signs of the disease might be absent, go away without treatment, or be confused with those of other diseases. Because syphilis can be hard to diagnose, you should take the following precautions:

- Visit your health care provider if you have a lesion (sore) in your genital area or a widespread rash.

- Get tested periodically for syphilis if your sexual behaviors put you at risk for STIs.
- Get tested to be sure you do not also have syphilis if you have been treated for another STI such as gonorrhea or HIV infection.

Your health care provider can diagnose early syphilis by seeing a chancre or rash and then confirming the diagnosis with laboratory tests. Because latent syphilis has no symptoms, it is diagnosed only by laboratory tests.

There are two laboratory methods for making the diagnosis.

- Identifying the bacteria under a microscope in a sample taken from a lesion.
- Performing a blood test for syphilis.

If your doctor thinks you might have neurosyphilis, your spinal fluid will be tested as well.

Treatment

Syphilis is easy to cure in its early stages. Penicillin, an antibiotic, injected into the muscle is the best treatment for syphilis. If you are allergic to penicillin, your health care provider may give you another antibiotic to take by mouth.

If you have neurosyphilis, you may need to receive daily doses of penicillin intravenously (in the vein) and may need to be treated in the hospital.

If you have late syphilis, damage done to your body organs cannot be reversed.

While you are being treated, you should abstain from sex until your sores are completely healed. You should also notify your sex partners so they can be tested for syphilis and treated if necessary.

For updated information on treatment for syphilis, read the Centers for Disease Control and Prevention Sexually Transmitted Diseases Treatment Guidelines at www.cdc.gov/std/treatment/.

Prevention

To prevent getting syphilis, you must avoid contact with infected tissue (a group of cells) and body fluids of an infected person. Usually syphilis is transmitted from people who have no visible sores or rashes and who do not know they are infected, however.

If you are not infected with syphilis and are sexually active, having mutually monogamous sex with only one uninfected partner is the best way to prevent syphilis. Using condoms properly and consistently during sexual intercourse reduces the risk of getting syphilis.

Washing or douching after sex will not prevent syphilis. Even if you have been treated for syphilis and cured, you can be reinfected by having sex with an infected partner.

The risk of a mother transmitting syphilis to her unborn baby during pregnancy declines with time but persists during latent syphilis. To prevent passing congenital syphilis to her unborn baby, all pregnant women should be tested for syphilis.

Complications

Pregnancy

Untreated syphilis results in a high-risk pregnancy. There are an estimated 8,000 pregnant women with syphilis in the United States. Untreated early syphilis results in death of the unborn baby in up to 40% of cases. Studies show that if a woman contracts syphilis during the four years before her pregnancy, untreated early syphilis may lead to infection of her unborn baby in more than 70% of cases. Therefore, if you are pregnant, you should be tested for syphilis.

Syphilis can cause miscarriages, premature births, stillbirths, or deaths of newborn babies. Some infants with congenital syphilis have symptoms at birth, but most develop symptoms later.

Untreated babies with congenital syphilis can have deformities, delays in development, or seizures along with many other problems such as rash, fever, swollen liver and spleen, anemia, and jaundice. Sores on infected babies are infectious. Rarely, the symptoms of syphilis go unseen in infants so that they later develop the symptoms of late-stage syphilis, including damage to their bones, teeth, eyes, ears, and brains.

HIV Infection

There is an estimated two- to five-fold increased risk of getting infected with HIV when syphilis is present. Substantial biological evidence shows the increased likelihood that getting and transmitting HIV is linked to the presence of sexually transmitted infections. You should discuss this and other STIs with your health care provider.

Research

Developing better ways to diagnose and treat syphilis is an important research goal of scientists supported by the National Institute of Allergy and Infectious Diseases (NIAID).

In the largest major clinical trial of syphilis since the 1950s, NIAID-supported researchers have shown that treating syphilis with oral azithromycin is just as effective as the current standard treatment, which is a series of injections of penicillin. Oral azithromycin has several advantages over injected penicillin: easy-to-take pills instead of a series of painful injections at a health facility; the treatment does not need to be kept cold (which is difficult in many developing areas); and it is less expensive. This study lends support for a potential alternative treatment option for managing syphilis, especially in developing countries where it is difficult to ensure drug delivery.

Scientists are developing new tests that may provide better ways to diagnose syphilis and define the stage of infection. Efforts to develop a diagnostic test that would not require a blood sample are a high priority. For example, researchers are evaluating saliva and urine to see whether they would work as well as blood. Researchers also are trying to develop other diagnostic tests for detecting infection in babies.

In an effort to stem the spread of syphilis, scientists are conducting research that could lead to the development of a vaccine. Molecular biologists are learning more about the various surface parts of the syphilis bacterium that stimulate the immune system to respond to it.

NIAID-funded researchers have also sequenced the genetic blueprint, or genome, of the bacterium that causes syphilis. The DNA sequence represents an encyclopedia of information about the bacterium. Researchers have identified clues in the genome that may help better diagnose, treat, and vaccinate against syphilis, fueling intensive research efforts.

Section 30.2

Syphilis Rates on the Rise in the United States

Armed with more than a decade's worth of statistics, researchers are sounding a new alarm about growing rates of syphilis among gay and bisexual men.

The overall number of syphilis cases in the United States fell from 50,578 in 1990 to just 7,177 in 2003 perhaps because of a nationwide prevention campaign aimed at heterosexuals. Nevertheless, gay men have seen their rates rise significantly in this decade.

"The entire nation was caught unawares," said study lead author James Heffelfinger, MD, a medical epidemiologist with the Centers for Disease Control and Prevention. "You're concentrating on one population, but the next thing you know, you start seeing a large increase among another group."

It is still easy to cure syphilis, but it can cause serious medical problems, including death if untreated. In addition, officials worry that gay men will get syphilis and become more susceptible to HIV infection, although statistics have not made it clear if that is actually happening.

The study authors looked at syphilis rates from 1990 to 2003 and reported the changes during that time. The *American Journal of Public Health* released the findings online in April 2007, and they also appeared in the June 2007 print edition.

Between 1990 and 2000, syphilis rates fell by a whopping 90%, from a rate of 20.3 cases per 100,000 people to 2.1 cases per 100,000. Among other factors, public health officials think the rates dropped because fewer people were selling sex to get crack cocaine as the decade went by.

However, the syphilis rate rose by 19% between 2000 and 2003.

During that period, the rates among women continued to slide—by 53%—while rates among men jumped by 62%. While syphilis statistics do not identify the gender of the sex partners of infected people, the study authors infer that a large number of those infected—62% in 2003—are gay or bisexual, in part, because so few women become infected.

The study does not look past 2003, but statistics suggest the trends continued through 2005, Heffelfinger said. There were 8,724 new cases of syphilis recorded in 2005.

Khalil Ghanem, MD, assistant professor of medicine at Johns Hopkins University School of Medicine, said rates among gay men could be going up for several reasons, including illicit drug use and "safe-sex fatigue." In addition, he said, prevention messages might have been "drowned out" by talk about how medications are doing a great job of keeping AIDS patients alive.

"We've been seduced by these amazing drugs and we've fallen behind in our prevention efforts," Ghanem said. "We have to get back on track with prevention messages. That's the only way we will curb this outbreak."

Heffelfinger JD, et al. Trends in primary and secondary syphilis in the United States: The reemergence of syphilis among men who have sex with men. *Am J Public Health* 97(6), 2007.

Section 30.3

Increasing Impact of Syphilis on MSM, Women, and African Americans

"New Data Reveal 7th Consecutive Syphilis Increase in the U.S. and Opportunities to Improve STD Screening and Prevention for Gay and Bisexual Men," 2008 National STD Prevention Conference, Centers for Disease Control and Prevention (www.cdc.gov), April 7, 2008.

The U.S. syphilis rate increased for the seventh consecutive year in 2007, largely reflecting continued increases among men who have sex with men (MSM), according to preliminary data from the Centers for Disease Control and Prevention (CDC) presented at the 2008 National STD Prevention Conference.

Other studies released at the conference indicate that many MSM with sexually transmitted diseases (STDs) remain undiagnosed due to inadequate STD testing.

"STDs remain a major threat to the health of gay and bisexual men, in part because having an STD other than HIV can increase the risk of transmitting or acquiring HIV," said Kevin Fenton, MD, director of CDC's National Center for HIV/AIDS, Viral Hepatitis, STD, and TB Prevention. "The resurgence of syphilis among MSM represents a formidable challenge to our STD prevention efforts, but one that is surmountable. The solution comes down to making STD screening and treatment a central part of medical care for gay and bisexual men, while finding innovative ways to help MSM avoid STD infections—including HIV—in the first place."

Syphilis Increases Pose Continuing Prevention Challenge

The preliminary 2007 syphilis data show that the national rate of primary and secondary syphilis—the most infectious stages of the disease—increased 12% between 2006 and 2007, from 3.3 to 3.7 cases per 100,000 population. As in recent years, this overall increase was driven by continued increases among males (from 5.7 per 100,000 in 2006 to 6.4 per 100,000 in 2007). Several sources of data indicate that substantial increases in syphilis among MSM since 2000 largely account for the overall trend in males.

The rate among females also increased between 2006 and 2007, from 1.0 to 1.1 cases per 100,000 population. While the reasons for the third consecutive annual increase among females are still being examined, this emerging trend deepens concerns about a potential resurgence of syphilis among women, after more than a decade of declining rates.

Rates among African Americans also remain much higher than rates among whites—six times higher for African American men and 13 times higher for African American women. Reported syphilis rates among African American men increased 25% from 2006 and 2007 (17.1 to 21.5 cases per 100,000 population). The rate among African American women rose 12% from 2006 and 2007 (4.8 to 5.4 cases per 100,000 population).

Studies Show Need for Increased Uptake of STD Screening Guidelines for MSM

Since 2002, CDC has recommended that sexually active MSM be tested at least annually for syphilis, chlamydia, and gonorrhea—at all anatomic sites of reported STD exposure (oral, anal, and/or urethral). CDC also recommends at least annual STD testing for all individuals with HIV infection. However, three new studies indicate the urgent need to continue increasing STD screening rates among MSM.

The first, an eight-city STD clinic study led by CDC's Kristen Mahle, found that as many as one-third of gonorrhea infections among MSM who were not HIV-infected were missed because MSM were not tested at all relevant anatomical sites. MSM were tested at all three sites only about half (52%) of the time. In another study, led by CDC researcher Eric Tai, only 49% of MSM surveyed in 15 cities in 2003–2005 reported being tested for syphilis, 35% reported being tested for gonorrhea and only 32% were screened for chlamydia in the past year. The third study, led by CDC's Karen Hoover, found that 82% of HIV-infected MSM in eight cities were tested for syphilis in the past year, but only 22% or fewer were tested for gonorrhea or chlamydia.

Another study, led by Julius Schachter of the University of California, San Francisco, could help pave the way for more thorough STD screening among MSM. The researchers found that a DNA testing method called a nucleic acid amplification test, which is already widely used to screen for genital gonorrhea and chlamydia infections, was able to detect at least twice as many gonorrhea and chlamydia infections in the throat and rectum as a traditional bacterial culture test, which is the current standard of diagnosing infections at extra-genital sites.

"While STD screening is by no means the only weapon in our STD prevention arsenal, it is certainly one of our best tools for ensuring prompt diagnosis and treatment and slowing the transmission of these diseases," said John M. Douglas, Jr., MD, director of CDC's Division of STD Prevention. "We are committed to supporting the efforts of physicians in the community as they work to increase screening among their patients. At the same time, we're working to support broader STD prevention programs for MSM, women, African Americans, and others who remain at risk."

CDC and Partners Intensifying Syphilis Elimination Efforts through Novel Approaches

In light of recent challenges in syphilis prevention, CDC has been working with public health, medical, and community partners since 2006 to implement an updated National Plan to Eliminate Syphilis. These efforts are designed to sustain progress made since the early 1990s in populations traditionally at risk, including African Americans and women of all races, and to support innovative solutions to fight the resurgence of syphilis among MSM. Recent examples of new strategies include the following:

- A revised formula for allocating federal syphilis elimination funding to states and cities, allowing CDC to respond more rapidly to emerging geographical trends in syphilis cases
- Use of a new program evaluation approach to more rapidly modify prevention programs to meet the changing epidemic
- Released new surveillance tool designed to capture behavioral data (such as the gender of sex partners of people infected with syphilis) that provides local and national information to direct our responses to the syphilis epidemic
- Guidance to public health programs about the use of the internet to more effectively reach at-risk populations with prevention approaches, such as health communication to increase community awareness and outreach to encourage testing and partner services

At the conference, one new modeling study underscores the potential for syphilis elimination funding to have an impact on disease rates.

Led by CDC's Harrell Chesson, researchers examined the correlation between state-level syphilis rates and federal syphilis elimination funding from 1999–2005 in the 28 states that were first provided with the funding, beginning in 1998. The researchers found that, in aggregate, these 28 states had either larger decreases or smaller increases in syphilis rates throughout the period than did other states, which either received syphilis elimination funding in later years or not at all.

Section 30.4

Syphilis and HIV/AIDS Co-Infection

"Syphilis lowers CD4 cell count and increases viral load in HIV-positive men," by Michael Carter. © 2004 NAM (www.aidsmap.com). Reprinted with permission.

Syphilis infection in HIV-positive men is associated with an increase in viral load and reduction in CD4 cell count, according to an American study published in the October 21, 2004 edition of *AIDS*. The study investigators believe that their findings indicate that HIV-positive men with syphilis are potentially more infectious and call for integrated public health campaigns to prevent the spread of both HIV and syphilis.

Although it is known that syphilitic ulcers can facilitate HIV transmission, the effect of syphilis on HIV viral load and CD4 cell count has been little studied. Other sexually transmitted infections have been linked to changes in immune status, and investigators in San Francisco wished to see if infection with syphilis had an impact on the viral load and CD4 cell counts of HIV-positive men.

In common with many other cities in the United States and Europe, there has been a substantial increase in the number of cases of primary and secondary syphilis diagnosed in gay men in San Francisco in recent years. Surveillance data for other sexually transmitted infections and behavioral studies also suggest an increase in risky sexual behavior amongst gay men.

Using a retrospective review of public health records, investigators identified a total of 52 cases of primary or secondary syphilis in

HIV-positive men in San Francisco between early 2001 and spring 2003. The men had a median age of 36 years.

In total, 35 men (67%) had secondary syphilis, and 30 (58%) were taking highly active antiretroviral therapy (HAART) at the time of their syphilis diagnosis. The overwhelming majority of men received between one and three injections of benzathine penicillin to treat their syphilis and this therapy was successful in all but two patients.

A total of 36 men had their HIV viral load measured before and during their infection with syphilis. The investigators noted that during syphilis infection viral load in these men increased significantly by a mean 0.21 $\log_{10}$ ($p = 0.02$). In men with secondary syphilis viral load increased by a mean of 0.33 $\log_{10}$, and amongst men not taking HAART the mean increase in viral load was 0.25 $\log_{10}$. Among the 10 men who had secondary syphilis and were not taking HAART, viral load was increased by a mean of 0.34 $\log_{10}$ during syphilis infection ($p = 0.05$).

Of the 26 men who had a detectable viral load before infection with syphilis, 13 experienced an increase in their viral load during infection with syphilis, and 12 of these men had an increase of 0.50 $\log_{10}$. However, of the 10 men taking HAART who had an undetectable viral load before syphilis was diagnosed, only two men had a detectable viral load during infection with syphilis.

For 35 men, data were available on viral load during and after infection with syphilis. Amongst these men, viral load did not decrease significantly after syphilis was treated (mean fall in viral load 0.10 $\log_{10}$).

In further analysis, the investigators looked at viral load in men for whom data were available on viral load before, during, and after syphilis. The mean increase in viral load was 0.10 $\log_{10}$ during infection with syphilis, and viral load fell by 0.3 $\log_{10}$ after syphilis was treated. Viral load increased by a mean of 0.007 $\log_{10}$ after syphilis compared to the level of viral load before syphilis infection. None of these changes in viral load was statistically significant.

The investigators also looked at the effect of syphilis infection on CD4 cell count. Amongst the 31 men who had before and during CD4 cell measurements available, the investigators noted a mean drop in CD4 cell count of 62 cells/mm^3 ($p = 0.04$). The decreases in CD4 cell count were most notable in men who had secondary syphilis and were not taking HAART. Although CD4 cell count increased by a mean of 33 cells/mm^3 after syphilis was treated, this change was not statistically significant ($p = 0.23$).

For 15 men, data on CD4 cell count before, during, and after syphilis infection were available. No significant changes in CD4 cell count were seen in this subset of individuals.

"Syphilis infection was associated with a significant increase in the plasma viral load and a significant decrease in CD4 cell counts in HIV-infected men," write the investigators. They point out that these changes were most notable in men with secondary infection, which could be the result of greater immune activation.

The investigators admit that their study has several limitations, not least that data on CD4 cell count and viral load before, during, and after syphilis infection were available for only 19 men. The investigators call for larger confirmatory studies.

"Syphilis infection in HIV-infected men was associated with a significant increase in viral load and a significant decrease in CD4 cell count...Integrated public health efforts to prevent new syphilis infections [are required]...to reduce the spread of both diseases within affected communities," conclude the investigators.

Reference

Buchacz K et al. Syphilis increases HIV viral load and decreases CD4 cell counts in HIV-infected patients with new syphilis infections. *AIDS* 18: 2075–2079, 2004.

Chapter 31

Trichomoniasis

What is trichomoniasis?

Trichomoniasis is a common sexually transmitted disease (STD) that affects both women and men, although symptoms are more common in women.

How common is trichomoniasis?

Trichomoniasis is the most common curable STD in young, sexually active women. An estimated 7.4 million new cases occur each year in women and men.

How do people get trichomoniasis?

Trichomoniasis is caused by the single-celled protozoan parasite, *Trichomonas vaginalis*. The vagina is the most common site of infection in women, and the urethra (urine canal) is the most common site of infection in men.

The parasite is sexually transmitted through penis-to-vagina intercourse or vulva-to-vulva (the genital area outside the vagina) contact with an infected partner. Women can acquire the disease from infected men or women, but men usually contract it only from infected women.

"Trichomoniasis Fact Sheet," Centers for Disease Control and Prevention (www.cdc.gov), December 19, 2007.

What are the signs and symptoms of trichomoniasis?

Most men with trichomoniasis do not have signs or symptoms; however, some men may temporarily have an irritation inside the penis, mild discharge, or slight burning after urination or ejaculation.

Some women have signs or symptoms of infection which include a frothy, yellow-green vaginal discharge with a strong odor. The infection also may cause discomfort during intercourse and urination, as well as irritation and itching of the female genital area. In rare cases, lower abdominal pain can occur. Symptoms usually appear in women within 5 to 28 days of exposure.

What are the complications of trichomoniasis?

The genital inflammation caused by trichomoniasis can increase a woman's susceptibility to HIV infection if she is exposed to the virus. Having trichomoniasis may increase the chance that an HIV-infected woman passes HIV to her sex partner(s).

How does trichomoniasis affect a pregnant woman and her baby?

Pregnant women with trichomoniasis may have babies who are born early or with low birth weight (low birth weight is less than 5.5 pounds).

How is trichomoniasis diagnosed?

For both men and women, a health care provider must perform a physical examination and laboratory test to diagnose trichomoniasis. The parasite is harder to detect in men than in women. In women, a pelvic examination can reveal small red ulcerations (sores) on the vaginal wall or cervix.

What is the treatment for trichomoniasis?

Trichomoniasis can usually be cured with prescription drugs, either metronidazole or tinidazole, given by mouth in a single dose. The symptoms of trichomoniasis in infected men may disappear within a few weeks without treatment. However, an infected man, even a man who has never had symptoms or whose symptoms have stopped, can continue to infect or re-infect a female partner until he has been treated. Therefore, both partners should be treated at the same time to eliminate the parasite. Persons being treated for trichomoniasis should avoid sex until they and their sex partners complete treatment and have no symptoms. Metronidazole can be used by pregnant women.

Having trichomoniasis once does not protect a person from getting it again. Following successful treatment, people can still be susceptible to re-infection.

How can trichomoniasis be prevented?

The surest way to avoid transmission of sexually transmitted diseases is to abstain from sexual contact, or to be in a long-term mutually monogamous relationship with a partner who has been tested and is known to be uninfected.

Latex male condoms, when used consistently and correctly, can reduce the risk of transmission of trichomoniasis.

Any genital symptom such as discharge or burning during urination or an unusual sore or rash should be a signal to stop having sex and to consult a health care provider immediately. A person diagnosed with trichomoniasis (or any other STD) should receive treatment and should notify all recent sex partners so that they can see a health care provider and be treated. This reduces the risk that the sex partners will develop complications from trichomoniasis and reduces the risk that the person with trichomoniasis will become re-infected. Sex should be stopped until the person with trichomoniasis and all of his or her recent partners complete treatment for trichomoniasis and have no symptoms.

Sources

Centers for Disease Control and Prevention. Sexually transmitted diseases treatment guidelines 2006. *MMWR.* 2006: 55 (No. RR-11).

Krieger JN and Alderete JF. Trichomonas vaginalis and trichomoniasis. In: K. Holmes, P. Markh, P. Sparling et al (eds). *Sexually Transmitted Diseases*, 3rd Edition. New York: McGraw-Hill; 1999, 587–604.

Weinstock H, Berman S, Cates W. Sexually transmitted disease among American youth: Incidence and prevalence estimates, 2000. *Perspectives on Sexual and Reproductive Health.* 2004;36: 6–10.

Chapter 32

Vaginosis Caused by Bacteria

Chapter Contents

Section 32.1

Understanding Bacterial Vaginosis

"Bacterial Vaginosis," National Institute for Allergy and Infectious Diseases (www3.niaid.nih.gov), September 1, 2008.

According to the Centers for Disease Control and Prevention (CDC), bacterial vaginosis (BV) is the most common cause of vaginitis symptoms among women of childbearing age. It previously was called nonspecific vaginitis, or Gardnerella-associated vaginitis. Health experts are not sure what role sexual activity plays in developing BV.

Cause

BV is a sign of a change in the growth of vaginal bacteria. The resulting chemical imbalance occurs when different types of bacteria outnumber the normal "good," or beneficial, ones. Instead of *Lactobacillus* (a type bacteria that normally lives in the vagina) being most common, increased numbers of bacteria such as *Gardnerella vaginalis*, *Bacteroides*, *Mobiluncus*, and *Mycoplasma hominis* inhabit the vaginas of women with BV.

Transmission

Although health experts are not sure what role sexual activity plays in developing BV, a change in sexual partners or having multiple sexual partners may increase a woman's chances of getting the infection. Using an IUD (intrauterine device) and douching also may increase her risk of getting BV.

Symptoms

The main symptom of BV is an abnormal, foul-smelling vaginal discharge. Some women describe it as a fish-like odor that is most noticeable after having sex.

Other symptoms may include the following:

- Thin vaginal discharge, usually white or gray in color
- Pain during urination
- Itching around the vagina

Some women who have signs of BV, such as increased levels of certain harmful bacteria, have no symptoms. A health care provider who sees these signs during a physical examination can confirm the diagnosis by doing lab tests of vaginal fluid.

Diagnosis

A health care provider can examine a sample of vaginal fluid under a microscope, either stained or in special lighting, to look for bacteria associated with BV. Then, they can diagnose BV based on the following symptoms:

- Absence of lactobacilli
- Presence of numerous "clue cells" (cells from the vaginal lining that are coated with BV germs)
- Fishy odor
- Change from normal vaginal fluid

Treatment

Health care providers use antibiotics such as metronidazole or clindamycin to treat women with BV. Generally, male sex partners will not be treated. For updated information about the treatment for BV and other sexually transmitted infections, read the Centers for Disease Control and Prevention Sexually Transmitted Diseases Treatment Guidelines (http://www.cdc.gov/std/treatment/).

Complications

In most cases, BV causes no complications. There have been documented risks of BV, however, such as an association between BV and pelvic inflammatory disease (PID). PID is a serious disease in women that can cause infertility and tubal (ectopic) pregnancy.

BV also can cause other problems such as premature delivery and low-birth-weight babies. Therefore, some health experts recommend that all pregnant women who previously have delivered a premature baby be checked for BV, whether or not they have symptoms. A pregnant woman who has not delivered a premature baby should be treated if she has symptoms and laboratory evidence of BV.

BV also is associated with increased chances of getting one or more sexually transmitted infections (STIs), including chlamydia, gonorrhea, or HIV infection.

Section 32.2

Vaginosis and the Risk of AIDS

"Common vaginal infection may double HIV acquisition risk," by Edwin J. Bernard. © 2005 NAM (www.aidsmap.com). Reprinted with permission.

Bacterial vaginosis, the most common vaginal infection in women of childbearing age, may double a woman's susceptibility to HIV infection, according to the results of a South African study published in the October 15, 2005 edition of the *Journal of Infectious Diseases,* which is now available online. If more effective diagnosis and treatment were available, argues an accompanying editorial, HIV infection rates in the developing world could be substantially reduced.

Bacterial vaginosis (BV) is a condition in women where the normal balance of bacteria in the vagina is disrupted, resulting in a change from an acidic to an alkaline environment. Although it is sometimes accompanied by symptoms such as discharge, odor, pain, itching, or burning, it is often asymptomatic. Although no pathogen has been isolated as the cause, it is considered to be a sexually transmitted infection, and, since it affects between 20%–25% of the general population, and up to 50% of women attending sexual health clinics, it is the most common STI worldwide. BV has been implicated in premature delivery in pregnant women and in the development of pelvic inflammatory disease.

Several—but not all—epidemiological and prospective studies have found an association between BV and HIV infection. In addition, in-vitro studies suggest that BV has the potential to increase susceptibility to HIV infection, possibly through increased production of interleukin (IL)-10 and/or increased secretion of tumor necrosis factor-alpha (TNF-α) and IL-1β.

Given the high prevalence of BV and HIV in many parts of sub-Saharan Africa, identifying and treating BV could have significant implications for HIV prevention. Consequently, investigators at the University of Cape Town, South Africa, sought to ascertain whether there was indeed an association between BV and HIV acquisition.

They conducted a case-control study, nested within a randomized controlled trial evaluating cervical cancer screening in Khayelitsha, near Cape Town. Of the 5,110 women who were HIV-negative at enrollment (between June 2000 and December 2002), the investigators selected all women who had seroconverted by December 2003 (n=86; overall incidence rate, 2.1/100 person-years) for this study. The majority of seroconversions (64%) were identified at the six-month follow-up visit, although the investigators report that risk of seroconversion remained constant throughout the 36-month follow-up period (data not shown).

A further 324 age-matched women were selected at random from the cohort as controls.

Women who seroconverted were significantly more likely to be unmarried, to report having had more than one sex partner in the month before enrollment, and to report having a new sex partner at the six-month follow-up visit.

BV was assessed only once, during the enrollment visit, by gynecological examination (Amsel criteria). Blinded microbiologic assessment (Nugent scoring) of Gram-stained slides also assessed BV status.

Using Amsel criteria, only 20% of the HIV-positive women were found to have BV, compared with 16% of the controls. However, using Nugent scoring, 74% of the seroconverters with suitable samples (n=59) had a BV diagnosis (Nugent scores between 7–10) compared with 62% of controls (n=189). Compared to the women with normal vaginal flora, the women who seroconverted were significantly more likely to have BV, as diagnosed by Nugent scoring (summary odds ratio [OR], 1.83; 95% CI, 1.00–3.85).

In multivariate analysis, after adjusting for demographic characteristics, other STIs and sexual behaviors, women with BV diagnosed by Nugent scoring were significantly more likely to seroconvert than women with normal vaginal flora (adjusted OR, 2.01; 95% CI, 1.12–3.62).

The investigators point out several limitations to their study, including the fact that BV was assessed only once and HIV seroconversions were identified over three years. During this time, vaginal flora may have changed, and a baseline BV assessment may not accurately reflect presence of BV at the time of seroconversion. The investigators also did not assess the presence of ulcerative STIs, including herpes simplex virus 2 (HSV-2), which have been found to increase HIV acquisition risk. It is also possible that other unknown confounding measures may have inflated the association between BV and HIV acquisition.

However, they conclude "if BV increases women's susceptibly to HIV infection, interventions to reduce the occurrence of BV may have an impact on the spread of HIV at a population level. The high prevalence of BV in our study population means that almost one-third of all new HIV infections in women in this setting might be prevented if all cases of BV could be cured."

Nevertheless, an accompanying editorial by Dr. Jane Schwebke of the University of Alabama at Birmingham points out that "present achievable BV cure rates, combined with high recurrence rates make this solution impracticable."

Although many of the women in the study (27% of seroconverters and 23% of controls) were treated for BV with the antibiotic metronidazole, this made no difference to HIV seroconversion rates. Indeed, a recent study from Kenya found that antibiotic prophylaxis failed to reduce HIV seroconversions.

In order to make a difference, more research into the cause, diagnosis, and treatment of BV is urgently required, argues Dr. Schwebke. "Until efficacious therapy, as well as an understanding of prevention methods, for BV is available," she concludes, "it will not be feasible to go forward with studies aimed at preventing the complications of this common vaginal infection."

References

Myer L et al. Bacterial vaginosis and susceptibility to HIV infection in South African women: a nested case-control study. *JID* 192: 000–000, 2005.

Schwebke JR. Abnormal vaginal flora as a biological risk factor for acquisition of HIV infection and sexually transmitted diseases. *JID* 192: 000–000, 2005.

Chapter 33

Less Common STDs and Their Treatments

Chapter Contents

Section 33.1

Candidiasis (Yeast Infections)

"Genital/Vulvovaginal Candidiasis (VVC)," excerpted from "Candidiasis," Centers for Disease Control and Prevention (www.cdc.gov), March 27, 2008.

What is genital candidiasis/VVC?

Candidiasis, also known as a "yeast infection" or VVC, is a common fungal infection that occurs when there is overgrowth of the fungus called *Candida*. *Candida* is always present in the body in small amounts. However, when an imbalance occurs, such as when the normal acidity of the vagina changes or when hormonal balance changes, *Candida* can multiply. When that happens, symptoms of candidiasis appear.

What are the symptoms of genital candidiasis/VVC?

Women with VVC usually experience genital itching or burning, with or without a "cottage cheese-like" vaginal discharge. Males with genital candidiasis may experience an itchy rash on the penis.

How is genital candidiasis/VVC transmitted?

Nearly 75% of all adult women have had at least one genital "yeast infection" in their lifetime. On rare occasions, men may also experience genital candidiasis. VVC occurs more frequently and more severely in people with weakened immune systems. The following are some other conditions that may put a woman at risk for genital candidiasis:

- Pregnancy
- Diabetes mellitus
- Use of broad-spectrum antibiotics
- Use of corticosteroid medications

What are the symptoms of genital candidiasis/VVC?

Most cases of *Candida* infection are caused by the person's own *Candida* organisms. *Candida* yeasts usually live in the mouth, gastrointestinal tract, and vagina without causing symptoms. Symptoms develop only when *Candida* becomes overgrown in these sites. Rarely, *Candida* can be passed from person to person, such as through sexual intercourse.

How is genital candidiasis/VVC diagnosed?

The symptoms of genital candidiasis are similar to those of many other genital infections. Usually the diagnosis is made by taking a sample of the vaginal secretions and looking at it under a microscope to see if *Candida* organisms are present.

How is genital candidiasis/VVC treated?

Several antifungal drugs are available to treat genital candidiasis/VVC. Antifungal vaginal suppositories or creams are commonly used. The duration of the treatment course of suppositories and creams ranges from single dose therapy to seven days of therapy. Uncomplicated VVC may also be treated with single-dose, oral fluconazole. Oral fluconazole should be avoided in pregnancy. These drugs usually work to cure the infection (80%–90% success rate), but some people will have recurrent or resistant infections. Short-course treatments should be avoided in recurrent or resistant infection.

What is the difference between the three-day treatments and the seven-day treatments for genital candidiasis/VVC?

The only difference between these is the length of treatment. Three-day and seven-day treatments may both be effective.

Are over-the-counter (OTC) treatments for genital candidiasis/VVC safe to use?

Over-the-counter treatments for VVC are available. As a result, more women are diagnosing themselves with VVC and using one of a family of drugs called "azoles" for therapy. However, misdiagnosis is common, and studies have shown that as many as two-thirds of all OTC drugs sold to treat VVC were used by women without the disease. Using these drugs when they are not needed may lead to a resistant infection. Resistant infections are very difficult to treat with the currently available medications for VVC.

Can Candida *infections become resistant to treatment?*

Overuse of these antifungal medications can increase the chance that they will eventually not work (the fungus develops resistance to medications). Therefore, it is important to be sure of the diagnosis before treating with over-the-counter or other antifungal medications.

What will happen if a person does not seek treatment for genital candidiasis/VVC?

Symptoms, which may be very uncomfortable, may persist. There is a chance that the infection may be passed between sex partners.

How can someone tell the difference between genital candidiasis/VVC and a urinary tract infection?

Because VVC and urinary tract infections share similar symptoms, such as a burning sensation when urinating, it is important to see a doctor and obtain laboratory testing to determine the cause of the symptoms and to treat effectively.

Section 33.2

Granuloma Inguinale (Donovanosis)

What is granuloma inguinale?

Granuloma inguinale is a chronic bacterial infection of the genital region, generally regarded to be sexually transmitted.

Who gets granuloma inguinale?

Granuloma inguinale is a relatively rare disease occurring in people living in tropical and subtropical areas. It occurs more frequently in males. In the United States, while homosexuals are at greater risk, it is relatively rare in heterosexual partners of those infected.

How is granuloma inguinale spread?

Granuloma inguinale is thought to be spread by sexual contact with an infected individual.

What are the symptoms of granuloma inguinale?

The disease begins with the appearance of lumps or blisters in the genital area. The blister becomes a slowly enlarging open sore.

How soon do symptoms appear?

The incubation period appears to be between eight and 80 days after infection.

When and for how long is a person able to spread granuloma inguinale?

Granuloma inguinale is communicable as long as the infected person remains untreated and bacteria from lesions are present.

Does past infection with granuloma inguinale make a person immune?

Past infection does not make a person immune. Susceptibility is variable. There is no evidence of natural resistance.

What is the treatment for granuloma inguinale?

There are several antibiotics that will effectively cure granuloma inguinale. Response to the antibiotic should be evident within seven days and total healing usually occurs within three to five weeks.

What complications can result from granuloma inguinale?

If left untreated, granuloma inguinale can result in extensive destruction of genital organs and may also spread to other parts of the body.

How can the spread of granuloma inguinale be prevented?

- Limit the number of sex partners.
- Use a condom.
- Carefully wash the genitals after sexual relations.

- If you think you are infected, avoid any sexual contact and visit your local sexually transmitted disease (STD) clinic, a hospital, or your doctor.
- Notify all sexual contacts immediately so they can obtain medical care.

Section 33.3

Lymphogranuloma Venereum (LGV)

"Lymphogranuloma Venereum (LGV) Fact Sheet," Centers for Disease Control and Prevention (www.cdc.gov), January 4, 2008.

What is LGV?

LGV (*Lymphogranuloma venereum*) is a sexually transmitted disease caused by three strains of the bacterium *Chlamydia trachomatis.* The visual signs include genital papule(s) (e.g., raised surface or bumps) and or ulcers, and swelling of the lymph glands in the genital area. LGV may also produce rectal ulcers, bleeding, pain, and discharge, especially among those who practice receptive anal intercourse. Genital lesions caused by LGV can be mistaken for other ulcerative STDs such as syphilis, genital herpes, and chancroid. Complications of untreated LGV may include enlargement and ulcerations of the external genitalia and lymphatic obstruction, which may lead to elephantiasis of the genitalia.

How common is LGV?

Signs and symptoms associated with rectal infection can be mistakenly thought to be caused by ulcerative colitis. While the frequency of LGV infection is thought to be rare in industrialized countries, its identification is not always obvious, so the number of cases of LGV in the United States is unknown. However, outbreaks in the Netherlands and other European countries among men who have sex with men (MSM) have raised concerns about cases of LGV in the U.S.

How do people get LGV?

LGV is passed from person to person through direct contact with lesions, ulcers, or other area where the bacteria is located. Transmission of the organism occurs during sexual penetration (vaginal, oral, or anal) and may also occur via skin-to-skin contact. The likelihood of LGV infection following an exposure is unknown, but it is considered less infectious than some other STDs. A person who has had sexual contact with a LGV-infected partner within 60 days of symptom onset should be examined, tested for urethral or cervical chlamydial infection, and treated with doxycycline, twice daily for seven days.

What are the signs and symptoms?

LGV can be difficult to diagnose. Typically, the primary lesion produced by LGV is a small genital or rectal lesion, which can ulcerate at the site of transmission after an incubation period of 3–30 days. These ulcers may remain undetected within the urethra, vagina, or rectum. As with other STDs that cause ulcers, LGV may facilitate transmission and acquisition of HIV.

How is LGV diagnosed?

Because of limitations in a commercially available test, diagnosis is primarily based on clinical findings. Direct identification of the bacteria from a lesion or site of the infection may be possible through testing for chlamydia but, this would not indicate if the chlamydia infection is LGV. However, the usual chlamydia tests that are available have not been U.S. Food and Drug Administration (FDA) approved for testing rectal specimens. In a patient with rectal signs or symptoms suspicious for LGV, a health care provider can collect a specimen and send the sample to his/her state health department for referral to CDC, which is working with state and local health departments to test specimens and validate diagnostic methods for LGV.

What is the treatment for LGV?

There is no vaccine against the bacteria. LGV can be treated with three weeks of antibiotics. CDC STD Treatment Guidelines recommend the use of doxycycline, twice a day for 21 days. An alternative treatment is erythromycin base or azithromycin. The health care provider will determine which is best.

If you have been treated for LGV, you should notify any sex partners you had sex with within 60 days of the symptom onset so they can be evaluated and treated. This will reduce the risk that your partners will develop symptoms and/or serious complications of LGV. It will reduce your risk of becoming re-infected as well as reduce the risk of ongoing transmission in the community. You and all of your sex partners should avoid sex until you have completed treatment for the infection and your symptoms and your partners' symptoms have disappeared.

Note: Doxycycline is not recommended for use in pregnant women. Pregnant and lactating women should be treated with erythromycin. Azithromycin may prove useful for treatment of LGV in pregnancy, but no published data are available regarding its safety and efficacy. A health care provider (like a doctor or nurse) can discuss treatment options with patients.

Persons with both LGV and HIV infection should receive the same LGV treatment as those who are HIV-negative. Prolonged therapy may be required, and delay in resolution of symptoms may occur among persons with HIV.

How can LGV be prevented?

The surest way to avoid transmission of sexually transmitted diseases is to abstain from sexual contact, or to be in a long-term mutually monogamous relationship with a partner who has been tested and is asymptomatic and uninfected.

Male latex condoms, when used consistently and correctly, may reduce the risk of LGV transmission. Genital ulcer diseases can occur in male or female genital areas that may or may not be covered (protected by the condom).

Having had LGV and completing treatment does not prevent re-infection. Effective treatment is available and it is important that persons suspected of having LGV be treated as if they have it. Persons who are treated for LGV treatment should abstain from sexual contact until the infection is cleared.

Section 33.4

Nongonococcal Urethritis (NGU)

What is NGU?

Non-gonococcal urethritis is a term that describes a combination of symptoms that occur in men, most often causing "urethritis" or an inflammation of the opening into the bladder. It is not a "bladder infection" and can be caused by several different sexually transmitted bacteria. Men should be tested for gonorrhea and chlamydia first, before diagnosing the symptoms as NGU.

What are the symptoms?

- Pain when urinating
- Discharge from the penis, usually clear
- Burning or itching around the opening of the penis

Often there are only mild or occasional symptoms. Some men have no symptoms at all.

Can women get NGU?

Yes, although in women it often causes problems in the reproductive tract (uterus, fallopian tubes) instead of the urethra. If a man is treated for NGU, his sexual partner(s) should be treated also.

Anal to vaginal sex without changing condoms can introduce bacteria from the rectum into the vagina. This can lead to an infection. There is no specific lab test for NGU.

How is it spread?

- NGU is spread through anal, oral, and vaginal sex with an infected partner.

- For men, having anal sex without a condom can result in these symptoms. The bacteria from the rectum can get into the urethra and bladder, causing an infection.

How is it treated?

- NGU is treated with antibiotics.
- Take all the medications as prescribed, even if you start to feel better and the symptoms are gone.
- Your sex partner(s) need to be seen and treated.
- Early treatment can prevent lasting damage to your body.

Are there long-term complications?

Yes. If left untreated, NGU may lead to:

- infertility;
- problem pregnancies (miscarriage, premature deliveries);
- infections in newborns;
- pelvic inflammatory disease (PID);
- chronic pelvic pain; and
- epididymitis (inflammation of the testicles).

How is it prevented?

- Don't have sex. You cannot give or get a sexually transmitted disease if there is no contact with the penis, vagina, mouth or anus.
- Limit your number of sexual partners. The more people you have sex with, the greater the chance of getting an STD.
- If you choose to have sex, be prepared. Have condoms with a water-based lubricant on hand and use a new condom every time you have sex.
- Have regular exams if you are sexually active. If you think you have an STD, get tested. Ask your partner(s) to get tested.
- Remember: a Pap smear is not an STD test. Ask to be tested for STDs if you are at risk.
- Telling your partner. If you are diagnosed with NGU, tell anyone you have recently had sex with that they should be treated.

Section 33.5

Sexually Transmitted Intestinal and Enteric Infections: Proctitis, Proctocolitis, and Enteritis

This section excerpted from "Canadian Guidelines on Sexually Transmitted Infections, 2006 Edition," Public Health Agency of Canada, 2006. Reproduced with permission of the Minister of Public Works and Government Services Canada, 2008.

Definitions

Proctitis: Inflammation limited to the rectal mucosa, not extending beyond 10–12 cm of the anal verge. Transmission of the involved pathogens is usually due to direct inoculation into the rectum during anal intercourse.

Proctocolitis: Inflammation of the rectal mucosa and of the colon extending above 10–12 cm of the anal verge; generally has an infectious etiology different from proctitis. Transmission is usually fecal-oral.

Enteritis: Inflammation of the duodenum, jejunum, and/or ileum. Transmission is usually fecal-oral.

Etiology

- Sexually transmitted intestinal syndromes involve a wide variety of pathogens at different sites of the gastrointestinal tract.
- The diversity of sexually transmissible pathogens responsible for intestinal disease remains a challenge for the clinician.
- Polymicrobial infection often occurs, causing an overlap of symptoms.
- Infections of the anus and rectum are often sexually transmitted and typically occur in men and women who engage in unprotected receptive anal intercourse.

- Sexually transmitted infections (STIs) should always be considered, but trauma and foreign bodies may result in findings suggestive of proctitis or proctocolitis.
- Some anorectal infections in women are secondary to the contiguous spread of the pathogens from the genitalia.
- Infections with pathogens traditionally associated with food- or water-borne acquisition are known to occur via sexual transmission, most often via the fecal-oral route.
- Infections are often more severe in persons infected with HIV, and the list of potential causes is greater.
- In persons with advanced HIV infection, consider cryptosporidium and microsporidium.

Table 33.1 lists the pathogens involved in the common sexually transmitted gastrointestinal syndromes and their modes of acquisition.

Epidemiology

- Sexual practices of individuals often involve direct or indirect contact with the rectal mucosal membranes (i.e., sharing sex toys).

Table 33.1. Common sexually transmitted gastrointestinal syndromes

Syndrome	Pathogen(s)	Mode of acquisition
Proctitis	• *Neisseria gonorrhoeae* • *Chlamydia trachomatis* (LGV and non-LGV serovars) • *Treponema pallidum* • Herpes simplex virus	Receptive anal intercourse in the majority of cases
Proctocolitis	• *Entamoeba histolytica* • *Campylobacter* species • *Salmonella* species • *Shigella* species • *C. trachomatis* (LGV serovars)	Direct or indirect fecal-oral contact
Enteritis	• *Giardia lamblia*	Direct or indirect fecal-oral contact

LGV=lymphogranuloma venereum

- Sexually transmitted intestinal syndromes occur commonly in men who have sex with men who engage in unprotected anal intercourse or oral-anal and oral-genital sexual activities.
- Heterosexual men and women can also be at risk for acquiring enteric infections by oral-anal sexual activities.
- Women can acquire sexually transmitted anorectal pathogens by unprotected anal intercourse.
- Unprotected anal intercourse is being reported more frequently among several subpopulations, such as sexually active adolescents and street youth.

Prevention

- Since anal intercourse is the main mode of sexual transmission for pathogens that cause proctitis, clinicians should identify barriers to prevention practices and discuss means to overcome them.
- Since oral-anal sexual activities are the main mode of acquisition for sexually transmitted proctocolitis and enteritis, the risks of fecal-oral contamination should be discussed, particularly with sex trade workers and men who have sex with men.

Manifestations

- Typical presenting symptoms of the different sexually transmitted intestinal syndromes are listed in Table 33.2.
- Asymptomatic infections are also prevalent.
- Clinicians should routinely inquire about specific sexual activities, regardless of the patient's reported sexual preference.

Diagnosis

- If a symptomatic patient reports any anorectal sexual activities, anoscopic evaluation should be a routine part of the physical examination.
- Specimen collection should be adapted to the clinical presentation and history, including possible exposure to lymphogranuloma venereum. For example, in some cases of enteric infections, evaluation for sexually transmitted pathogens might not be relevant.

- Anoscopic examination for proctitis:
  - Obtain rectal swabs for culture, preferably under direct vision through an anoscope, for appropriate diagnostic testing for *Neisseria gonorrhoeae*, *Chlamydia trachomatis* (further testing is required for positive cultures to differentiate between Chlamydia and LGV infections), and herpes simplex virus (HSV).
  - A specimen from the lesions should also be collected for a diagnostic test for HSV.
  - Syphilis serology should also be performed in all patients.
  - Although nucleic acid amplification tests (NAATs) are available for detection of gonococcal and chlamydial infections in urogenital specimens, they have not been extensively studied for rectal specimens.
- If indicated by clinical presentation and/or history: collect stool specimen for culture for enteric pathogens and examination for ova and parasites.

Management and Treatment

- Treatment of sexually transmitted intestinal infections should be based on physical findings.

Table 33.2. Possible symptoms of sexually transmitted intestinal syndromes

Syndrome	List of possible symptoms
Proctitis	• Anorectal pain • Tenesmus • Constipation • Hematochezia (bloody stools) • Mucopurulent discharge
Proctocolitis	• Proctitis symptoms • Diarrhoea • Cramps • Abdominal pain • Fever
Enteritis	• Diarrhoea • Cramps • Bloating • Nausea

- A high index of suspicion concerning the different etiological agents should be maintained by the clinician.
- Most often, treatment of suspected proctitis will be empirical and should not await test results.

Consideration for Other STIs

- Proctitis is associated with specific high-risk sexual activities; therefore, patients presenting with symptoms should be evaluated for other STIs.
- Counselling and testing for HIV are recommended.
- Screening for hepatitis B markers may be considered in certain high-risk individuals before considering immunization.
- Immunization against hepatitis A and B is recommended.
- Serologic testing for syphilis should be strongly considered in all individuals presenting with proctitis.
- For women, discuss HPV vaccine as per the recommendations outlined in the Canada Communicable Disease Report, Volume 33 ACS-2, (2007) *National Advisory Committee on Immunization (NACI) statement on human papillomavirus vaccine*.

Reporting and Partner Notification

- Patients with conditions that are notifiable according to provincial and territorial laws and regulations should be reported to the local public health authority.
- When treatment for proctitis is indicated, all partners who have had sexual contact with the index case within 60 days prior to onset of symptoms or date of diagnosis (if asymptomatic) should be located, clinically evaluated, and treated with the same regimen as the index case regardless of clinical findings and without waiting for test results.
- Local public health authorities are available to assist with partner notification and help with appropriate referral for clinical evaluation, testing, treatment, and health education.

Follow-up

- Follow-up should be arranged for every patient. If a recommended treatment regimen has been given and properly taken, symptoms and signs have disappeared and there has been no re-exposure to any untreated partner, then repeat diagnostic testing for *N. gonorrhoeae* and *C. trachomatis* is not routinely recommended.

- In cases of confirmed syphilis, appropriate serological follow-up according to syphilis recommendations should be carried out.

Special Considerations

- Despite movement toward more social consciousness and awareness of STIs and diversity in sexual practices, real and perceived prejudice on the part of some clinicians against anorectal activities may contribute to a reluctance to seek medical care or to disclose sexual behaviours.

Children

- All persons named as suspects in child sexual abuse cases should be located and clinically evaluated; prophylactic treatment may or may not be offered and the decision to treat or not should be based on history, clinical findings, and test results.

Part Four

Testing and Diagnosing Sexually Transmitted Diseases

Chapter 34

Who Should Get Tested for STDs

Who should be tested for sexually transmitted diseases (STDs)?

Note: Your doctor may recommend additional STD tests based on your sexual history, signs, symptoms, etc.

Sexually active women 25 years and older.

- Chlamydia testing every year

Sexually active men or women, who are not in a long term, mutually monogamous relationship.

- Hepatitis B vaccination
- Annual HIV testing
- Chlamydia, as recommended by your health care provider

All men who have sex with men (MSM).

- Hepatitis A vaccination
- Hepatitis B vaccination

"Frequently Asked Questions," National HIV and STD Testing Resources, a service of the Centers for Disease Control and Prevention (www.hivtest.org), undated. Accessed December 22, 2008. Reviewed in January 2009 by Dr. David A. Cooke, M.D., Diplomate, American Board of Internal Medicine.

Sexually active men who have sex with men, who are not in a long term, mutually monogamous relationship.

- Hepatitis A vaccination
- Hepatitis B vaccination

At least once every year for the following tests:

- HIV
- Syphilis
- Chlamydia
- Gonorrhea

Pregnant women.

- Chlamydia, at first prenatal visit
- Syphilis, at first prenatal visit
- HIV, as early as possible in the pregnancy
- Hepatitis B, during an early prenatal visit
- Hepatitis C, as recommended by your health care provider
- Gonorrhea, as recommended by your health care provider

Any person seeking STD evaluation or treatments.

- Testing for HIV
- Hepatitis B vaccination
- Testing for syphilis, gonorrhea, chlamydia, as recommended by your health care provider

Should I get an HIV test?

The following are behaviors that increase your chances of getting HIV. If you answer yes to any of them, you should definitely get an HIV test. If you continue with any of these behaviors, you should be tested every year. Talk to a health care provider about an HIV testing schedule that is right for you.

- Have you injected drugs or steroids or shared equipment (such as needles, syringes, works) with others?

- Have you had unprotected vaginal, anal, or oral sex with men who have sex with men, multiple partners, or anonymous partners?
- Have you exchanged sex for drugs or money?
- Have you been diagnosed with or treated for hepatitis, tuberculosis (TB), or a sexually transmitted disease, like syphilis?
- Have you had unprotected sex with someone who could answer yes to any of the above questions?

If you have had sex with someone whose history of sex partners and/or drug use is unknown to you or if you or your partner has had many sex partners, then you have more of a chance of being infected with HIV. Both you and your new partner should get tested for HIV, and learn the results, before having sex for the first time.

For women who plan to become pregnant, testing is even more important. If a woman is infected with HIV, medical care and certain drugs given during pregnancy can lower the chance of passing HIV to her baby. All women who are pregnant should be tested during each pregnancy.

Chapter 35

Getting Tested for STDs If You Have Been Sexually Assaulted

Sexual assault can be an extremely traumatic experience. You may have been hurt both physically and emotionally. Feelings of anger, guilt, shame, and fear are common reactions. In addition to dealing with these strong emotions, you may also be concerned about being infected with a sexually transmitted disease or HIV, the virus that causes AIDS.

This chapter provides you with information about sexually transmitted diseases (STDs) and available medical counseling services to help you deal with your concerns. Remember: It is not your fault. You are not alone.

Testing for STDs and HIV

If you did not get immediate medical attention after the sexual assault, get a full check up for STDs, including HIV, right away. A rape examination usually includes STD tests. If STD and HIV testing are not available, you should go to another clinic for a test as soon as possible.

Most medical clinics, hospitals, and private physicians will test for STDs and HIV. Some clinics and public hospitals will do the testing free of charge. If the case is being investigated or prosecuted by a Federal Government agency, you are entitled to testing at no cost to

---

"Sexual Assault," United States Attorney's Office (www.usdoj.gov/usao), undated. Accessed November 26, 2008. Reviewed in January 2009 by Dr. David A. Cooke, M.D., Diplomate, American Board of Internal Medicine.

you. Certain requirements apply. Check with the Victim Witness Assistance Program with the investigative agency investigating your case, or the Victim Witness Assistance Program at the U.S. Attorney's Office, for details and procedures. Many STDs take several days to several months to show up. If an STD is diagnosed at an exam done right after the assault, you probably had the STD before the assault. The infection could be from past sexual contact or drug use. Talk to your health care provider about taking medicine and telling partners. If your first tests are negative, you may be able to rule out the possibility that you had an STD before the assault.

Even if your tests are negative, get tested again in three to six months. You cannot be sure if you have HIV or another STD unless you get tested at least three months after the assault. It can take up to six months after infection for antibodies to show up on a test. Victim assistance staff can assist you in obtaining this second test at no cost to you. Your health and peace of mind are worth it.

While waiting for the test results, it is normal to feel anxious and worried. Your counselor or doctor may be able to help. During this time, you need to protect your health and your loved ones from infection.

Testing and Confidentiality

It is important to be tested in a facility that offers counseling and protects your confidentiality. STD and HIV tests usually are free in public health clinics. You have the right to have up to two confidential and anonymous tests following a sexual assault that poses a risk of transmission of HIV virus or an STD. Test results are not given over the phone or sent in the mail. The nurse who drew your blood will give you the test results on your second visit and explain them to you in private.

Counseling and Information

Most sexual assault crisis centers have hotlines operated by trained counselors who understand sexual assault and will talk to you confidentially. Most medical centers also provide counseling. Or, a victim witness advocate from the investigative agency or U.S. Attorney's Office will help you make arrangements for counseling.

HIV Testing and the Perpetrator of Sexual Assault

A judge can order a person charged with a sexual assault to be tested for HIV if the victim requests this through the Assistant U.S.

Attorney. You will be given the results; however, you are allowed to share this information ONLY with your doctor, counselor, family members, and any sexual partners you may have had after the assault. Regardless of the perpetrator's test, you still need to have your own HIV test. Even if the perpetrator has HIV, you may not have been infected during the sexual assault. If the perpetrator's HIV test is negative, the perpetrator could still have HIV. Recent infections (within three to six months) may not show up on his test. People with HIV can infect others at any time, even before their own blood shows signs of HIV.

What You Need to Know about HIV and Other Sexually Transmitted Diseases

- There are many common sexually transmitted diseases, including gonorrhea, syphilis, chlamydia, genital warts, herpes, and HIV (the AIDS virus).
- Proper testing is the only way to know if you are infected.
- STDs, including HIV, usually are passed through vaginal, oral, or anal intercourse. However, some STDs can be passed from skin-to-skin contact in the genital area.
- An infected woman can pass HIV to her baby through breast milk.
- Many STDs can be cured easily especially if they are found early.
- HIV is fairly hard to get from a single sexual act.
- There are only a few cases of HIV infection from sexual assault.
- You are more likely to get other STDs from a single contact with an infected person.
- Signs of STDs may not show up right away. Some people never notice any signs of infection. This is especially true for women.

Clinics and Support

Your private doctor can test you for HIV and other STDs or you can go to a clinic. Referral numbers that may help include the following:

- The Rape, Abuse & Incest National Network, at 800-656-4673, provides an automatic link to your local rape crisis center.

- HIV/AIDS Nightline, at 800-273-2437, offers after-hours emotional support and crisis intervention services.
- Center for Disease Control National Hotline, at 800-342-2437, provides information on HIV and other sexually transmitted diseases.

Chapter 36

Tests for HIV

Chapter Contents

Section 36.1

HIV Testing Options

"Ways to Test for HIV," © 2007 Project Inform. Reprinted with permission. For more information, contact the National HIV/AIDS Treatment Hotline, 1-800-822-7422, or visit our website at www.projectinform.org.

About four to six weeks after you've been exposed to HIV, you will want to test for it with a standard HIV antibody test. You can get this test at anonymous HIV testing sites. You can also get it through your doctor's office, at public health clinics, some AIDS service organizations, and through an in-home collection kit.

A standard antibody test does not look directly for HIV. Rather, it checks for antibodies—proteins your body makes in response to having HIV. If you have these antibodies, you are considered to be HIV-positive. That means you have HIV, the virus that causes AIDS.

If your result comes back positive, some people take a second test to confirm the result. For some, taking another test eases their doubts about the result. However, labs normally test your blood two different ways to confirm a positive result. So, when you get a positive test result, your blood or saliva has already been tested twice.

If you do not have these antibodies, you are considered HIV-negative. However, it can take up to six months after you've been exposed to HIV for you to develop antibodies. If you test negative, then you should screen again three months and again at six months after the exposure to confirm that you're HIV-negative. You won't know for certain if you are negative until you confirm it with another test after six months from the original exposure.

In some cases, the test result may come back indeterminate. Usually this occurs when the test is taken too early after the exposure. When this happens, you should repeat the test awhile later. Rarely, it can take several months before the test gives a definitive answer.

The standard antibody test, however, is not used for newborn babies. It is not reliable in detecting if a baby—born to an HIV-positive woman—is infected with HIV. In this case, babies are born with their mother's antibodies, so special tests must be used to tell if a baby is infected.

Depending on where you live, you may have several screening options available to you. It's important that you think about and choose the one that's right for you. HIV screening will be part of your first nPEP [non-occupational post-exposure prophylaxis] visit. You doctor may have rapid testing available, and thus be able to get immediate results. These results can only tell you if you have HIV from a previous exposure. They cannot tell you if you've recently been exposed to HIV and if that has led to an established HIV infection. The basic HIV screening options are explained below. Other options may be available to you through your doctor or site where you are getting nPEP services.

Going to Your Doctor's Office

If you have a doctor that you usually see, you might choose to call for an appointment. He or she can order HIV screening for you. Your doctor will either take a sample of your blood or saliva in the office or send you to a lab to get it done.

The benefit of going to your doctor is that you may already have a good relationship and feel at ease talking to her or him about HIV. The drawback is that he or she may not be well trained in providing counseling before and after testing. A well-trained counselor can help answer questions you might have about HIV and can often provide you with referrals to local resources.

Going to a Local Testing Site

When you test for HIV, you may decide you don't want to see your regular doctor. Or, you may prefer to have a trained testing counselor on hand for you. In this case, you could look in the phone book to find the number of your local Department of Public Health. They can direct you to a local anonymous or confidential testing site or public health clinic that provides HIV screening.

These sites usually provide counseling free of charge along with the screening. You could then talk one-on-one with the counselor who can answer the questions you might have. They usually can refer you to HIV prevention resources in your area and provide you with emotional support. And, if you do test positive, they can help you cope with the news and direct you to local resources for more support. Some sites use standard blood draws or saliva swabs, where results are often available in a week or two after being sent to a lab and processed. Some sites have saliva-based rapid tests available (called OraQuick). These test results may be read in about 20 minutes.

Using an In-Home Kit

Perhaps you feel uneasy talking to someone face-to-face or fear going to an HIV testing site. In this case, you can test by using an in-home collection kit. The Home Access kit can be bought online (www.homeaccess.com) and at many drug stores, but it's not available in every state.

The kit includes a booklet that discusses and answers some questions about HIV screening. It also contains a needle, a small blotter pad, and a postage-paid envelope. You will also find a unique ID code that you must keep in order to get your results.

To use the kit, prick your finger with the needle and put a few drops of blood on the blotter pad, as directed. Mail the blotter pad in the postage-paid envelope. The booklet gives you a toll-free phone number to call for your results.

When you call, an automated machine will ask you to enter your ID code. After you do, you will be passed to a counselor who will explain your test results and answer your questions. Over the phone, the counselor can give you a list of referrals for HIV prevention or other services in your area. If you want, they often can link you directly by phone to them.

The kit costs in the $45–60 range (depending on how quickly you request your results). But before you choose to test this way, consider how you feel about being counseled over the phone, how you feel about getting information about your HIV status over the phone, and whether you may benefit more from face-to-face counseling.

Several in-home HIV test kits are advertised on the internet. Only one is approved by the U.S. Food and Drug Administration (FDA). That is the Home Access Express HIV-1 Test System, made by Home Access Health Corporation. Other tests are not proven reliable and should be avoided. The FDA offers the warning below to consumers about other HIV testing options.

The advertisers of the unapproved HIV home test kits claim that the presence of a visual indicator, such as a red dot, within 5–15 minutes of taking the test shows a positive result for HIV infection. These unapproved test kits use a simple finger prick process for home blood collection or a special sponge device for saliva collection. The blood or saliva sample is then added to a plastic testing device containing a special type of paper. A developing solution is added to determine if the sample is positive for HIV. The samples are not sent to a laboratory for professional analysis. Although this approach may seem faster and simpler, it may provide a less accurate result than can be achieved using an approved test, which is analyzed under more controlled conditions than is possible in the home.

Why Not Use More Sensitive Tests?

Other types of HIV tests are available, called HIV RNA tests. Rather than looking for antibodies, these tests look for the actual virus. Several tests are available, including Amplicor, bDNA [branched DNA], and NASBA [nucleic acid sequence-based amplification]. These are routinely used to monitor people with HIV infection, find out their risk of disease progression, and monitor the effect of anti-HIV therapy.

These tests are not routinely used to check for HIV infection. First, they cost a lot more than antibody tests. Second, a number of problems occur when using them to screen for the presence of HIV. The major problem is that they have a significant false positive rate. That means the test sometimes suggests that someone is infected when in fact they are not. Using these tests to screen for HIV has caused people emotional unrest. As well, antibody tests are more than 99.9% accurate.

Section 36.2

Privacy, Insurance, and the Cost of HIV Testing

This section excerpted from "Questions and Answers for the General Public: Revised Recommendations for HIV Testing of Adults, Adolescents, and Pregnant Women in Healthcare Settings," Centers for Disease Control and Prevention (www.cdc.gov), January 2007.

Will my test results become part of my medical records?

Yes, your test results will become part of your medical records. It is important for your doctor or other health care provider to know whether you are infected in order to give you the best care.

How will my privacy be protected?

HIV test results fall under the same strict privacy rules as all of your medical information, including those for other sexually transmitted diseases. Information about your HIV test cannot be released without your permission. If your test shows you are infected with HIV, this information will be reported to the state health department, like other sexually transmitted disease (STD) results. After all personal information about you (name, address, etc.) is removed, this information, in turn, is forwarded to the Centers for Disease Control and Prevention (CDC). CDC uses this information to keep track of HIV/AIDS in the United States and to direct funding and resources where they are needed the most. CDC does not share this information with anyone else, including insurance companies.

Will my test results be given to my insurance company?

Generally, testing laboratories are not required to share test results with insurance plans and can only share them with the "authorized person" who can be the patient and/or the individual or laboratory (i.e., referral testing) who ordered the test and is responsible for using the results. However, this may vary from state to state and between insurance plans. If you file insurance claims for treatment for HIV or AIDS, your insurance company will know you are infected with HIV.

Will my insurance company drop me if I've been tested for HIV?

An insurance company should not drop you for being tested for HIV. Companies should also not drop you if you are infected with HIV. Certain insurance plans have restrictions on what they will pay for, including pre-existing conditions, but they should not drop you for receiving an HIV test.

Will screening increase fear and anxiety surrounding HIV testing?

By making HIV testing part of routine care, CDC believes that fear and anxiety surrounding HIV testing will decrease. If health care providers test all of their patients, then no one is singled out. A negative HIV test result will not imply that you are at high risk, just that you were tested.

Who will pay for my HIV test?

If you have insurance coverage, your insurer may pay for an HIV test, if it is ordered as part of your routine medical care. Insurance companies usually pay for tests that are ordered as a routine part of medical care, unless they have included a specific provision related to that test. If you have a question about your coverage, please refer to your policy for details.

If your insurance will not pay for an HIV test, there are places where you can get an HIV test at a reduced cost or for free. Visit www.hivtest.org or call 1-800-CDC-INFO to find a testing site in your area. Your public health department or local community-based organizations may also provide that information.

Who will pay for my treatment if the test shows I have HIV?

If you have insurance, your insurer may pay for treatment. If you do not have insurance, or your insurer will not pay for treatment, there are government programs, such as Medicaid, Medicare, Ryan White Care Act treatment centers, and community health centers, that may be able to assist if you meet their eligibility criteria (usually income and/or disability). CDC is working with its federal partners that oversee these programs to make sure that all people who need treatment can get it. Your health care provider or local public health department can direct you to HIV treatment programs.

Section 36.3

Over-the-Counter and Home Test Kits for HIV

"Vital Facts About HIV Home Test Kits," Food and Drug Administration (www.fda.gov), January 29, 2008.

Privacy and confidentiality are main factors that lead people to choose home testing kits to find out if they are infected with human immunodeficiency virus (HIV), which causes AIDS.

It is important that consumers know there is only one product currently approved by FDA and legally sold in the United States as a "home" testing system for HIV.

This product is a kit marketed as either "The Home Access HIV-1 Test System" or "The Home Access Express HIV-1 Test System." The kit is a home collection-test system that requires users to collect a blood specimen, and then mail it to a laboratory for professional testing. No test kits allow consumers to interpret the results at home.

Beware of False Claims

Numerous HIV home test systems that have not been approved by FDA are currently being marketed online and in newspapers and magazines.

Manufacturers of unapproved systems have falsely claimed that their products can detect antibodies to HIV in blood or saliva samples, and that they can provide results in the home in 15 minutes or less. Some have even claimed that their systems are approved by FDA or are manufactured in a facility that is registered with FDA.

FDA takes appropriate action against people or firms that sell unapproved and ineffective tests.

About the Approved Product

The FDA-approved Home Access System kits allow people to collect a blood sample. Using a personal identification number (PIN), they then mail the sample anonymously to a laboratory for testing. The PIN can then be used to obtain results.

The kits, manufactured by Illinois-based Home Access Health Corp., can be purchased at pharmacies, by mail order, or online. They only allow testing for the presence of antibodies of the virus known as HIV-1. They do not provide the ability to test for HIV-2, a less common cause of AIDS.

The Home Access System offers users pre- and post-test, anonymous and confidential counseling through both printed material and telephone interaction. It also provides the user with an interpretation of the test result.

Checking for Antibodies to HIV

Like most HIV tests, the approved Home Access testing system checks for the presence of antibodies to HIV that are produced once the virus enters the body. The rate at which individuals infected with HIV produce these antibodies differs.

There's a "window period" between the time someone is infected with HIV and the time the body produces enough antibodies to be detected through testing. During this time, an HIV-infected person will still get a negative test result.

According to FDA's Center for Biologics and Research (CBER), which regulates all HIV tests, detectable antibodies usually develop within two to eight weeks. The average is about 22 days.

Still, some people take longer to develop detectable antibodies. Most will develop antibodies within three months following infection. In very rare cases, it can take up to six months to develop detectable antibodies to HIV.

Rapid Tests: A Clinical Option

Consumers do have the option of taking a rapid test, some of which test for both HIV-1 and HIV-2. These tests are run where the sample is collected, and produce results within 20 minutes.

Because HIV testing requires interpretation and confirmation, rapid antibody tests are only approved and available in a professional health care setting, such as doctors' offices, clinics, and outreach testing sites.

According to the CDC, there are tests that look for HIV's genetic material directly, but these are not in widespread use. Tests using saliva or urine are also available, although not for "at-home" use.

If you are unsure whether a certain type of HIV test is FDA-approved, look for the test on the agency's list at www.fda.gov/cber/products/testkits.htm. You can also contact CBER by phone at 800-835-4709, or e-mail at OCTMA@CBER.FDA.GOV.

Chapter 37

Tests for Other STDs

Chapter Contents

Section 37.1

Laboratory Tests for Chlamydia

How is it used?

The test is used:

1. to diagnose the cause of symptoms,
2. to screen sexually active people for the microorganism, or
3. to document that a person has been sexually abused.

A definitive diagnosis is important because chlamydia can resemble gonorrhea, and the two infections require different antibiotic treatment.

The preferred method of testing currently is the molecular test also known as nucleic acid amplification tests (NAAT). This test is based on amplification of the DNA that is present in *Chlamydia trachomatis*. Molecular testing for *Chlamydia trachomatis* is currently the standard and is widely utilized. The advantage of molecular tests is that they are generally more sensitive and specific than conventional culture and can therefore identify more positive specimens. Molecular tests should not be used to diagnose or verify cases with legal implications. Until the legal system changes, only a positive culture result proving infection with chlamydia is admissible in court. All positive molecular tests for *Chlamydia trachomatis* should be verified by the same or another methodology for confirmation. Molecular tests need to be validated for different sources of specimens. They have not been FDA approved for performance with ocular, pharyngeal, or rectal sites.

Testing for *Neisseria gonorrhoeae* (gonorrhea) and *Chlamydia trachomatis* is generally done simultaneously as the two organisms have similar clinical presentations.

When is it ordered?

A doctor may order the test if you have symptoms such as vaginal discharge and abdominal pain (for women) or unusual discharge from the penis or pain on urination (for men). However, about 75% of infected women and 50% of infected men show no active symptoms, so the Centers for Disease Control recommend testing in the following cases:

- All sexually active females under 20 years of age (test at least once a year).
- Women ages 20 and older who have one or more risk factors (test annually). Risk factors include having new or multiple sex partners, having sex with someone who has other partners, and not using barrier contraceptives, such as condoms.
- All women with an infection of the cervix.
- All pregnant women.
- Men with painful and frequent urination (dysuria), penile discharge, infection of the prostate (prostatitis), or inflammation involving the anus and rectum (proctitis).

What does the test result mean?

A positive test indicates an active infection that requires treatment with a course of antibiotics.

Is there anything else I should know?

Chlamydia is often called "the silent epidemic" because infections are so prevalent yet many people do not know that they are infected. An estimated three million cases occur annually in the U.S. Chlamydia is especially widespread among young people and most common in women between the ages of 19 and 25. It is four times as common as gonorrhea and six times as common as herpes.

Chlamydia is easily treated, but if left untreated, it can cause severe reproductive and other health problems. If you are infected, your sexual partner(s) should also be tested and treated as well.

People who are infected have a higher risk of developing other sexually transmitted diseases, including a three to five times greater risk of acquiring HIV if exposed to it.

Section 37.2

Laboratory Tests for Gonorrhea

How is it used?

The test is used in two ways:

- to diagnose the cause of symptoms, and
- to screen sexually active people.

A definitive diagnosis is important because symptoms of gonorrhea can resemble chlamydia clinically, and the two disorders require different treatment.

The preferred method of testing currently is the molecular test, also known as Nucleic acid amplification tests (NAAT). This test is based on amplification of the DNA that is present in *Neisseria gonorrhoeae*. Molecular testing for *Neisseria gonorrhoeae* is currently the standard and is widely utilized. The advantage of molecular tests is that they are generally more sensitive and specific than conventional culture and can therefore identify more positive specimens. Molecular tests should not be used to diagnose or verify cases with legal implications. Until the legal system changes, only a positive culture result proving infection with gonorrhea is admissible in court. All positive molecular tests for *Neisseria gonorrhoeae* should be verified by the same or another methodology for confirmation. Molecular tests need to be validated for different sources of specimens.

Testing for *Neisseria gonorrhoeae* and *Chlamydia trachomatis* is generally done simultaneously as the two organisms have similar clinical presentations.

When is it ordered?

A doctor may order the test if you have symptoms such as (for women) a yellow or bloody vaginal discharge, bleeding associated with vaginal intercourse, or burning/painful urination; or (for men) pus discharging from the penis, a burning sensation during urination, prostatitis (infection of the prostate), or proctitis (inflammation of the rectal or anal area). Pregnant women should be tested at least once during the pregnancy.

What does the test result mean?

A positive test indicates an active infection that requires treatment with a course of antibiotics.

Is there anything else I should know?

Many people contract gonorrhea without knowing it, because symptoms are very mild or even absent. If you test positive for gonorrhea, you should also be screened for other sexually transmitted diseases and your sexual partner(s) should be tested and treated as well.

If you are infected, your risk of contracting other sexually transmitted diseases increases, including HIV, the virus that causes AIDS.

Section 37.3

Laboratory Tests for HBV and HCV

This section includes "Hepatitis B" and "Hepatitis C," © 2008 American Association for Clinical Chemistry. Reprinted with permission. For additional information about clinical lab testing, visit the Lab Tests Online website at www.labtestonline.org.

Hepatitis B Test

How is it used?

There are several tests used to detect the presence of hepatitis B antibodies. Antibodies are produced by the body to offer protection from antigens (foreign proteins). There are also several tests that detect the presence of viral antigens.

The hepatitis B surface antibody (anti-HBs) is the most common test. Its presence indicates previous exposure to hepatitis B virus

(HBV), but the virus is no longer present and the person cannot pass on the virus to others. The antibody also protects the body from future HBV infection. In addition to exposure to HBV, the antibodies can also be acquired from successful vaccination. This test is done to determine the need for vaccination (if anti-HBs is absent), or following the completion of vaccination against the disease, or following an active infection.

Hepatitis B surface antigen (HBsAg) is a protein antigen produced by HBV. This antigen is the earliest indicator of acute hepatitis B and frequently identifies infected people before symptoms appear. HBsAg disappears from the blood during the recovery period. In some people (particularly those infected as children or those with a weak immune system, such as those with AIDS), chronic infection with HBV may occur and HBsAg remains positive.

Sometimes, HBV goes into "hiding" in the liver and other cells and does not produce new viruses that can infect others, or produces them in such low amounts that they cannot be found in the blood. People who have this form are said to be carriers. In other cases, the body continues to make viruses that can further infect the liver and can be spread to other people. In both these cases, HBsAg will be positive. The next test is helpful for distinguishing these two states.

Hepatitis B e-antigen (HBeAg) is a viral protein associated with HBV infections. Unlike the surface antigen, the e-antigen is found in the blood only when there are viruses also present. When the virus goes into "hiding," the e-antigen will no longer be present in the blood. HBeAg is often used as a marker of ability to spread the virus to other people (infectivity). Measurement of e-antigen may also be used to monitor the effectiveness of HBV treatment; successful treatment will usually eliminate HBeAg from the blood and lead to development of antibodies against e-antigen (anti-HBe). There are some types (strains) of HBV that do not make e-antigen; these are especially common in the Middle East and Asia. In areas where these strains of HBV are common, testing for HBeAg is not very useful.

Anti-HBe is an antibody produced in response to the Hepatitis B e-antigen. In those who have recovered from acute hepatitis B infection, anti-HBe will be present along with anti-HBc and anti-HBs. In those with chronic hepatitis B, usually anti-HBe becomes positive when the virus goes into hiding or is eliminated from the body. In strains that do not make HBe antigen, anti-HBe is also positive.

Anti-hepatitis B core antigen (anti-HBc) is an antibody to the hepatitis B core antigen. The core antigen is found on virus particles but disappears early in the course of infection. This antibody is produced during and after an acute HBV infection and is usually found in chronic HBV carriers as well as those who have cleared the virus, and usually persists for life. Anti-HBc testing is either specific for the IgM antibody, anti-HBc, IgM, which indicates acute infection, or measures total antibody, anti-HBc, which indicates past infection, either acute or chronic.

HBV DNA is a more sensitive test than HBeAg for detecting viruses in the blood stream. It is usually used in conjunction with—rather than instead of—the regular serologic tests. It may be used to monitor antiviral therapy in patients with chronic HBV infections.

When is it ordered?

These tests are used to determine whether the vaccine has produced the desired level of immunity as well as to diagnose and follow the course of an infection.

In a patient with acute hepatitis, anti-HBc IgM and HBsAg are usually ordered together to detect recent infection by HBV. In persons with chronic hepatitis, or with elevated ALT (alanine aminotransferase) or AST (aspartate aminotransferase), HBsAg and anti-HBc are usually done to see if the liver damage is due to HBV. If so, HBsAg and HBeAg are usually measured on a regular basis (every six months to a year), since in some people HBeAg (and, less commonly, HBsAg) will go away on their own. Recent evidence suggests that many of those who have anti-HBc but no HBsAg may have very low levels of HBV DNA in their blood and/or in their liver. The significance of this is still being debated. In those who are being treated for chronic HBV, HBeAg and HBV DNA can be used to determine whether the treatment is successful (in which case, both will become undetectable). If a person is given the HBV vaccine, anti-HBs is used to see if it successful; if levels of the antibody are over 10 IU/mL, the person is probably protected for life from infection by HBV, unless they have or develop problems with their immune system (such as HIV infection, renal failure, or treatment with drugs that suppress the immune system).

All donated blood is tested for the presence of the HBsAg before being distributed.

What does the test result mean?

- Hepatitis B surface antibody (anti-HBs): A positive result indicates immunity to hepatitis B from the vaccination or recovery from an infection.

- Hepatitis B surface antigen (HBsAg): A negative result indicates that a person has never been exposed to the virus or has recovered from acute hepatitis and has rid themselves of the virus (or has, at most, an occult infection). A positive (or reactive) result indicates an active infection but does not indicate whether the virus can be passed to others.
- Hepatitis B e-antigen (HBeAg): A positive (or reactive) result indicates the presence of virus that can be passed to others. A negative result usually means the virus cannot be spread to others, except in parts of the world where infection with strains that cannot make this protein are common.
- Anti-hepatitis B core antigen (anti-HBc): If it is present with a positive anti-HBs, it usually indicates recovery from an infection and the person is not a carrier or chronically infected. In acute infection, the first type of antibody to HBc to appear is an IgM antibody. Testing for this type of antibody can prove whether a person has recently been infected by HBV (where anti-HBc, IgM would be positive) or for some time (where anti-HBc, IgM would be negative).
- HBV DNA: A positive (or reactive) result indicates the presence of virus that can be passed to others. A negative result usually means the virus cannot be spread to others, especially if tests that can pick up as few as 200 viruses (copies) in one mL of blood are used.

Is there anything else I should know?

While the tests described above are specific for HBV, other liver function tests such as AST, ALT, and gamma-glutamyl transferase (GGT) may be used to monitor the progress of the disease. In some cases, a liver biopsy may be performed for confirmation.

Hepatitis C Test

How is it used?

Each of the five most common tests has a slightly different purpose:

- Anti-HCV tests detect the presence of antibodies to the virus, indicating exposure to hepatitis C virus (HCV). These tests cannot tell if you still have an active viral infection, only that you were exposed to the virus in the past. Usually, the test is reported as "positive" or "negative." There is some evidence that, if your test is "weakly positive," it may not mean that you have been exposed to the HCV virus. The Centers for Disease Control and Prevention (CDC) revised its guidelines in 2003 and suggests that weakly positive tests be confirmed with the next test before being reported.

- HCV RIBA (recombinant immunoblot assay) test is an additional test to confirm the presence of antibodies to the virus. In most cases, it can tell if the positive anti-HCV test was due to exposure to HCV (positive RIBA) or represents a false signal (negative RIBA). In a few cases, the results cannot answer this question (indeterminate RIBA). Like the anti-HCV test, the RIBA test cannot tell if you are currently infected, only that you have been exposed to the virus.
- HCV-RNA (ribonucleic acid) test identifies whether the virus is in your blood, indicating that you have an active infection with HCV. In the past, it was usually performed by a test called a qualitative HCV. Qualitative HCV RNA is reported as a "positive" or "detected" if any HCV viral RNA is found; otherwise, the report will be "negative" or "not detected." The test may also be used after treatment to see if the virus has been eliminated from the body.
- Viral load or quantitative HCV tests measure the number of viral RNA particles in your blood. Viral load tests are often used before and during treatment to help determine response to treatment by comparing the amount of virus before and after treatment (usually after three months); successful treatment causes a decrease of 99% or more (2 logs) in viral load soon after starting treatment (as early as 4–12 weeks), and usually leads to viral load being not detected. Some newer viral load tests can detect very low amounts of viral RNA, and some laboratories no longer do qualitative HCV RNA tests if they use one of these versions of viral load testing.
- Viral genotyping is used to determine the kind, or genotype, of the virus present. There are six major types of HCV; the most common (genotype 1) is less likely to respond to treatment than genotypes 2 or 3 and usually requires longer therapy (48 weeks, versus 24 weeks for genotype 2 or 3). Genotyping is often ordered before treatment is started to give an idea of the likelihood of success and how long treatment may be needed.

When is it ordered?

Hepatitis C infection is the most common cause of chronic liver disease in North America; about 2% of all adults in the United States have been exposed to the virus, and 75–85% of those are chronically infected. The CDC recommends HCV testing in the following cases:

- If you have ever injected illegal drugs
- If you received a blood transfusion or organ transplant before July 1992*
- If you have received clotting factor concentrates produced before 1987
- If you were ever on long-term dialysis
- For children born to HCV-positive women
- For health care, emergency medicine, and public safety workers after needlesticks, sharps, or mucosal exposure to HCV-positive blood
- For people with evidence of chronic liver disease

* The blood supply has been monitored in the U.S. since 1990, and any units of blood that test positive for HCV are rejected for use in another person. The current risk of HCV infection from transfused blood is about one case per two million transfused units.

A positive anti-HCV test may be confirmed with an HCV RIBA test, especially if the test is "weakly positive." Qualitative HCV-RNA is often used when the antibody test is positive to see if the infection is still present. HCV viral load and genotyping may be done to plan treatment; viral load and qualitative HCV RNA are also used to monitor response to treatment.

What does the test result mean?

If the antibody test result is positive, you have probably been infected with hepatitis C, even if it was so mild you did not realize you had it.

A positive RIBA confirms that you had been exposed to the virus, while a negative RIBA indicates that your first test was probably a false positive and you have never been infected by HCV.

A positive (or detectable) HCV RNA means that you are currently infected by HCV.

Is there anything else I should know?

HCV antibodies usually do not appear until several months into an infection but will always be present in the later stages of the disease.

Section 37.4

Laboratory Tests for Herpes

"Herpes," © 2008 American Association for Clinical Chemistry. Reprinted with permission. For additional information about clinical lab testing, visit the Lab Tests Online website at www.labtestonline.org.

How is it used?

Herpes simplex virus (HSV) testing is used to detect the presence of the herpes simplex virus in those who have genital sores, encephalitis, and in newborns suspected of having neonatal herpes (a rare but serious condition where herpes is contracted during birth). A pregnant woman who has been diagnosed with herpes may be monitored regularly prior to delivery to identify a reactivation of her infection (which would indicate the necessity for a caesarean section to avoid infecting the baby). The primary methods of testing for the virus are the herpes culture and HSV DNA testing.

Although it is not as sensitive, HSV antibody testing can be used to help diagnose an acute HSV infection if acute and convalescent blood samples are collected. The convalescent blood sample is collected several weeks after the acute sample, and HSV IgG antibody levels are compared to see if they have risen significantly (indicating a current infection). Antibody testing may also be used to screen certain populations, such as sexually active people, potential organ transplant recipients, and those with HIV/AIDS, for a previously contracted HSV infection.

When is it ordered?

A herpes culture (or HSV DNA testing) may be ordered when a patient has a blister or vesicle on their genitals. HSV DNA testing is ordcred when a patient has encephalitis that the doctor suspects may be caused by a virus. HSV testing may be ordered regularly when a pregnant woman has herpes. A mother and newborn may be tested for HSV when a baby shows signs of HSV infection (such as meningitis or skin lesions).

HSV antibody testing is ordered primarily when a patient is being screened for a previous exposure to HSV. Occasionally, acute and convalescent HSV antibody testing may be ordered when a current infection is suspected.

What does the test result mean?

A positive herpes simplex culture or HSV DNA test from a vesicle scraping indicates an active HSV-1 or HSV-2 infection. A negative test result indicates that the herpes simplex virus was not isolated but does not definitely rule out the presence of virus. This is because if the specimen taken does not contain actively replicating virus or if the sample was not transported under optimum conditions, no viable virus may be detectable, resulting in a false negative result. For example, viruses can be readily inactivated and if the sample was taken from an older lesion, not a fresh blister, or if transport of the sample was delayed, there may not be sufficient virus to detect even though the patient is infected.

The presence of HSV-1 or HSV-2 IgM antibodies indicates an active or recent infection. HSV-1 or HSV-2 IgG antibodies indicate a previous infection. A significant increase in HSV IgG antibodies, measured by comparing acute and convalescent samples, indicates an active or recent infection. Negative HSV antibody results mean that it is unlikely that the patient has been exposed to HSV, or that the body has not had time to begin HSV antibody production.

Is there anything else I should know?

The most serious, or life-threatening, HSV infections can occur in newborns after perinatal infection and in immunocompromised individuals. The lesions tend to be more extensive and persist longer than in immunocompetent individuals. Infection with HSV can increase HIV viral load. HSV-2 infection is a significant opportunistic infection in HIV-infected individuals; up to 90% of HIV-infected individuals are co-infected with HSV-2.

HSV, in combination with human papilloma virus (HPV) infection, has been associated with a higher risk of developing cervical cancer.

Section 37.5

Laboratory Tests for HPV

How is it used?

For women younger than 30 years of age, the Pap smear and pelvic exam are the primary cervical cancer screening tools. If results indicate abnormal changes that may be due to a high-risk type of HPV, then DNA HPV testing may be ordered as a follow-up test. It is not routinely used as a screening tool in this age group because HPV is very common and rarely causes cancer in those under 30.

The American College of Obstetricians and Gynecologists (ACOG) released guidelines in August 2003 recommending that women 30 years or older be offered the HPV DNA test in addition to their Pap smear and pelvic exam. If the HPV DNA test and Pap smear are negative and the woman does not have an underlying health condition, such as HIV or immunosuppression, then the guidelines suggest that she may wait three years before having another Pap smear and HPV DNA test.

The HPV DNA test and Pap smear may be ordered on a more frequent basis to monitor positive HPV tests, abnormal Pap smear changes, and those patients who have underlying medical conditions, such as HIV or immunosuppression.

During an exam, a doctor can detect warts and other lesions through visual inspection that may warrant further investigation. Some otherwise invisible warts in the genital tissue may be identified by applying acetic acid to areas of suspected infection. This process makes the infected areas whiten when they are examined by a procedure called colposcopy.

A doctor might also take a small piece of tissue (called a biopsy) from the cervix and examine it under a microscope. When either the Pap smear or the biopsy indicates a condition that could lead to cancer in some women (called intraepithelial neoplasia), the DNA HPV test can determine if the patient is infected with a high-risk strain of HPV that increases the chance that cancer might develop if not treated.

When is it ordered?

Women who are sexually active with more than one partner—or whose partner has more than one sex partner—should have regular exams for sexually transmitted diseases, including HPV. The American Cancer Society recommends that women over the age of 18 and all sexually active women have a Pap smear yearly to screen for cancer or situations that may develop into cancer. When results indicate abnormal changes that may be due to a high-risk type of HPV, then DNA HPV testing may be ordered as a follow-up test.

Doctors may order the HPV DNA test as a cervical cancer screening test, along with the Pap smear test, when a woman is 30 years old or older and at intervals of three years if initial testing is negative. Patients who are positive for high-risk HPV, have abnormal cell changes on their Pap smear, or have underlying medical conditions should be screened more frequently, with the frequency to be determined by the patient and their doctor on an individual basis.

Some doctors will test men who fall into a high-risk category. Men who have sex with men and those who have HIV may be tested for HPV. Evaluating the risk of HPV-related diseases of the anal canal in men is becoming more common.

What does the test result mean?

On a Pap smear, "low-grade" changes indicate the likely presence of HPV and the need for further testing. A positive HPV DNA test indicates the presence of a high-risk type of HPV, but the test does not specify which type is present. If both are negative, it is unlikely that there is a high-risk HPV infection. If the Pap smear is abnormal but the HPV DNA test is negative, then follow-up testing and further monitoring are indicated.

Typing of the HPV is not usually necessary. However, if it is done, then common findings may include:

- HPV types 6 and 11 typically cause venereal warts and (along with types 42, 43, and 44) have a low risk of progressing to cancer.
- HPV types 16, 18, 31, 33, and 39 have a higher risk of progressing to cancer.

Recently, some doctors have screened men who are at a high risk for sexually transmitted diseases for HPV-related anal cancer. The test is similar to a cervical Pap smear where the anal lining is swabbed and the cells are examined under a microscope. HPV DNA tests can also be performed on these samples. As in cervical samples, positive results will need to be followed up by your doctor with further testing, including a more thorough exam and possible biopsy.

Is there anything else I should know?

HPV is one of the most commonly transmitted sexually transmitted diseases (STDs) in the world. In 90% of women who have cervical HPV infection, the infection becomes undetectable within two years. A few women have persistent infection, which is a key risk factor for cervical cancer. Regular Pap smears and HPV screening can monitor this risk and provide an early warning that you might need treatment.

Section 37.6

Laboratory Tests for Syphilis

How is it used?

The test is used to diagnose infection with syphilis in sexually active persons. Pregnant women also are screened, and many states in the U.S. require a blood test for syphilis when applying for a marriage license to prevent the spread of infection to others, especially a newborn baby.

When is it ordered?

A doctor may order the test:

- if you have symptoms, such as a chancre (sore) on the genitals or throat;

- if you are being treated for another sexually transmitted disease, such as gonorrhea;
- if you are pregnant, because untreated syphilis can infect and even kill a developing fetus; or
- if you complain of non-specific symptoms that resemble those of syphilis, to determine the exact cause of your illness.

What does the test result mean?

If a scraping reveals presence of the syphilis bacterium (a positive test), you have an infection that requires treatment with a course of antibiotics.

The blood test detects the antibodies that the body produces to combat infection, so a positive test indicates that you have either a current or past infection. The blood test might not find antibodies for up to three months after exposure to the bacteria. In addition, the antibodies remain in the body for years, so if you have had a past infection with syphilis and were treated, your test results could still be positive. Therefore, to avoid being retreated, keep a record of the previous treatment and show it to your doctor.

Is there anything else I should know?

Screening tests for syphilis are not highly specific and may give a false positive result. Positive tests should be confirmed with a more specific test method.

If you are sexually active, you should consult your doctor about any suspicious rash or sore in the genital area.

If you are infected, tell your sexual partner(s) to get tested and treated.

If you are infected, your risk of contracting other sexually transmitted diseases increases, including the risk of being infected with HIV, the virus that causes AIDS.

Part Five

Discussing and Living with Sexually Transmitted Diseases

Chapter 38

Sharing Your Sexual History

Sharing Sexual Histories with a New Partner

Sharing your sexual history with a new partner is very important before you engage in any sexual behavior. You may wonder whether your new partner really needs to know the whole truth about your past, especially how many partners you have had, but the truth is that partners need to share their sexual histories honestly so that both can assess the risk factors for sexually transmitted diseases. The sexual risks you took in the past affect your new partner's life now. This means that before participating in sexual behaviors with a new partner you should sit down and discuss each of your sexual histories openly and honestly. Many sexual behaviors other than penile-vaginal sex put you and your partner at risk for sexually transmitted diseases (STDs), including oral sex, among the others. This means that it is important to talk to your partner about more than just the partners they have had penile-vaginal sex with. There are a few tips to keep in mind when talking to your partner about this sensitive subject.

Location

It is a good idea to try to choose a neutral, yet private location where you and your partner can openly speak about each of your histories.

This section includes "Sharing Sexual Histories with a New Partner" and "How to Tell Your Partner If You Have an STD," reprinted with permission from the website SexInfo, www.soc.ucsb.edu/sexinfo. Copyright © 2007 University of California, Santa Barbara. All rights reserved.

Having this conversation in your or your partner's home gives one of you the advantage in feeling more comfortable, so try to choose common ground. You also want to choose a location where there will be no interruptions, this includes making sure any cell phones and pagers are turned off. Make sure that before you sit down and have this conversation you allow plenty of time to talk. Make sure that you and your partner have no prior engagements to ensure the proper amount of time needed to have the conversation.

Bringing up the Topic of Discussion

Sometimes it may be hard to start this conversation by just jumping into the topic at hand. It may be easier to start off with a more general discussion of sex. You could start to talk about how the topic of sex was handled by your parents or maybe by sharing each of your first sexual experiences—even first kissing experiences. Topics like these slowly lead you into more intimate topics because you are both already starting to self-disclose personal information about your pasts. Eventually you want to lead your conversation to deal with both of your past sexual experiences. You may want to start by openly and honestly sharing your sexual past. After sharing your sexual history you may want to explain why you think it is important to share each of your past experiences. For instance, you might mention that you want both of you to be safe and not to have to worry about STDs. This way your partner feels that you care about his or her safety too. By showing your partner that you are comfortable with discussing your past, your partner may in turn feel more comfortable sharing.

Listening to Your Partner's Sexual History

It is important to use effective listening skills when your partner shares with you. Try not to interrupt your partner when he or she is talking, except when you want to clarify information just told to you. This will allow your partner to speak freely and comfortably.

Controlling Nonverbal Cues

One other general tip is to try to control your expression of nonverbal cues, such as posture, facial cues, and sounds. According to Albert Mehrabian, who has conducted many studies on communication, words only count for 7% of what we communicate. The next 38% is paralanguage (things like tone, pitch, and tempo of your voice) and 55% is body language (including facial expressions and body posture).

When you are expressing to your partner why it is important to share each of your sexual histories, you want to make sure that your body language and tone of voice correspond to what you are saying. Closing off your body and acting shy may demonstrate to your partner that you are insecure about talking about the subject or that you are not serious. When your partner shares his or her sexual past, it is important that you do not respond with facial expressions of disgust or shock. If your facial expressions show that you are comfortable and understanding of your partner's sexual past, he or she will be more likely to be open and honest with you.

How to Tell Your Partner If You Have an STD

There are two main situations in which one person might have to tell a partner that the first person has a sexually transmitted disease. The first person has an incurable STD (such as HIV, herpes, or human papillomavirus [HPV]) and needs to tell a new partner before engaging in any sexual behavior. One of the two people finds out that he or she has an STD (curable or incurable) during an existing relationship. In both of these situations, it can be frightening to tell a partner for the fear of rejection. However, finding the best way to communicate this information to a partner may help the partner be more understanding, no matter how he or she finally reacts to it.

Telling a New Partner about an Incurable STD

Living with a sexually transmitted disease is not easy. Since there is a stigma in our society (of being dirty or sexually promiscuous) that is associated with having an STD, many individuals who have an STD fear rejection by new partners. Yet it is still very important that you share this information with a new partner, and in some states it is a crime to engage in sexual activity without informing your partner of an STD. Finding a good location where you and your potential partner can talk is important in starting the conversation. Be honest in telling him or her about your STD and in how you believe to have contracted it. Also sharing information about the specific STD that you have may help him or her feel more informed and comfortable. Explain how it is transmitted, and what the symptoms are like for you individually. Try to be understanding of your partner's initial reaction: It could be shock, confusion, and not knowing how to react. If your partner needs time to think about the situation, be willing to give the time, do not expect anyone to be immediately accepting of this information. Also do not be quick to jump to the conclusion that they are planning to reject you just because they do not accept you with your STD right away (even though this of course is a possibility). Forming a strong friendship with your partner may help him or her see past your STD and decide to be with you. If your partner decides to accept the STD and if you choose to engage in sexual activities you both should try to find out information about ways to have safe sex so your partner does not contract the disease.

Finding out You Have an STD in an Existing Relationship and Telling Your Partner

Finding out you have an STD can be very frightening and confusing when you are currently in what you thought was a monogamous relationship. Some people allow their fear to turn into anger and accuse their partner of cheating and giving them an STD. Blaming your partner does not help you gain anything, instead you should focus on you and your partner getting proper medical care. Also keep in mind that some STDs may lack symptoms (such as HIV and chlamydia), so you or your partner may have contracted it before entering your current relationship. In telling your partner about the STD be honest and straightforward about how you discovered you had the STD and the need for your partner to obtain a medical evaluation. Remembering to control for nonverbal cues, try to be sensitive to how they might react. Keep in mind some of your initial thoughts and reactions when you discovered you had the STD. Your partner may react with anger or resentment. Try not to become defensive and listen to your partner's feeling: These are the best ways to deal with this situation. Before resuming any sexual activity make sure that you are both properly treated for the STD (if it is curable) and are clear of the infection. By communicating to your partner honestly and clearly you may be able to deal with and overcome a problematic situation.

Real Life Situation

Mary had been dating John for about a month and could tell that they both cared for each other a lot. For a while she had been shying away from any type of sexual encounter because she knew she would have to tell him that she had genital warts and carried the human papillomavirus (HPV), which could infect him if they did any sort of risky sexual behavior. Mary feared that the great friendship that they had formed and the romantic feelings that they shared would all end with rejection because she had an STD. John and Mary would talk about sex in general, their sexual histories, and even STDs, yet Mary still was too scared to tell John about her own STD. After time John started to sense from Mary's nonverbal cues that there was something that Mary was hiding from him. Mary knew that she could no longer hide her secret from John and finally at her home sat down with John and told him about her situation. John was initially a little shocked, but knew that whatever Mary had been hiding from him was important, so he had expected something big and was able to show Mary that he understood her situation. For the rest of the conversation he let Mary speak about how she contracted HPV and provided support by attentively listening to what she had to say and rubbing her arm to show compassion. John and Mary were able to move past Mary's STD and continue their relationship while being careful to use protection when engaging in any sort of sexual behavior.

Assessing John and Mary's Situation

Mary and John were lucky. Things do no always go right when discussing STDs. John might have gotten very upset when feeling that Mary was hiding something from him. He might have reacted negatively when she explained her STD. Hopefully when talking about an STD with a partner, you should begin with an open and honest discussion of the topic since openness and honesty are often highly respected by others, John did attentively listen to Mary and use correct nonverbal cues to show that he cared and understood what Mary was telling him.

Chapter 39

Talking to Your Partner about STDs

Sexually transmitted diseases (STDs) are common infections you can get from sexual contact. One out of five adults has an STD. It is normal to feel embarrassed or upset if you learn you have an STD, but there are still advantages to talking about the infection with your sex partner(s) and health care provider. All STDs can be treated, and many can be cured. With time, information, and support, most people are able to put their infection in perspective.

Asking your partner(s) about their sexual history, and telling your partners about your own, are excellent ways to help yourself stay safe and healthy. Just KNOWING the HIV status of your partner(s) decreases your HIV risk by 50%.

It is important that you don't make assumptions about the sexual history of your partner(s). You can't tell by looking at someone whether or not they have an STD. Don't assume your partner is clean, or let them assume those things about you without having a discussion. The following tips are designed to help you tell your partner that you have an infection.

If you are ready to tell your partner about your infection: There are certain things you should do before the conversation, like:

- get the facts about your STD;

"Do Ask, Do Tell: Talk to Your Partner about STDs," © 2004 Safeguards LGBT Health Resource Center (www.safeguards.org). Reprinted with permission. Reviewed in January 2009 by Dr. David A. Cooke, M.D., Diplomate, American Board of Internal Medicine.

- get treatment for your STD;
- come to terms with the fact that you have an STD; DON'T put yourself down for it; and
- remember to speak calmly, and talk with confidence.

When should I tell my partner?

You should tell your partner before you become sexually intimate—although it is never too late to tell them!

What STDs should I tell my partner about?

ANY active STDs that you have, or are receiving treatment for. STDs that don't go away, even after they've been treated, which are:

- genital warts (HPV);
- herpes (HSV);
- hepatitis (HBV); and
- HIV/AIDS.

If you are thinking about telling your partner about your infection: It may be difficult to tell your partner you have an infection, but you should give some thought to these reasons why it's important that your infection is not a secret.

If you are beginning a relationship:

- Telling shows you have respect for your partner's well-being.
- Telling helps build honesty and trust—essential elements of all good relationships.
- Telling will begin an important discussion about sexual health.
- Your honesty may encourage your partner to share sexual information with you.
- Telling will allow you and your partner to make decisions together about how to reduce risk.

If you are having casual relationships:

- Telling helps prevent the spread of infections.
- Telling will prevent further misunderstandings.

- Telling allows you to get rid of your secrets. Since secrets take a lot of energy to hide, being dishonest may make you feel more tired, anxious, and worried.
- Telling may also help you feel less guilt.

How might my partner react?

Some partners may overreact, but some may not react at all. Many people have heard a lot about STDs, so they may not be surprised.

- Your partner may need some time to think about the information.
- A few people may react negatively, but if your partner doesn't want to continue a relationship because of your infection, you need to know that right away. Good relationships are built on honesty and good communication. Telling shows you have those qualities—you deserve someone else who does too.
- It makes sense to feel bad if your partner rejects you after you tell them. But rejection is not the end of the world, it's part of life. We all get rejected at times—from jobs, loans, even partners. Most of us have experienced rejection, have survived, and moved on.
- If you are having casual sex, and your partner refuses you after you tell them—chances are that you can easily find another casual relationship.

If you are not ready to tell your partner about your infection: It is not easy to tell your partner about an infection. It is normal to be scared of the possible rejection it can cause. If you are not ready to tell your partner(s) about your infection, you should be careful and safe. You should also think about making a plan to talk to your partner(s) when you are ready.

How can I protect my partner?

All STDs are different, so protecting your partner depends on what infection you have. If your STD is curable, both you and your partner should get treated. If your infection will not go away, there are ways to reduce your risk. Condoms help prevent the spread of most STDs. Regular check-ups and practicing healthy behaviors will also help protect you and your partners.

Chapter 40

Disclosure Assistance Services

Why assistance for disclosure?

After more than 20 years of the HIV epidemic, with advances in treatment and increases in understanding and acceptance of HIV, getting an HIV+ diagnosis still can be a traumatic experience. HIV+ persons must come to terms with their own infection and be concerned with possible infection in past and future partners. Talking to partners about HIV is especially hard because even though it is a manageable disease, HIV still is not curable.

Disclosure assistance services (also known as partner counseling and referral services or PCRS) are an array of voluntary and confidential services available to persons living with HIV and their exposed sex and/or needle-sharing partner(s). Disclosure assistance is cost effective and can play a critical role in identifying those individuals most at risk for HIV infection, and linking those who are infected to early medical care and treatment.[1,2,3]

Most HIV+ persons make the decision to disclose or not disclose to their partners on their own. But HIV+ persons may want support for telling their partners about HIV, whether by encouragement for self-disclosure or by having someone who is well-trained carefully and confidentially notify a partner for them. In one study, persons who received disclosure assistance were over three times more likely to have informed a partner of their risk.[4]

In the past few years, HIV counseling and testing programs across the U.S. have shifted their emphasis from testing anyone, to finding and testing persons at greatest risk for HIV infection.[5] At general HIV testing sites, around 1% of clients tested are found to be HIV+, whereas 8–39% of clients tested through disclosure assistance are found to be HIV+.[2]

What is disclosure assistance?

Often, disclosure assistance or PCRS mistakenly has been seen as only provider disclosure, but there are three forms of assistance:

Self disclosure: The client chooses to notify a partner him/herself. The disclosure assistance provider guides and prepares the client before disclosure. Currently, most HIV+ persons choose this method.

Dual disclosure: The client chooses to notify a partner in the presence of a provider. The provider supports the client during disclosure and acts as a resource for the partner. This method is rarely chosen and requires highly skilled providers.

Provider disclosure (anonymous third party): The client prefers a professional to notify a partner, and gives his/her provider identifying and locating information for partner(s). Most often, providers give this info to Disease Intervention Specialists (DIS) who then locate and notify the named partners, keeping client identity strictly confidential. This method is chosen less often, yet it is the only one with client anonymity.

For the partners of an HIV+ client, disclosure assistance services can include: being notified of exposure to HIV, HIV prevention counseling, HIV testing options, referrals for HIV medical evaluation if positive, and referrals for other social or medical services.[6]

How does it work?

Disclosure assistance services are first offered when a person receives a positive HIV test result. It is not a one-time only service, but should be offered as clients' risk circumstances and needs change. The main element is helping HIV+ persons tell their sexual and/or needle-sharing partners about possible HIV exposure.

The quality and use of disclosure assistance services can vary widely. Services differ from state to state: some have legal mandates to provide it, some offer it through HIV, STD, or combined HIV/STD programs, and states can receive referrals from clinicians, health departments, or testing sites.[7]

Services can be provided by HIV service agencies, health departments, and most clinics and hospitals. Most service agencies can provide coaching and support for self or dual disclosure and gather partner identifying and locating information which is forwarded to DIS staff. Most notification of partners has been done by DIS at local health departments because they have the capacity, expertise, trained staff, and protection from liability.

Good provider disclosure depends on DIS staff who are properly trained and have enough experience and knowledge of the populations they serve. DIS staff should be evaluated regularly to assure quality and be provided with support and ongoing training.[6]

What are the concerns?

Public health messages have traditionally urged disclosure to all sexual and drug using partners. In reality, disclosure is complex and difficult. Some HIV+ persons may fear that disclosure will bring partner or familial rejection, limit sexual opportunities, reduce access to drugs of addiction, or increase risk for physical and sexual violence. Because of this, some HIV+ persons choose not to disclose. Programs need to accept that not disclosing is a valid option.

Many HIV service agencies and testing and counseling sites routinely offer self disclosure and dual disclosure, working with HIV+ clients by preparing and supporting them to disclose to partners on their own.

Although provider disclosure services have been used for many years with other STDs, there is a wide variety in rates of acceptance of provider disclosure in HIV: in North Carolina, 87% of newly diagnosed HIV+ persons accepted provider disclosure,[8] in Florida 63.1%,[9] Los Angeles, CA 60%,[10] New York State 32.9%,[11] Seattle, WA 32%[12] and among anonymous testers in San Francisco, CA 3.1%.[13] In Los Angeles, the most common reasons for refusal were: already notified partner (23.4%), not being ready to disclose (15.3%), being abstinent (15%), and having an anonymous partner (11%).[10]

Disclosing HIV status to partners can be scary, but also can be empowering. In one study, HIV+ injection drug users who disclosed their status found increased social support and intimacy with partners, reaffirmation of their sense of self, and the chance to share experiences and feelings with sexual partners.[14] Another study of HIV+ persons and their partners who received disclosure assistance found that emotional abuse and physical violence decreased significantly after notification.[15]

What's being done?

Florida utilizes trained DISs to deliver disclosure assistance for all reported new HIV infections. In 2004, 63.1% of all newly infected HIV+ persons accepted provider disclosure, identifying 4,460 sex or needle-sharing partners. Among those, 21.8% had previously tested HIV+. Of the 2,518 persons notified, 84.2% agreed to counseling and testing and 11.5% were HIV+.[9]

The Massachusetts Department of Public Health piloted a client-centered model of disclosure assistance that is integrated into the client's routine prevention, care, and support services. The program required significant changes to the standard model of DIS provider disclosure, building close relationships between service providers and DIS to better support clients' disclosure needs while protecting confidentiality.[16]

California instituted a voluntary disclosure assistance program that includes counseling and preparing HIV+ persons for self disclosure; anonymous third party provider notification; counseling, testing, and referrals for notified partners; and training and technical assistance to providers in public and private medical sites. About one-third of patients opted for provider disclosure and 85% referred partners. Of the partners located, 56% tested for HIV and half had never tested before. Overall, 18% of partners tested HIV+.[4]

What needs to be done?

New HIV testing technologies can be useful with disclosure assistance services. Improved rapid testing is a potential invaluable tool for offering HIV tests in the field to notified partners. Nucleic acid amplification testing (NAAT) can determine acute infections, that is, new HIV infections that do not show up during the window period of other HIV tests. Combining these testing strategies with disclosure assistance can help identify newly infected persons and provide immediate counseling, support, and referrals to medical or social services as needed.[17]

Disclosure assistance services, and particularly provider disclosure, may need extensive changes from the traditional DIS model in order to work well and be accepted within HIV services. Health departments could forge closer ties between their STD and HIV programs and with outside service agencies. HIV staff also can be trained to be DIS providers to broaden access to and comfort with disclosure services.

Disclosure assistance services should be made available not only upon HIV diagnosis, but on an ongoing basis as HIV+ persons' circumstances and needs change. It is not the role of providers to decide if a client will need or want disclosure assistance, but to offer clients support and choices, whether or not a client chooses to disclose.

Says who?

1. Landis SE, Schoenbach VJ, Weber DJ, et al. Results of a randomized trial of partner notification in cases of HIV infection in North Carolina. *New England Journal of Medicine.* 1992;326: 101–106.

2. Golden MR. Editorial: HIV partner notification, a neglected prevention intervention. *Sexually Transmitted Diseases.* 2002;29:472–475.

3. Varghese B, Peterman TA, Holtgrave DR. Cost-effectiveness of counseling and testing and partner notification: a decision analysis. *AIDS.* 1999;13:1745–1751.

4. Eckert V. Utilization of voluntary HIV partner counseling and referral services. California Office of AIDS & STD Control Branch. Presented at the Statewide PCRS Conference, May 2004.

5. Centers for Disease Control and Prevention. Advancing HIV Prevention: New Strategies for a Changing Epidemic—U.S., 2003. *Morbidity and Mortality Weekly Report.* 2003:52;329–332. http://www.cdc.gov/mmwr/preview/mmwrhtml/mm5215a1.htm (accessed April 2006).

6. HIV partner counseling and referral services guidance. Centers for Disease Control and Prevention. 1998. www.cdc.gov/hiv/pubs/pcrs.htm

7. Aldridge C, Randall L. Implementing partner counseling and referral services programs. Presented at the National HIV Prevention Conference, Atlanta, GA. 2005. Abst #TO-057.

8. Centers for Disease Control and Prevention. Partner counseling and referral services to identify persons with undiagnosed

HIV–North Carolina, 2001. *Morbidity and Mortality Weekly Report.* 2003;52:1181–1184. http://www.cdc.gov/mmwr/preview/mmwrhtml/mm5248a4.htm (accessed April 2006).

9. George D. Partner counseling and referral services (PCRS): the Florida experience. Presented at the National HIV Prevention Conference, Atlanta, GA. 2005. Abst #M3-B1605.
10. Aynalem G, Hawkins K, Smith LV, et al. Who and why? Partner counseling and referral service refusal: implication for HIV infection prevention in Los Angeles. Presented at the National HIV Prevention Conference, Atlanta, GA. 2005. Abst #MP-036.
11. Birkhead G. HIV partner counseling and referral services in New York state. Presented at the National HIV Prevention Conference, Atlanta, GA. 2005. Abst #M3-B1603.
12. Golden MR. Partner notification: where do we stand and outstanding barriers. Presented at the National HIV Prevention Conference, Atlanta, GA. 2005. Abst #T3-D1302.
13. Schwarcz S, McFarland W, Delgado V, et al. Partner notification for persons recently infected with HIV: experience in San Francisco. *Journal of Acquired Immune Deficiency Syndrome.* 2001;28:403–404.
14. Parsons JT, Vanora J, Missildine W, et al. Positive and negative consequences of HIV disclosure among seropositive injection drug users. *AIDS Education and Prevention.* 2004;16: 459–475.
15. Kissinger PJ, Niccolai LM, Magnus M, et al. Partner notification for HIV and syphilis: effects on sexual behaviors and relationship stability. *Sexually Transmitted Diseases.* 2003;30:75–82.
16. Cranston K. Planning for HIV partner counseling and referral services in the third decade. Presented at the National HIV Prevention Conference, Atlanta, GA. 2005. Abst #T3-D1301.
17. Pilcher CD, Fiscus SA, Nguyen TQ, et al. Detection of acute infections during HIV testing in North Carolina. *New England Journal of Medicine.* 2005;352:1873–1883.

Chapter 41

Revealing Your HIV Status

What Are the Issues?

When you test positive for HIV, it can be difficult to know who to tell about it, and how to tell them.

Telling others can be good because:

- You can get love and support to help you deal with your health.
- You can keep your close friends and loved ones informed about issues that are important to you.
- You don't have to hide your HIV status.
- You can get the most appropriate health care.
- You can reduce the chances of transmitting the disease to others.
- In many states, you can be found guilty of a felony for not telling a sexual partner you are HIV-positive before having intimate contact.

Telling others may be bad because:

- Others may find it hard to accept your health status.

"Telling Others You are HIV Positive," Fact Sheet #204, © 2008 AIDS InfoNet. Reprinted with permission. Fact Sheets are regularly updated. Check http://www.aidsinfonet.org for the most recent information.

- Some people might discriminate against you because of your HIV.
- You may be rejected in social or dating situations.

You don't have to tell everybody. Take your time to decide who to tell and how you will approach them. Be sure you're ready. Once you tell someone, they won't forget you are HIV-positive.

General Guidelines

Here are some things to think about when you're considering telling someone that you're HIV-positive:

- Know why you want to tell them. What do you want from them?
- Anticipate their reaction. What's the best you can hope for? The worst you might have to deal with?
- Prepare by informing yourself about HIV disease. You may want to leave articles or a hotline phone number for the person you tell.
- Get support. Talk it over with someone you trust, and come up with a plan.
- Accept the reaction. You can't control how others will deal with your news.

Special Situations

People you may have exposed to HIV: It can be very difficult to disclose your status to sexual partners or people you shared needles with. However, it is very important that they know so they can decide to get tested and, if they test positive, get the health care they need. The Department of Health can tell people you might have exposed, without using your name.

Employers: You may want to tell your employer if your HIV illness or treatments interfere with your job performance. Get a letter from your doctor that explains what you need to do for your health (taking medications, rest periods, etc.). Talk with your boss or personnel director. Tell them you want to continue working, and what changes may be needed in your schedule or workload. Make sure they understand if you want to keep your HIV status confidential.

People with disabilities are protected from job discrimination under the Americans with Disabilities Act (ADA). As long as you can do the essential functions of your job, your employer cannot legally discriminate against you because of your HIV status. When you apply for a new job, employers are not allowed to ask about your health or any disabilities. They can only legally ask if you have any condition that would interfere with essential job functions.

Family members: It can be difficult to decide whether to tell your parents, children, or other relatives that you are HIV-positive. Many people fear that their relatives will be hurt or angry. Others feel that not telling relatives will weaken their relationships and may keep them from getting the emotional support and love that they want. It can be very stressful to keep an important secret from people you are close to.

Family members may want to know how you were exposed to HIV. Decide if or how you will answer questions about how you got infected.

Your relatives may appreciate knowing that you are getting good health care, that you are taking care of yourself, and about your support network.

Health care providers: It's your decision whether or not to tell a health care provider that you have HIV. If your providers, including dentists, know you have HIV, they should be able to give you more appropriate health care. All providers should protect themselves from diseases carried in patients' blood. If providers are likely to come in contact with your blood, you can remind them to put gloves on.

Social contacts: Dating can be very threatening for people with HIV. Fear of rejection keeps many people from talking about their HIV status. Remember, every situation is different and you don't have to tell everybody. If you aren't going to be in a situation where HIV could be transmitted, there's no need to tell. Sooner or later in a relationship, it will be important to talk about your HIV status. The longer you wait, the more difficult it gets.

An HIV-positive child's school: It is best to have good communication about your child's HIV status. Meet with the principal and discuss the school's policy and attitude on HIV. Meet with the nurse and your child's teacher. Be sure to talk about your child's legal right to confidentiality.

Getting Help

You can get help with telling others about your HIV status from the counselors at the HIV anonymous test sites, or your HIV case manager.

Chapter 42

Building a Doctor/Patient Relationship

For the Patient...

Sharing Your Point of View with Your Doctor

Share your point of view. If something is or isn't working for you, it's important you let your doctor know. Being honest about your viewpoint is especially important if you're considering enrolling in a study or using experimental treatments.

Explain why you are considering a particular decision and listen to what your doctor has to say. While some doctors feel uncomfortable recommending certain studies or unapproved medications, many are willing to work with and support patients who have clearly put some thought and time into their decisions.

Whether or not agreement is reached on the use of a particular treatment, cooperation in the form of proper monitoring through examinations and lab tests should be secured. In turn, you should agree to heed reasonable warnings suggested by the monitoring process.

When requesting prescriptions for existing approved medications, a friendly and firm request is likely to work best. If the doctor is opposed, you are entitled to know why, in clear terms. The doctor's concerns and knowledge should be given due respect, whether or not you agree with them.

This section is excerpted from "Building a Cooperative Doctor/Patient Relationship," © 2007 Project Inform. Reprinted with permission. For more information, contact the National HIV/AIDS Treatment Hotline, 1-800-822-7422, or visit our website at www.projectinform.org.

Choosing a Relationship Style

Choose a relationship style and discuss it with your doctor. People have different styles of relating to doctors, and those styles may change at different times or for different illnesses. In the "traditional" doctor-patient relationship, the doctor leads and the patient follows. For some, this is effective because they feel secure and cared for.

Others may view the doctor-patient relationship as more of a partnership, where both doctor and patient contribute to the decision-making process. Some prefer to make decisions and use a doctor primarily as a consultant. This relationship style will require diplomacy on the part of the patient; many doctors have not adjusted to the role of consultant.

None of these relationship styles is right or wrong, but they are all different choices that make different demands upon the relationship. It is important that you let your doctor know which style you prefer. Realize that as time passes and you become more familiar with HIV/AIDS and as you experience different health challenges, the doctor-patient relationship style that works best for you may change.

Learning the Information

Knowledge makes a world of difference. Generally, the more you know before a medical appointment, the more you can benefit from each visit. Obtaining information on your own doesn't need to be difficult or overwhelming. In fact, the education process can begin right at home. Many websites, hotlines, and community organizations are dedicated to answering questions about HIV/AIDS—from transmission to treatment.

If you're comfortable with some of the basics of HIV disease and treatment, you will be better able to ask your doctor specific questions during your visit. Do realize that you can't learn everything at once, so concentrate on the information that is most important to your health right now. Remember that while self-learning is great, it should not be a substitute for using your doctor as a source of information.

Preparing for Appointments

Come prepared for appointments. Both the patient and doctor benefit when a visit is well-planned. It takes only a few minutes to write down key questions ahead of time. Get in the habit of writing down symptoms and side effects you've been experiencing, the changes in meds (including complementary therapies), the missed doses, and any questions that come up between visits in a medical journal. Use this record to update your doctor at the start of the visit.

The limited time in the doctor's office should be used to focus on the most critical issues, rather than everything that comes to mind. Preparation might include bringing along treatment literature to be discussed in the visit. This allows the doctor to know your sources of information and how to evaluate them.

Show your written list of questions to your doctor at the beginning of the visit, so they can be incorporated into the overall visit. Don't wait until the end of the visit to ask questions, as there may not be enough time to address them all.

Getting Emotional News

Be prepared for the emotional content of the visit. Most doctors are sensitive, caring people who respond emotionally to their patients. They have seen an enormous amount of suffering. When fear is written all over a patient's face, no one should fault the doctor for using the "kid gloves" gentle treatment, perhaps even shielding the patients temporarily from the harshest implications.

If you prefer a more straightforward approach, let your doctor know. But don't expect him or her to also serve as your therapist if news is unusually hard to hear. By choosing a more direct approach, you also choose a path that requires greater inner support.

In any case, there is only so much emotional support a doctor can give in the short time allotted for most visits. Plan in advance to make use of other support resources.

If Disagreements Occur...

When disagreements occur despite a cooperative relationship, it's difficult to know what to do. In consideration of active disease states, such as a bout of PCP (Pneumocystis pneumonia), the doctor's expertise must lead the way because the course of treatment is better known and, in many instances, there is a degree of medical consensus. Exceptions may occur in institutions or areas of the country where expertise with HIV is not at a state-of-the-art level, or when bureaucratic procedures may hamper the quality of care. In these cases, a second opinion should always be sought from doctors in the leading AIDS hospitals, and doctors can be referred to the WARMline.

When considering treatment of HIV infection and immune deficiency, disagreements about treatments often occur in a very different context. When patients may have as much information as the doctor about some therapies, each may arrive at different conclusions based on similar data. This presents a challenge for both.

A doctor must feel that he or she is practicing sound medicine, yet the patient may feel s/he cannot compromise on a treatment option s/he considers essential to his or her health or survival. In this instance, both must strive to listen and understand the other's views. Rather than butting heads, both must seek to find ways to satisfy the other's needs and concerns. Both must begin by acknowledging a common goal of keeping the patient alive and maintaining health. Sometimes, it's possible to find new alternatives that neither party had expected before the discussion began.

The patient might ask: "What will it take for you to feel comfortable with what I want to do? More careful monitoring? Reviewing the decision in a month or two? More review of available data? Discussion with other doctors? A statement releasing you from liability?"

Similarly, the doctor might ask: "What can I do to help you better understand the risks and why I'm concerned with what you want to do?" or "What other options, if any, have you considered?" or "Will you wait while I review the matter more carefully?"

While this type of dialogue is very productive, it won't overcome every obstacle. Patients cannot expect doctors to heartily support the use of remedies for which there is no supporting evidence of any kind. Nor can patients realistically expect doctors to give the same credence to highly experimental approaches as they would to better proven therapies. And doctors can't realistically expect patients to "wait and see" indefinitely while the research proceeds.

At the very least, both parties must take the time to fully understand each other's beliefs and the reasoning behind them. Simple confrontation over opposing conclusions is unproductive for both.

If, in the final analysis, the doctor cannot feel comfortable cooperating with unapproved or unorthodox treatment strategies, and the patient is equally firm in his or her convictions, then doctors and patient must question whether it's possible to continue having a mutually acceptable relationship. In many instances, it is possible to maintain the relationship while disagreeing and continuing to communicate over the differences. The option of changing doctors should be reached only as a last resort, and only when it is clear that the parties cannot accept each other's approach to the relationship. Each of us must ultimately find the combination of patient + doctor + approach that makes a cooperative relationship possible.

Chapter 43

Caring for Someone with HIV/AIDS

Giving Care

People living with AIDS should take care of themselves as much as they can for as long as they can. They need to be and feel as independent as possible. They need to control their own schedules, make their own decisions, and do what they want to do as much as they are able. They should develop their own exercise program and eating plan. In addition to regular visits to the doctor, many people with AIDS work at staying healthy by eating properly, sleeping regularly, doing physical exercises, praying or meditating, or other things. If the person you are caring for finds something that helps them, encourage them to keep it up. An exercise program can help maintain weight and muscle tone and can make a person feel better if it is tailored to what the person can do. Well-balanced, good-tasting meals help people feel good, give them energy, and help their body fight illness. People with HIV infection are better off if they don't drink alcoholic drinks, smoke, or use illegal drugs. Keeping up-to-date on new treatments and understanding what to expect from treatments the person is taking are also important.

There are some simple things you can do to help someone with AIDS feel comfortable at home.

- Respect their independence and privacy.

This section contains excerpts from "Caring for Someone with AIDS at Home," Centers for Disease Control and Prevention (www.cdc.gov), June 21, 2007.

- Give them control as much as possible. Ask to enter their room, ask permission to sit with them, etc. Saying "Can I help you with that?" lets them keep control.
- Ask them what you can do to make them comfortable. Many people feel shy about asking for help, especially help with things like using the toilet, bathing, shaving, eating, and dressing.
- Keep the home clean and looking bright and cheerful.
- Let the person with AIDS stay in a room that is near a bathroom.
- Leave tissues, towels, a trash basket, extra blankets, and other things the person might need close by so these things can be reached from the bed or chair.

If the person you are caring for has to spend most of their time in bed, be sure to help them change position often. If possible, a person with AIDS should get out of bed as often as they can. A nurse can show you how to help someone move from a bed to a chair without hurting yourself or them. This helps prevent stiff joints, bedsores, and some kinds of pneumonia. They may also need your help to turn over or to adjust the pillows or blankets. A medical "trapeze" over the bed can help the person shift position by themselves if they are strong enough. If they are so weak they can't turn over, have a nurse show you how to use a sheet to help roll the person in bed from side to side. Usually a person in bed needs to change position at least every four hours.

Bedsores

Bedsores or other broken skin can be serious problems for someone with AIDS. In addition to changing position in bed often, to help keep skin healthy, put extra-soft material (sheepskin, "egg crate" foam, or water mattresses) under the person, keep the sheets dry and free from wrinkles, and massage the back and other parts of the body (like hips, elbows, and ankles) that press down on the bed. Report any red or broken areas on the skin to the doctor or nurse right away.

Exercises

Even in bed, a person can do simple arm, hard, leg, and foot exercises. These are usually called "range of motion" exercises. These exercises help prevent stiff, sore points and help keep the blood moving. A doctor, nurse, or physical therapist can show you how to help.

Breathing

If someone is having trouble breathing, sitting them up may help. Raise the head of a hospital-type bed or use extra pillows or some other soft back support. If they have severe trouble breathing, they need to see a doctor.

Comfort

A good back rub can help a person relax as well as help their circulation. A nurse, physical therapist, or book on massage can give you some tips on how to give a good back rub. Put books, remote controls, water, tissues, and a bell to call for help within easy reach. If the person can't get up, put a urinal or bedpan within easy reach.

Providing Emotional Support

You are caring for a person, not just a body; their feelings are important too. Since every person is different, there are no rules about what to do or say, but here are some ideas that may help.

- Keep them involved in their care. Don't do everything for them or make all their decisions. Nobody likes feeling helpless.
- Have them help out around the house if they can. Everybody likes to feel useful. They want to be part of the group, contributing what they can.
- Include them in the household. Make them part of normal talk about books, TV shows, music, what is going on in the world, and so on. Many people will want to feel involved in the things that are happening around them. But you don't always have to talk, just being there is sometimes enough. Just watching TV together or sitting and reading in the same room is often comforting.
- Talk about things. Sometime they may need to talk about AIDS or talk through their own situation as a way to think out loud. Having AIDS can make a person angry, frustrated, depressed, scared, and lonely, just like any other serious illness. Listening, trying to understand, showing you care, and helping them work through their emotions is a big part of home care. A support group of other people with AIDS can also be a good place for them to talk things out. Contact the National Association of People with AIDS for information about support groups in your area. If they want professional counseling, help them get it.

- Invite their friends over to visit. A little socializing can be good for everyone.
- Touch them. Hug them, kiss them, pat them, hold their hands to show that you care. Some people may not want physical closeness, but if they do, touch is a powerful way of saying you care.
- Get out together. If they are able, go to social events, shopping, riding around, walking around the block, or just into the park, yard, or porch to sit in the sun and breathe fresh air.

Guarding against Infections

People living with AIDS can get very sick from common germs and infections. Hugging, holding hands, giving massages, and many other types of touching are safe for you, and needed by the person with AIDS. But you have to be careful not to spread germs that can hurt the person you are caring for.

Wash Your Hands

Washing your hands is the single best way to kill germs. Do it often. Wash your hands after you go to the bathroom and before you fix food. Wash your hands again before and after feeding them, bathing them, helping them go to the bathroom, or giving other care. Wash your hands if you sneeze or cough; touch your nose, mouth, or genitals; handle garbage or animal litter; or clean the house. If you touch anybody's blood, semen, urine, vaginal fluid, or feces, wash your hands immediately. If you are caring for more than one person, wash your hands after helping one person and before helping the next person. Wash your hands with warm, soapy water for at least 15 seconds. Clean under your fingernails and between your fingers. If your hands get dry or sore, put on hand cream or lotion, but keep washing your hands frequently.

Cover Your Sores

If you have any cuts or sores, especially on your hands, you must take extra care not to infect the person with AIDS or yourself. If you have cold sores, fever blisters, or any other skin infection, don't touch the person or their things. You could pass your infection to them. If you have to give care, cover your sores with bandages, and wash your hands before touching the person. If the rash or sores are on your hands, wear disposable gloves. Do not use gloves more than one time;

throw them away and get a new pair. If you have boils, impetigo, or shingles, if at all possible, stay away from the person with AIDS until you are well.

Keep Sick People Away

If you or anybody else is sick, stay away from the person with AIDS until you're well. A person with AIDS often can't fight off colds, flu, or other common illnesses. If you are sick and nobody else can do what needs to be done for the person with AIDS, wear a well-fitting, surgical-type mask that covers your mouth and nose and wash your hands before coming near the person with AIDS.

Watch Out for Chickenpox

Chickenpox can kill a person with AIDS. If the person you are caring for has already had the chickenpox, they probably won't get it again. But follow these precautions just to be on the safe side:

- Never let anybody with chickenpox in the same room as a person with AIDS, at least not until all the chickenpox sores have completely crusted over.
- Don't let anybody who recently has been near somebody with chickenpox in the same room as a person who has AIDS. After three weeks, the person who was exposed to the chickenpox can visit, if they aren't sick. Most adults have had chickenpox, but you have to be very careful about children visiting or living in the house if they have not yet had chickenpox. If you are the person who was near somebody with chickenpox and you have to help the person with AIDS, wear a well-fitting, surgical-type mask, wash your hands before doing what you have to do for the person with AIDS, and stay in the room as short a time as you can. Tell the person with AIDS why you are staying away from them.
- Don't let anybody with shingles (herpes zoster) near a person with AIDS until all the shingles have healed over. The germ that causes shingles can also cause chickenpox. If you have shingles and have to help the person with AIDS, cover all the sores completely and wash your hands carefully before helping the person with AIDS.
- Call the doctor as soon as possible if the person with AIDS does get near somebody with chickenpox or shingles. There is

a medicine that can make the chickenpox less dangerous, but it must be given very soon after the person has been around someone with the germ.

Get Your Shots

Everybody living with or helping take care of a person with AIDS should make sure they took all their "childhood" shots (immunizations). This is not only to keep you from getting sick, but also to keep you from getting sick and accidentally spreading the illness to the person with AIDS. Just to be sure, ask your doctor if you need any shots or boosters for measles, mumps, or rubella since these shots may not have been available when you were a child. Discuss any vaccinations with your doctor and the doctor of the person with AIDS before you get the shot. If the person with AIDS is near a person with measles, call the doctor that day. There is a medicine that can make the measles less dangerous, but it has to be given very soon after the person is around the germ.

Children or adults who live with someone with AIDS and who need to get vaccinated against polio should get an injection with "inactivated virus" vaccine. The regular oral polio vaccine has weakened polio virus that can spread from the person who got the vaccine to the person with AIDS and give them polio.

Everyone living with a person with AIDS should get a flu shot every year to reduce the chances of spreading the flu to the person with AIDS. Everyone living with a person with AIDS should be checked for tuberculosis (TB) every year.

Be Careful with Pets and Gardening

Pets can give love and companionship. Having a pet around can make a person with AIDS feel better and enjoy life more. However, people with HIV or AIDS should not touch pet litter boxes, feces, bird droppings, or water in fish tanks. Many pet animals carry germs that don't make healthy people sick, but can make the person with AIDS very sick. A person with AIDS can have pets, but must wash their hands with soap and water after handling the pet. Someone who does not have HIV infection must clean the litter boxes, cages, fish tanks, pet beds, and other things. Wear rubber gloves when you clean up after pets and wash your hands before and after cleaning. Empty litter boxes every day, don't just sift. Just like the people living with AIDS, pets need yearly checkups and current vaccinations. If the pet gets sick, take it to the veterinarian right away. Someone with AIDS should not touch a sick animal.

Gardening can also be a problem. Germs live in garden or potting soil. A person with AIDS can garden, but they must wear work gloves while handling dirt and must wash their hands before and after handling dirt. You should do the same.

Personal Items

A person with HIV infection should not share razors, toothbrushes, tweezers, nail or cuticle scissors, pierced earrings or other "pierced" jewelry, or any other item that might have their blood on it.

Laundry

Clothes and bed sheets used by someone with AIDS can be washed the same way as other laundry. If you use a washing machine, either hot or cold water can be used, with regular laundry detergent. If clothes or sheets have blood, vomit, semen, vaginal fluids, urine, or feces on them, use disposable gloves and handle the clothes or sheets as little as possible. Put them in plastic bags until you can wash them. You can but you don't need to add bleach to kill HIV; a normal wash cycle will kill the virus. Clothes may also be dry cleaned or hand washed. If stains from blood, semen, or vaginal fluids are on the clothes, soaking them in cold water before washing will help remove the stains. Fabrics and furniture can be cleaned with soap and water or cleansers you can buy in a store; just follow the directions on the box. Wear gloves while cleaning.

Cleaning House

Cleaning kills germs that may be dangerous to the person with AIDS. You may want to clean and dust the house every week. Clean tubs, showers, and sinks often; use household cleaners, then rinse with fresh water. You may want to mop floors at least once a week. Clean the toilet often; use bleach mixed with water or a commercial toilet bowl cleaner. You may clean urinals and bedpans with bleach after each use. Replace plastic urinals and bedpans every month or so. About ¼ cup of bleach mixed with 1 gallon of water makes a good disinfectant for floors, showers, tubs, sinks, mops, sponges, etc. (or 1 tablespoon of bleach in 1 quart of water for small jobs). Make a new batch each time because it stops working after about 24 hours. Be sure to keep the bleach and the bleach and water mix, like other dangerous chemicals, away from children.

Food

Someone with AIDS can eat almost anything they want; in fact, the more the better. A well-balanced diet with plenty of nutrients, fiber, and liquids is healthy for everybody. Fixing food for a person with AIDS takes a little care, although you should follow these same rules for fixing food for anybody.

- Don't use raw (unpasteurized) milk.
- Don't use raw eggs. Be careful: Raw eggs may be in homemade mayonnaise, hollandaise sauce, ice cream, fruit drinks (smoothies), or other homemade foods.
- All beef, pork, chicken, fish, and other meats should be cooked well done, with no pink in the middle.
- Don't use raw fish or shellfish (like oysters).
- Wash your hands before handling food and wash them again between handling different foods.
- Wash all utensils (knives, spatulas, mixing spoons, etc.) before reusing them with other foods. If you taste food while cooking, use a clean spoon every time you taste; do not stir with the spoon you taste with.
- Don't let blood from uncooked beef, pork, or chicken, or water from shrimp, fish, or other seafood, touch other food.
- Use a cutting board to cut things on and wash it with soap and hot water between each food you cut.
- Wash fresh fruits and vegetables thoroughly. Cook or peel organic fruits and vegetables because they may have germs on the skins. Don't use organic lettuce or other organic vegetables that cannot be peeled or cooked.

A person living with AIDS does not need separate dishes, knives, forks, or spoons. Their dishes don't need special cleaning either. Just wash all the dishes together with soap or detergent in hot water.

A person with AIDS can fix food for other people. Just like everybody else who fixes food, people with AIDS should wash their hands first and not lick their fingers or the utensils while they are cooking. However, no one who has diarrhea should fix food.

To keep food from spoiling, serve hot foods hot and cold foods cold. Cover leftover food and store it in the refrigerator as soon as possible.

Protect Yourself

A person who has AIDS may sometimes have infections that can make you sick. You can protect yourself, however. Talk to the doctor or nurse to find out what germs can infect you and other people in the house. This is very important if you have HIV infection yourself.

For example, diarrhea can be caused by several different germs. Wear disposable gloves if you have to clean up after or help a person with diarrhea and wash your hands carefully after you take the gloves off. Do not use disposable gloves more than one time.

Another cause of diarrhea is the cryptosporidiosis parasite. It is spread from the feces of one person or animal to another person or animal, often by contaminated water, raw food, or food that isn't cooked well enough. Again, wash your hands after using the bathroom and before fixing food. You can check with your local health department to see if cryptosporidiosis is in the water. If you hear that the water in your community may have cryptosporidiosis parasites, boil your drinking water for at least one minute to kill the parasite, then let the water cool before drinking. You may want to buy bottled (distilled) water for cooking and drinking if the cryptosporidiosis parasite or other organisms that might make a person with HIV infection sick could be in the tap water.

If the person with AIDS has a cough that lasts longer than a week, the doctor should check them for TB. If they do have TB, then you and everybody else living in the house should be checked for TB infection, even if you aren't coughing. If you are infected with TB germs, you can take medicine that will prevent you from developing TB.

If the person with AIDS gets yellow jaundice (a sign of acute hepatitis) or has chronic hepatitis B infection, you and everybody else living in the house and any people the person with AIDS has had sex with should talk to their doctor to see if anyone needs to take medicine to prevent hepatitis. All children should get hepatitis B vaccine whether or not they are around a person with AIDS.

If the person with AIDS has fever blisters or cold sores (herpes simplex) around the mouth or nose, don't kiss or touch the sores. If you have to touch the sores to help the person, wear gloves and wash your hands carefully as soon as you take the gloves off. This is especially important if you have eczema (allergic skin) since the herpes simplex virus can cause severe skin disease in people with eczema. Throw the used gloves away; never use disposable gloves more than once.

Many persons with or without AIDS are infected with a virus called cytomegalovirus (CMV), which can be spread in urine or saliva. Wash your hands after touching urine or saliva from a person with AIDS. This is especially important for someone who may be pregnant because a pregnant woman infected with CMV can also infect her unborn child. CMV causes birth defects such as deafness.

Remember, to protect yourself and the person with AIDS from these diseases and others, be sure to wash your hands with soap and water before and after giving care, when handling food, after taking gloves of, and after going to the bathroom.

Gloves

Because the virus that causes AIDS is in the blood of infected persons, blood or other body fluids (such as bloody feces) that have blood in them could infect you. You can protect yourself by following some simple steps. Wear gloves if you have to touch semen, vaginal fluid, cuts or sores on the person with AIDS, or blood or body fluids that may have blood in them. Wear gloves to give care to the mouth, rectum, or genitals of the person with AIDS. Wear gloves to change diapers or sanitary pads or to empty bedpans or urinals. If you have any cuts, sores, rashes, or breaks in your skin, cover them with a bandage. If the cuts or sores are on your hands, use bandages and gloves. Wear gloves to clean up urine, feces, or vomit to avoid all the germs, HIV and other kinds, that might be there.

There are two types of gloves you can use. Use disposable, hospital-type latex or vinyl gloves to take care of the person with AIDS if there is any blood you might touch. Use these gloves one time, then throw them away. Do not use latex gloves more than one time even if they are marked "reusable." You can buy hospital-type gloves by the box at most drug stores, along with urinals, bedpans, and many other medical supplies. Many insurance companies and Medicaid will pay for these gloves if the doctor writes a prescription for them. For cleaning blood or bloody fluids from floors, bed, etc., you can use household rubber gloves, which are sold at any drug or grocery store. These gloves can be cleaned and reused. Clean them with hot, soapy water and with a mixture of bleach and water (about 1/4 cup bleach to 1 gallon of water). Be sure not to use gloves that are peeling, cracked, or have holes in them. Don't use the rubber gloves to take care of a person with AIDS; they are too thick and bulky.

To take gloves off, peel them down by turning them inside out. This will keep the wet side on the inside, away from your skin and other people. When you take the gloves off, wash your hands with soap and water right away. If there is a lot of blood, you can wear an apron or smock to keep your clothes from getting bloody. (If the person with AIDS is bleeding a lot or very often, call the doctor or nurse.) Clean up spilled blood as soon as you can. Put on gloves, wipe up the blood with paper towels or rags, put the used paper towels or rags in plastic bags to get rid of later, then wash the area where the blood was with a mix of bleach and water.

Since HIV can be in semen, vaginal fluid, or breast milk just as it can be in blood, you should be as careful with these fluids as you are with blood.

If you get blood, semen, vaginal fluid, breast milk, or other body fluid that might have blood in it in your eyes, nose, or mouth, immediately pour as much water as possible over where you got splashed, then call the doctor, explain what happened, and ask what else you should do.

Needles and Syringes

A person with AIDS may need needles and syringes to take medicine for diseases caused by AIDS or for diabetes, hemophilia, or other illnesses. If you have to handle these needles and syringes, you must be careful not to stick yourself. That is one way you could get infected with HIV.

Use a needle and syringe only one time. Do not put caps back on needles. Do not take needles off syringes. Do not break or bend needles. If a needle falls off a syringe, use something like tweezers or pliers to pick it up; do not use your fingers. Touch needles and syringes only by the barrel of the syringe. Hold the sharp end away from yourself.

Put the used needle and syringe in a puncture-proof container. The doctor, nurse, or an AIDS service organization can give you a special container. If you don't have one, use a puncture-proof container with a plastic top, such as a coffee can. Keep a container in any room where needles and syringes are used. Put it well out of the reach of children or visitors, but in a place you can easily and quickly put the needle and syringe after they are used. When the container gets nearly full, seal it and get a new container. Ask the doctor or nurse how to get rid of the container with the used needles and syringes.

If you get stuck with a needle used on the person with AIDS, don't panic. The chances are very good (better than 99%) that you will not be infected. However, you need to act quickly to get medical care. Put the needle in the used needle container, then wash where you stuck yourself as soon as you can, using warm, soapy water. Right after washing, call the doctor or the emergency room of a hospital, no matter what time it is, explain what happened, and ask what else you should do. Your doctor may want you to take medicine, such as AZT. If you are going to take AZT, you should begin taking it as soon as possible, certainly within a few hours of the needlestick.

Wastes

Flush all liquid waste (urine, vomit, etc.) that has blood in it down the toilet. Be careful not to splash anything when you are pouring liquids into the toilet. Toilet paper and tissues with blood, semen, vaginal fluid, or breast milk may also be flushed down the toilet.

Paper towels, sanitary pads and tampons, wound dressings and bandages, diapers, and other items with blood, semen, or vaginal fluid on them that cannot be flushed should be put in plastic bags. Put the items in the bag, then close and seal the bag. Ask the doctor, nurse, or local health department about how to get rid of things with blood, urine, vomit, semen, vaginal fluid, or breast milk on them. If you can't have plastic bags handy, wrap the materials in enough newspaper to stop any leaks. Wear gloves when handling anything with blood, semen, vaginal fluids, or breast milk on it.

Sex

If you used to or still do have sex with a person with HIV infection, and you didn't use latex condoms the right way every time you had sex, you could have HIV infection, too. You can talk to your doctor or a counselor about taking an HIV antibody test. The idea of being tested for HIV may be scary. But, if you are infected, the sooner you find out and start getting medical care, the better off you will be. Talk to your sex partner about what will need to change. It is very important that you protect yourself and your partner from transmitting HIV infection and other sexually transmitted diseases. Talk about types of sex that don't risk HIV infection. If you decide to have sexual intercourse (vaginal, anal, or oral), use condoms. Latex condoms can protect you from HIV infection if they are used the right way every time you have sex. Ask your doctor, counselor, or call CDC-INFO 24 hours/day at 800-CDC-INFO (232-4636), 888-232-6348 (TTY), in English, en Español, for more information about safer sex, HIV antibody testing, and referrals to places in your area where you can get confidential or anonymous HIV testing.

Part Six

Sexually Transmitted Disease Vaccines and Research

Chapter 44

Overview of Significant Advances in STD Research

The prevention and treatment of sexually transmitted infections (STIs) are critical global and national health priorities because of their devastating impact on women and infants and their inter-relationships with HIV/AIDS. STIs and HIV are linked both by biological interactions and because both infections occur in the same populations. Infection with certain STIs can increase the risk of HIV acquisition and transmission as well as alter the course of disease progression. In addition, STIs can cause long-term health problems, particularly in women and infants. Some of the sequelae of STIs include pelvic inflammatory disease (PID), infertility, tubal or ectopic pregnancy, cervical cancer, and perinatal or congenital infections in infants born to infected mothers.

NIAID supports research for more effective prevention and treatment approaches to control STIs, including the following:

- Research for safe and effective vaccines, topical microbicides, therapeutics, and strategies for preventing and treating STIs and their sequelae
- Basic research on pathogenesis, immunity, molecular and structural biology of sexually transmitted pathogens, and the impact of STIs in various populations
- Development of better and more rapid diagnostics

This section excerpted from "2005–2006 Biennial Report on Women's Health Research," National Institute for Allergy and Infectious Diseases (www3.niaid.nih.gov).

Each year, an estimated 15 million Americans suffer the effects of STIs at a cost exceeding $16 billion. Recent studies indicate that the more prevalent STIs that cause non-ulcerative diseases (chlamydia, gonorrhea, and trichomoniasis), as well as the STIs that cause ulcerative diseases (syphilis and chancroid), increase the risk of HIV transmission by at least two- to five-fold.

Because some infectious agents (e.g., *Chlamydia trachomatis*) can ascend to the upper female genital tract, the long-term consequences of infection are also more severe for women and may result in PID, infertility, or tubal/ectopic pregnancy. The harmful effects on babies born to infected mothers may include stillbirth, premature birth, and perinatal and congenital infections. Moreover, many infections are often asymptomatic in women, resulting in a delay or lack of treatment. Women and children bear a disproportionate burden of the harm caused by STIs. Group B streptococci (GBS) also cause infections in mothers during pregnancy as well as in the neonate. During pregnancy, women can be afflicted with amnionitis, endometritis, sepsis, and meningitis. Intrauterine infections from GBS can lead to stillbirth or sepsis. In addition, infants can also be infected with GBS during passage through the birth canal resulting in sepsis, pneumonia, and/or meningitis.

NIAID supports a broad array of biomedical research focused on the STIs. Selected significant advances in sex- and gender-specific STI research are provided.

Genital Herpes

There are two types of herpes simplex virus (HSV) and both can cause genital herpes. HSV type 1 (HSV-1) most commonly infects the lips, causing sores known as fever blisters or cold sores, but it also can infect the genital area and produce sores. HSV type 2 (HSV-2) is the usual cause of genital herpes, but it can also infect the mouth. HSV-2 is more common in women (approximately one out of four women) than in men (almost one out of five). Genital HSV infections can present serious health consequences including lifelong recurrent episodes of painful, genital lesions, increased likelihood of HIV transmission and acquisition, and for women, possible transmission to fetus or neonate that can result in neonatal brain damage or death.

The 1994–2004 Center for Disease Control and Prevention's (CDC) surveillance results showed the overall seroprevalence of HSV-2 to be 17%, which is a substantial decrease from the seroprevalence rate of 21% in 1988–1994. Decreases in HSV-2 seroprevalence were prominent among the 14–19 age group and continued through the young adult age group, even after adjusting for changes in sexual behavior. This promising data shows the trajectory of increasing HSV-2 from the 1988–1994 has been reversed. [*JAMA*, 2006; (296 Vol. 8): 964–973].

Herpevac Clinical Trial for Women

A pivotal phase III double-blind clinical efficacy trial of an investigational vaccine for the prevention of genital herpes is enrolling 7,550 women at approximately 42 sites in the United States and Canada. This study, which is known as the Herpevac Trial for Women (http://www.niaid.nih.gov/dmid/stds/herpevac), is being conducted as a public private partnership with GlaxoSmithKline.

Human Papillomavirus

Human papillomavirus (HPV) is the name of a group of viruses that includes more than 100 different strains. More than 30 of these viruses are sexually transmitted, and they can infect the genital area of men and women. Most people who become infected with HPV will not have any symptoms and will clear the infection on their own. Some of the viruses are called "high risk" types and can lead to cancer of the cervix, vulva, vagina, anus, or penis in addition to Pap test abnormalities. "Low risk" types of HPV may cause mild Pap test abnormalities or genital warts.

HPV is of clinical and public health importance because persistent infection with certain oncogenic types can lead to cervical cancer. Cervical cancer is one of the most common cancers in women worldwide. On June 8, 2006, an HPV vaccine was licensed by the Food and Drug Administration (FDA) for use in females, ages 9–26 years. Gardasil is the first vaccine developed to prevent cervical cancer, precancerous genital lesions, and genital warts due to HPV types 6, 11, 16 and 18.

Scientific Advances

Condom use reduces risk of genital HPV infection in young women: NIAID-sponsored researchers evaluated whether the use of the male condom reduced the risk of male-to-female transmission of HPV infection. This study followed young women who reported their sexual activities just prior to and during the study period. Cervical and vulvovaginal samples for HPV DNA and Pap smear testing were collected and sexual behavior was recorded in electronic diaries. Research results suggest the incidence of genital HPV was lower among women whose partners used condoms for all instances of intercourse as compared with those women whose partners used condoms less than 5% of the time. These findings suggest that among newly sexually active women, consistent condom use by their partners appears to reduce the risk of cervical and vulvovaginal HPV infection. (*NEJM* 354(25):2645–2654, 2006)

Chlamydia

Chlamydia trachomatis infections are among the most prevalent of all STIs. In women, chlamydial infections may result in PID, which is a major cause of infertility, ectopic pregnancy, and chronic pelvic pain. The rate of reported chlamydial infection is greater among women than men, and adolescent women are at the highest risk of infection. Asymptomatic infection is common in both men and women. In the United States, the continuing increase in reported chlamydia cases is likely to represent expansion of screening for the infection, the development of more sensitive screening tests, and more complete national reporting.

Scientific Advances

Chlamydia protein offers a neutralizing antigen: *Chlamydia trachomatis* is the leading cause of bacterial sexually transmitted disease and infectious preventable blindness. Despite decades of effort, there is no vaccine against *C. trachomatis* diseases. In this study, researchers conducted an investigation of a protein, polymorphic membrane protein D (PmpD) that was described decades ago as being found across multiple chlamydia strains. The results from this study indicate antibodies specific to this particular protein are neutralizing *in vivo*, but this action is blocked *in vitro*, suggesting that a decoy-like immune evasion strategy may be active *in vivo*. These results suggest a vaccine protocol using this recombinant protein (PmpD) to elicit neutralizing antibodies might offer protection from many or all strains of Chlamydia and possibly surpass the level of protection achieved through natural immunity. This basic research may provide an important step towards the development of a vaccine against chlamydia infections. (*PNAS* 2006; 103; 1894–1899)

Chancroid

Chancroid is an acute ulcerative disease caused by *Haemophilus ducreyi*. It is endemic in many parts of the developing world and is an important risk factor for heterosexual spread of HIV. Chancroid usually occurs in discrete outbreaks in the United States, although the disease is endemic in some areas.

Scientific Advances

Immunization with the *Haemophilus ducreyi* hemoglobin receptor HgbA protects against infection in the swine model of chancroid: The sexually transmitted infection chancroid facilitates the spread of HIV in populations where both chancroid and AIDS are endemic. Thus, successful efforts to prevent chancroid may lower HIV infection rates in these populations. The etiologic agent of chancroid is *Haemophilus ducreyi.* Using a swine model of *H. ducreyi* infection, researchers demonstrated that an experimental HgbA vaccine prevents chancroid, as determined by several parameters including histological examination and measurement of antibody activity. Anti-HgbA immunoglobulin G blocked hemoglobin binding to *H. ducreyi's* HgbA receptor, suggesting a novel mechanism of protection that works by limiting iron acquisition by the pathogen. This study provides the first example of a vaccine for chancroid with significant efficacy in an animal model. Taken together, these data suggest continuing the development of an HgbA vaccine to prevent chancroid. Such a vaccine strategy might also be applied to other bacterial pathogens with strict iron requirements. (*Infection and Immunity* 74(4): 2224–2232, 2006.)

Trichomoniasis

Trichomoniasis is a sexually transmitted infection that affects both men and women and results in approximately 7.4 million new cases, in the United States. The trichomoniasis infection commonly occurs in a woman's vagina, resulting in a vaginal discharge, vaginal odor, discomfort during sexual intercourse and urination, irritation and itching of the genital area and, in rare cases, lower abdominal pain. Both men and women with trichomoniasis have an increased susceptibility to HIV infection and many transmit HIV to their sexual partners. Pregnant women with the infection may deliver a low weight or premature infant. Although prescription drugs cure trichomoniasis, drug resistance has become an increasing concern.

Scientific Advances

Scientists sequence genome of parasite responsible for trichomoniasis: NIAID-sponsored researchers have decoded the genetic makeup of the parasite that causes trichomoniasis, one of the most common STIs, revealing potential clues as to why the parasite has become increasingly drug resistant and suggesting possible pathways for new treatments, diagnostics, and a potential vaccine strategy. (JM Carlton et al. Draft genome of the sexually transmitted pathogen *Trichomonas vaginalis*. *Science* DOI:10.1126/Science.1132894(2007).)

Chapter 45

STD Vaccines and Vaccine Research

Chapter Contents

Section 45.1

Vaccines for Hepatitis A and B

This section begins with excerpts from "Hepatitis A: What You Need to Know," reprinted with permission of the Hepatitis C Support Project, http://www.hcvadvocate.org, © 2008. All rights reserved. Additional information from the Hepatitis B Foundation is cited separately within the section.

Hepatitis A Vaccine

The Hepatitis A (HAV) vaccine is considered safe and effective. The two-dose vaccine is administered by injection, with the second dose given 6–12 months after the first. Antibody testing after vaccination is not recommended since 97–100% of people given two doses of the HAV vaccine develop protective anti-bodies within one month of receiving the first dose and 100% have protective levels after the second dose. Experts believe that that the HAV vaccine will provide protection against hepatitis A for at least 20 years. Some experts believe that people with compromised immune systems (such as people with HIV or people taking immunosuppressants) may require more doses of the HAV vaccine.

There have been no serious adverse reactions attributed to the HAV vaccine. Common side effects may include soreness/tenderness at injection site, headache and malaise.

The vaccine is recommended for anyone at risk of exposure to HAV, including men who have sex with men, day care center workers, and certain international travelers. People with hepatitis B or C or other types of liver disease should receive the HAV vaccine to prevent fulminant hepatitis A.

Routine mandatory vaccination of school age children in some states has reduced the incidence of outbreaks among children. Vaccination programs have the potential to dramatically reduce future outbreaks, if not eliminate the disease altogether. There is also a combination HAV/HBV vaccine (Twinrix) that has been U.S. Food and Drug Administration (FDA) approved for an accelerated dosing schedule (three shots within 30 days and a booster shot after one year). People who have previously been infected with hepatitis A are immune and do not need to be vaccinated.

Hepatitis B Vaccine

"Hepatitis B Vaccine," © 2008 Hepatitis B Foundation (www.hepb.org). All rights reserved. Reprinted with permission.

It takes only three shots to protect yourself and your loved ones against hepatitis B for a lifetime.

In 1981, the Food and Drug Administration approved the first vaccine for hepatitis B, which was plasma-derived (i.e., made from blood products). This vaccine was discontinued in 1990 and is no longer available in the U.S.

The currently used hepatitis B vaccines are made synthetically (i.e., they do not contain blood products) and have been available in the U.S. since 1986. You cannot get hepatitis B from the vaccine.

This safe and effective vaccine is recommended for all infants at birth and for children up to 18 years. Adults, especially those who fall into a high-risk group, should also seriously consider getting the hepatitis B vaccine.

Vaccine Side Effects and Safety

Common side effects include soreness, swelling, and redness at the injection site. The vaccine may not be recommended for those with documented yeast allergies or a history of an adverse reaction to the vaccine.

The hepatitis B vaccine is considered one of the safest and most effective vaccines ever made. Numerous studies looking at the vaccine's safety have been conducted by the Centers for Disease Control, World Health Organization, and other professional medical associations. They have not found any evidence that the vaccine causes sudden infant death syndrome (SIDS), multiple sclerosis, or other neurological disorders.

Vaccine Recommendations

The hepatitis B vaccine is recommended specifically for all infants and children by the Centers for Disease Control and the American Academy of Pediatrics. The CDC also recommends that adults in high-risk groups be vaccinated.

The following list is a general guide for vaccination, but since every person is at some risk for infection, these guidelines should be individualized for each situation.

- All infants at birth and all children up to 18 years

- Health care professionals and emergency personnel
- Sexually active teens and adults
- Men who have sex with men
- Sex partners or close family/household members living with an infected person
- Families considering adoption, either domestic or international
- Travelers to countries where hepatitis B is common (Asia, Africa, South America, the Pacific Islands, Eastern Europe, and the Middle East)
- Patients with kidney disease or undergoing dialysis
- Residents and staff of correctional facilities and group homes
- Any person who may fall into a high risk group due to occupation or lifestyle choices

Vaccine Schedule

The vaccine is readily available at your doctor's office or local health clinic. Three doses are generally required to complete the hepatitis B vaccine series, although there is an accelerated two-dose series for adolescents.

- First injection: At any given time
- Second injection: At least one month after the first dose
- Third injection: Six months after the first dose

Cost of Vaccine

The three-shot vaccine series for children in the United States usually costs $75 to $165, but this can vary. Infants up to age 18 months, and sometimes older children, can receive the vaccine free of charge from most local public health clinics.

Insurance companies will usually cover the cost of vaccines for infants and children. There is also a federal program to help cover the cost of children's vaccines. For more information, contact the Vaccines for Children Program (http://www.cdc.gov/nip/vfc/default.htm).

The hepatitis B vaccine costs more for adults. If an adult is in a high-risk group, the cost may be also covered by insurance. Contact your insurance company for more information about the hepatitis B vaccine.

Approved Hepatitis B Vaccines

There are currently two commercial vaccines used to prevent hepatitis B infection among infants, children, and adults in the United States. They are both manufactured using recombinant technology and neither contains blood products. You cannot get hepatitis B from these vaccines.

- Engerix-B, produced by GlaxoSmithKline
- Recombivax HB, produced by Merck

There is also a combination vaccine for hepatitis A and B available for adults:

- Twinrix, produced by GlaxoSmithKline

Section 45.2

HPV Vaccine and Cervical Cancer

"HPV Vaccine Information for Young Women," Centers for Disease Control and Prevention (www.cdc.gov), June 26, 2008.

There is now a vaccine that prevents the types of genital human papillomavirus (HPV) that cause most cases of cervical cancer and genital warts. The vaccine, Gardasil®, is given in three shots over six months. The vaccine is routinely recommended for 11- and 12-year-old girls. It is also recommended for girls and women age 13 through 26 who have not yet been vaccinated or completed the vaccine series.

Why the HPV Vaccine Is Important

Genital HPV is a common virus that is passed on through genital contact, most often during sex. Most sexually active people will get HPV at some time in their lives, though most will never even know it. It is most common in people in their late teens and early 20s.

There are about 40 types of HPV that can infect the genital areas of men and women. Most HPV types cause no symptoms and go away on their own. But some types can cause cervical cancer in women and other less common genital cancers—like cancers of the anus, vagina, and vulva (area around the opening of the vagina). Other types of HPV can cause warts in the genital areas of men and women, called genital warts. Genital warts are not a life-threatening disease. But they can cause emotional stress and their treatment can be very uncomfortable.

Every year, about 12,000 women are diagnosed with cervical cancer and almost 4,000 women die from this disease in the U.S.

About 1% of sexually active adults in the U.S. (or one million people) have visible genital warts at any point in time.

Who Should Get the HPV Vaccine

The HPV vaccine is recommended for 11- and 12-year-old girls. (Note: The vaccine can also be given to girls 9 or 10 years of age.) It is also recommended for girls and women age 13 through 26 years of age who have not yet been vaccinated or completed the vaccine series.

Will sexually active females benefit from the vaccine?

Ideally females should get the vaccine before they become sexually active, when they may be exposed to HPV. Females who are sexually active may also benefit from the vaccine, but they may get less benefit from it. This is because they may have already gotten an HPV type targeted by the vaccine. Few sexually active young women are infected with all HPV types covered by the vaccine so they would still get protection from those types they have not yet gotten. Currently, there is no test available to tell if a girl/woman has had HPV in the past, or which types.

Can pregnant women get the vaccine?

The vaccine is not recommended for pregnant women. There has been limited research looking at vaccine safety for pregnant women and their unborn babies. So far, studies suggest that the vaccine does not cause health problems for pregnant women or their developing child. But more research is still needed. For now, pregnant women should wait until their pregnancy is over before getting the vaccine. If a woman finds out she is pregnant after she has started getting the vaccine series, she should wait until her pregnancy is over before finishing the three-dose series.

Should girls/women be screened for cervical cancer before getting vaccinated?

No. Girls/women do not need to get an HPV test or Pap test to find out if they should get the vaccine. Neither of these tests can tell the specific HPV type(s) that a woman has (or has had in the past), so there's no way to know if she has already had the HPV types covered by the vaccine.

Why is the HPV vaccine only recommended for girls/women through age 26?

The vaccine has been widely tested in girls/women 9 through 26 years of age. New research is being done on the vaccine's safety and efficacy in women older than 26 years of age. The FDA will consider licensing the vaccine for these women when there is enough research to show that it is safe and effective for them.

What about vaccinating boys and men?

We do not yet know if the vaccine is effective in boys or men. It is possible that vaccinating males will have health benefits for them by preventing genital warts and rare cancers, such as penile and anal cancer. It is also possible that vaccinating boys/men will have indirect health benefits for girls/women. Studies are now being done to find out if the vaccine works to prevent HPV infection and disease in males. When more information is available, this vaccine may be licensed and recommended for boys/men as well.

Effectiveness of the HPV Vaccine

This vaccine targets the types of HPV that most commonly cause cervical cancer and genital warts. The vaccine is highly effective in preventing those types of HPV and related diseases in young women.

The vaccine is less effective in preventing HPV-related disease in young women who have already been exposed to one or more HPV types. That is because the vaccine does not treat existing HPV infections or the diseases they may cause. It can only prevent HPV before a person gets it.

How long does vaccine protection last? Will a booster shot be needed?

Research suggests that vaccine protection will last a long time. More research is being done to find out if women will need a booster vaccine many years after getting vaccinated to boost protection.

What does the vaccine not protect against?

The vaccine does not protect against all types of HPV—so it will not prevent all cases of cervical cancer. About 30% of cervical cancers will not be prevented by the vaccine, so it will be important for women to continue getting screened for cervical cancer (regular Pap tests). Also, the vaccine does not prevent other sexually transmitted infections (STIs). So it will still be important for sexually active persons to lower their risk for other STIs.

Will girls/women be protected against HPV and related diseases, even if they don't get all three doses?

It is not yet known how much protection girls/women would get from receiving only one or two doses of the vaccine. For this reason, it is very important that girls/women get all three doses of the vaccine.

Safety of the HPV vaccine

This vaccine has been licensed by the FDA and approved by CDC as safe and effective. It was studied in thousands of females (ages 9 through 26 years) around the world and its safety continues to be monitored by CDC and the FDA. Studies have found no serious side effects. The most common side effect is soreness in the arm (where the shot is given). There have recently been some reports of fainting in teens after they got the vaccine. For this reason, it is recommended that patients wait in their doctor's office for 15 minutes after getting the vaccine.

Cost and Paying for the HPV vaccine

The retail price of the vaccine is about $125 per dose ($375 for full series).

Is the HPV vaccine covered by insurance plans?

While some insurance companies may cover the vaccine, others may not. Most large insurance plans usually cover the costs of recommended vaccines.

How can I get help paying for the vaccine?

Children age 18 and younger may be eligible to get vaccines, including the HPV vaccine, for free through the Vaccines for Children (VFC) program if they are: Medicaid eligible; uninsured; or American Indian or Alaska Native. Doctors may charge a small fee to give each shot. However VFC vaccines cannot be denied to an eligible child if the family cannot afford the fee.

Some states also provide free or low-cost vaccines at public health department clinics to people without health insurance coverage for vaccines. Contact your State Health Department to see if your state has such a program.

What Vaccinated Girls/Women Need to Know

Women will still need regular cervical cancer screening (Pap tests) because the vaccine will NOT protect against all HPV types that cause cervical cancer. Also, women who got the vaccine after becoming sexually active may not get the full benefit of the vaccine if they had already acquired HPV.

Other Ways to Prevent HPV and Cervical Cancer

Another HPV vaccine is now being considered for licensure by the FDA. This vaccine would protect against the types of HPV that cause most cervical cancers, but it would not protect against genital warts.

Are there other ways to prevent cervical cancer?

Regular cervical cancer screening and follow-up can prevent most cases of cervical cancer. The Pap test can detect cell changes in the cervix before they turn into cancer. Pap tests can also detect most, but not all, cervical cancers at an early, treatable stage. Most women diagnosed with cervical cancer in the U.S. have either never had a Pap test, or have not had a Pap test in the last five years. The HPV test can tell if a woman has HPV on her cervix. This test can be used with the Pap test to help your doctor determine next steps in cervical cancer screening.

Are there other ways to prevent HPV?

The only sure way to prevent HPV is to abstain from all sexual activity. For those who are sexually active, condoms may lower the chances of getting HPV, if used all the time and the right way. Condoms may also lower the risk of developing HPV-related diseases (genital warts and cervical cancer). But HPV can infect areas that are not covered by a condom—so condoms may not fully protect against HPV.

Sexually active adults can also lower their risk of HPV by being in a mutually faithful relationship with someone who has had no or few sex partners, or by limiting their number of sex partners. The fewer partners a person has had, the less likely he or she is to have HPV. But even persons with only one lifetime sex partner can get HPV, if their partner has had previous partners.

Sources

Food and Drug Administration (FDA). FDA News: FDA Licenses New Vaccine for Prevention of Cervical Cancer and Other Diseases in Females Caused by Human Papillomavirus.

FUTURE II Study Group. Prophylactic efficacy of a quadrivalent human papillomavirus (HPV) vaccine in women with virological evidence of HPV infection. *J Infect Dis*. 2007; 196:1438–1446.

FUTURE II Study Group. Quadrivalent vaccine against human papillomavirus to prevent high-grade cervical lesions. *N Engl J Med*. 2007; 356(19):1915–27.

Garland SM, Hernandez-Avila M, Wheeler CM, Perez G, Harper DM, Leodolter S, et al. Females United to Unilaterally Reduce Endo/Ectocervical Disease (FUTURE) I Investigators. Quadrivalent vaccine against human papillomavirus to prevent anogenital diseases. *N Engl J Med*. 2007; 356(19):1928–43.

Harper DM, Franco EL, Wheeler C, et al; HPV Vaccine Study Group. Sustained efficacy up to 4.5 years of a bivalent L1 virus-like particle vaccine against human papillomavirus types 16 and 18: follow-up from a randomised controlled trial. *Lancet*. 2006; 367(9518): 1247–1255.

Ho GY, Bierman R, Beardsley L, et al. Natural history of cervicovaginal papillomavirus infection as measured by repeated DNA testing in adolescent and young women. *N Engl J Med*. 1998; 338(7): 423–428.

Koutsky LA. Epidemiology of genital human papillomavirus infection. *Am J Med*. 1997; 102(5A):3–8.

National Institutes of Health (NIH). NIH Consensus Statement: Cervical Cancer. 1996; 14:1–38.

Paavonen J, Jenkins D, Bosch FX, Naud P, Salmeron J, Wheeler CM et al. Efficacy of a prophylactic adjuvanted bivalent L1 virus-like-particle vaccine against infection with human papillomavirus types 16 and 18 in young women: an interim analysis of a phase III double-blind, randomised controlled trial. *Lancet* 2007;370(9596):1414.

United States Cancer Statistics, National Program of Cancer Registries (NPCR). U.S. Cancers by Type.

Weinstock H, Berman S, Cates W, Jr. Sexually transmitted diseases among American youth: incidence and prevalence estimates, 2000. *Perspect Sex Reprod Health*. 2004; 36(1):6–10.

Winer R, Hughes JP, Feng Q, et al. Consistent condom use from time of first vaginal intercourse and the risk of genital human papillomavirus infection in young women. N Engl J Med. 2006;354: 2645–2654.

Section 45.3

HPV Vaccines for Children and State Mandates

The news that the governor of Texas signed a bill to mandate, or require, the HPV vaccine for school entry has met with much debate. The stories have included discussions of religion, parents' right to choose, and conspiracy. But, how can parents make a good decision if the story is all about the controversy? Little useful information has been provided and even if parents were thinking the vaccine would benefit their children, what will they think after the debate?

The Science behind the Vaccine

HPV is a cause of cervical cancer and genital warts. Two types of human papillomavirus cause about 70% of cervical cancers. Since the vaccine includes these two types of HPV, the vaccine will reduce, but not eliminate, cervical cancer.

- Although the vaccine is new, it was tested in about 21,000 girls and young women before it was approved for general use. The most common side effects were redness and tenderness at the site of the injection. Some people got a low-grade fever.
- The vaccine cannot cause HPV. There are several types of HPV and each type is made up of several proteins. The vaccine is made using only one protein from each of four types of HPV, two that commonly cause cervical cancer and two that commonly cause genital warts. Because the vaccine does not contain the whole virus or any genetic material, it cannot cause HPV.
- HPV is transmitted sexually. More than half of sexually active people will be infected with HPV at some time in their lives and about half of the new infections each year occur in people who are 15 to 24 years old.
- The HPV vaccine will not prevent all sexually transmitted diseases (STDs). This vaccine will only prevent HPV, but not other STDs, like chlamydia, herpes, syphilis, or gonorrhea.
- Pap tests are still necessary. Because only 7 of 10 cervical cancers will be prevented by the HPV vaccine, it is still necessary to have this screening exam.

Sexual Promiscuity

Some groups have proposed that giving teenagers a vaccine for an STD will cause them to be sexually promiscuous. The reality is that many teenagers are already sexually active.

- The 2005 Youth Risk Behavior Surveillance study found that about 47% of 9th through 12th graders had sexual intercourse. Rates were similar in both urban and suburban schools. About 6% of current high school students had sexual intercourse before they were 13 years old.
- About 14% of current high school students report having had four or more sexual partners.
- The goal in providing the vaccine to 11- and 12-year-olds is to protect as many girls as possible before they become sexually active. The HPV vaccine can offer protection for years before exposure to HPV, but once exposed to HPV, the vaccine will not work.

School Entry Mandates

Historically, mandates have been important in controlling the spread of infectious diseases and saving lives. Mandates promote widespread immunization and opportunities for herd immunity; allow some people to be immunized who could otherwise not afford it; and cause more people to be vaccinated because it is a requirement. As new vaccines become available, the role of mandates will continue to be a part of the conversation.

The HPV Vaccine

The time for the conversation about HPV is here. While people discuss mandates and sexual promiscuity, you can protect your daughter from cancer by having her get the vaccine.

Spotlight: Preventive Vs. Therapeutic Vaccines

Vaccines can be given for different reasons. A vaccine is preventive if it is given before a person gets a disease. Childhood vaccines are preventive because they are given before children are infected with certain diseases. Alternatively, therapeutic vaccines are given after a disease is already affecting someone. Currently, there are no therapeutic vaccines on the market, but vaccines in development for AIDS and multiple sclerosis would be of this type.

Section 45.4

Possibilities and Challenges in the Quest for an Effective HIV Vaccine

"The Quest for an Effective HIV Vaccine Presents New Possibilities, Challenges," National Institute for Allergy and Infectious Diseases (www3.niaid.nih.gov), May 16, 2007.

A vaccine that prevents HIV infection remains an important goal in the fight against AIDS, but the current top HIV vaccine candidates may not work in this way, say scientists at the National Institute of Allergy and Infectious Diseases (NIAID), part of the National Institutes of Health (NIH). Rather, the first successful preventive HIV vaccines, if administered prior to HIV infection, may reduce HIV levels in the body, thereby delaying the progression to AIDS and the need to start antiretroviral drugs. These vaccines may also reduce the chance that a person infected with HIV would pass the virus on to other people, according to NIAID Director Anthony S. Fauci, MD, and Margaret I. Johnston, PhD, director of NIAID's Vaccine Research Program in the Division of AIDS.

In a review article in the May 17, 2007 issue of the *New England Journal of Medicine*, Drs. Johnston and Fauci examine the daunting challenges posed by HIV, the evolution of HIV vaccine research, the role T cells may play in HIV vaccine effectiveness, and how the first successful HIV vaccine may fit into a comprehensive HIV/AIDS prevention effort.

Vaccines typically work by mimicking the effects of natural exposure to a specific microbe. Because of initial exposure, the immune system develops the ability to recognize the specific microbe and can protect the human body against it if it reappears. HIV, however, has thwarted scientists' efforts thus far to develop a classic preventive vaccine for the virus because of its ability to integrate into target cells and evade clearance by the immune system. The interaction between HIV and the immune system is complex, and how different HIV-specific immune responses help to control infection is only partially understood.

"The development of an HIV vaccine is a complex research challenge because the virus is unusually well-equipped to elude immune defenses," says Dr. Fauci. "Much progress has been made; however, we must continue research efforts to improve our understanding of HIV and how it evades the immune system, to design new vaccine candidates and to assess the most promising ones in clinical trials."

Dr. Johnston adds, "An important research challenge is to determine if these so-called T-cell vaccines that primarily induce a cellular immune response can have a beneficial effect by reducing viral levels and preserving critical cells needed to control infection. There will be a tremendous public health challenge as well, in an HIV vaccine that does not completely prevent the virus from establishing itself in the body."

Once HIV enters the body, it infects crucial CD4+ T cells, replicates, spreads throughout the body and establishes HIV reservoirs in lymphatic tissues. Within weeks of exposure, virus levels peak and then decline to levels that may remain low for months or years. It is believed that CD8+ T cells—so-called killer T-cells—are responsible for this reduction in HIV levels; however, their ability to continue to suppress the virus declines over time as the virus mutates and the immune system is progressively destroyed.

The infection of CD4+ T cells occurs very early in HIV disease, and virus persists indefinitely. Other viruses also replicate robustly but, unlike HIV, most do not establish a permanent reservoir of infected cells in the body. The window of opportunity to prevent long-term HIV infection may close permanently once a pool of latently infected cells is in place, Drs. Johnston and Fauci note. Neutralizing antibodies, which can attach to and eliminate free virus, only appear after HIV levels have declined substantially. Further, the effectiveness of these antibodies is stymied because of the rapid genetic changes that occur in HIV's outer envelope protein, which allow the virus to escape detection.

While early efforts to develop an HIV vaccine focused on the viral envelope, an improved understanding of how HIV causes disease has brought increased attention to the role that T cells could play in an HIV vaccine by spurring cellular immunity. Numerous animal and human studies have confirmed how important cellular immunity is in the early and later stages of HIV infection, even though the virus is never completely eliminated. Vaccines that induce strong cellular immune responses may have some benefits, say the authors. In non-human primate models of HIV infection, T-cell vaccines have reportedly decreased the total amount of virus produced during early infection, caused a reduction in virus levels following the acute stage of infection, or produced some combination of these effects. In many of these animals, disease progression was also delayed.

Based on the scientific evidence, several questions remain, say Drs. Johnston and Fauci: Can a vaccine that does not prevent HIV infection but reduces virus levels and preserves a segment of uninfected CD4+ T cells from destruction benefit the immunized individual? Might people immunized with T-cell vaccines before HIV exposure remain disease-free for a prolonged period once they are infected?

Additionally, T-cell vaccines may reduce secondary HIV transmission if they can help the immune system keep viral replication at a very low level for a long time. Studies have suggested that people with high levels of virus—namely those in the early and late stages of infection—are most likely to infect their sexual partners. A preventive vaccine given before exposure to HIV might stifle the initial burst of virus, better control virus levels and potentially reduce that person's ability to infect other people, Drs. Johnston and Fauci assert.

Vaccines of this type present several complications, however. T-cell-mediated control of HIV infection may not stave off disease forever. Additional human studies would be needed to determine if the vaccine also reduces the spread of HIV. Finally, an HIV vaccine that delays but does not completely prevent disease could not stand alone as a preventive measure; the public health community would need to include it as part of a broader HIV prevention program, so that recipients would minimize, or ideally, not engage in high-risk behaviors, according to the authors.

Currently, several vaccines that induce primarily T-cell responses are in or will soon enter expanded human clinical trials to determine if they impact HIV infection. Researchers also continue to give high priority to creating an HIV vaccine that induces broadly neutralizing antibodies, which might prevent the establishment of HIV infection. Although rare, such antibodies do exist, giving hope to scientists that a vaccine to induce such antibodies can be designed.

Drs. Johnston and Fauci conclude that a vaccine that prevents HIV infection by clearing the virus before cells become latently infected remains the goal. In addition, they believe that even a vaccine that does not prevent infection could prove beneficial if it prolongs the disease-free period and possibly even reduces virus transmission. If such a vaccine is shown to be successful and is eventually licensed, it would need to be delivered as part of a comprehensive, multifaceted HIV prevention program.

Section 45.5

Research on Preventive HIV Vaccines

"Preventive HIV Vaccines," AIDSinfo, U.S. Department of Health and Human Services (www.aidsinfo.nih.gov), May 2006.

What is a vaccine?

A vaccine is a medical product designed to stimulate your body's immune system in order to prevent or control an infection. An effective preventive vaccine trains your immune system to fight off a particular microorganism so that it can't establish a serious infection or make you sick.

What is the difference between a preventive HIV vaccine and a therapeutic HIV vaccine?

Therapeutic HIV vaccines are designed to control HIV infection in people who are already HIV positive. Preventive HIV vaccines are designed to protect HIV-negative people from becoming infected or getting sick. This section focuses on preventive HIV vaccines.

Although there is currently no vaccine to prevent HIV, researchers are developing and testing potential HIV vaccines. The goal is to develop a vaccine that can protect people from HIV infection, or at least lessen the chance of getting HIV or AIDS should a person be exposed to the virus.

How does a preventive vaccine work?

When your body encounters a microorganism, your immune system mounts an attack on the invader. After the microorganism is defeated, your immune system continues to "remember" how to quickly beat the invader should it try to infect you again.

A vaccine is designed to resemble a real microorganism. The vaccine trains your immune system to recognize and attack the real microorganism should you ever encounter it. If you've received an effective vaccine, your immune system will "remember" how to quickly attack and defeat a particular microorganism for many years.

Can an HIV vaccine give me HIV or AIDS?

The experimental HIV vaccines currently being studied in clinical trials do not contain any "real" HIV, and therefore cannot cause HIV or AIDS. However, some HIV vaccines in trials could prompt your body to produce antibodies against HIV. These HIV antibodies could cause you to test "positive" on a standard HIV test, even if you don't actually have HIV. Other tests are available that can distinguish between vaccinated and infected people. For more information about this issue, please visit http://www.hvtn.org/science/volunteerfaqs.html (click on "Will I test HIV-positive as a result of the vaccine?").

What are the different types of vaccine?

There are three main types of vaccines that are being studied for the prevention of HIV infection and AIDS:

- Subunit vaccines, also known as "component" or "protein" vaccines, contain only individual parts of HIV, rather than the whole virus. Instead of collecting these parts from the virus itself, the HIV subunits are made in the laboratory using genetic engineering techniques. These manmade subunits alone—without the rest of the virus—can prompt the body to produce an anti-HIV immune response, although that response may be too weak to actually protect against future HIV infection.
- Recombinant vector vaccines take advantage of non-HIV viruses that either don't cause disease in humans or have been deliberately weakened so that they can't cause disease. These weakened (attenuated) viruses are used as vectors, or carriers, to deliver copies of HIV genes into the cells of the body. Once inside cells, the body uses the instructions carried in the copies of HIV genes to produce HIV proteins. As with subunit vaccines, these HIV proteins can stimulate an anti-HIV immune response. Most of the recombinant vector vaccines for HIV deliver several HIV genes (but not the complete set) and may therefore create a stronger immune response.

  Some of the virus vectors being studied for HIV vaccines include ALVAC (a canarypox virus), MVA (a type of cowpox virus), VEE (a virus that normally infects horses), and adenovirus-5 (a human virus that doesn't usually cause serious disease) based vectors.
- DNA vaccines also introduce HIV genes into the body. Unlike recombinant vector vaccines, DNA vaccines do not rely on a

virus vector. Instead, "naked" DNA containing HIV genes is injected directly into the body. Cells take up this DNA and use it to produce HIV proteins. As with subunit and recombinant vector vaccines, the HIV proteins trigger the body to produce an immune response against HIV.

Again, none of these vaccines contain real HIV or anything else that could cause HIV infection or AIDS.

What is a prime-boost vaccination strategy?

A single type of HIV vaccine may be used alone, or it may be used in combination with another type of HIV vaccine. One approach to combined HIV vaccination is called the prime-boost strategy. In this approach, administration of one type of HIV vaccine (such as a DNA vaccine) is followed by later administration of a second type of HIV vaccine (such as a recombinant vector vaccine). The goal of this approach is to stimulate different parts of the immune system and enhance the body's overall immune response to HIV.

How can I participate in a vaccine clinical trial?

Clinical trial volunteers are tremendously important in the effort to develop a preventive HIV vaccine. To find an HIV vaccine trial near you, contact AIDSinfo toll-free at 800-448-0440 to speak to an information specialist, who will help you locate trials in your area. You can also locate research sites using the AIDSinfo vaccine webpage at http://aidsinfo.nih.gov/Vaccines/. On the left side of the screen, under "Preventive HIV Vaccine Trials," click "New and Recruiting Trials" for a complete list of currently recruiting preventive HIV vaccine studies.

Enrolling in a clinical trial isn't the only way to help the HIV vaccine effort—there are other ways to participate. Consider serving on an HIV vaccine community advisory board. Get involved with outreach and community education programs. Lobby your elected officials to support HIV vaccine research and development. Or volunteer in other HIV/AIDS prevention, treatment, and support efforts—all are valuable ways to contribute.

Resources for More Information about HIV Vaccines

http://www.vrc.nih.gov/VRC/

http://www.hvtn.org/

Or contact your doctor or an AIDSinfo Health Information Specialist at 800-448-0440 or http://aidsinfo.nih.gov.

Chapter 46

Topical Microbicides and STDs

What Are Microbicides?

Microbicides are anti-HIV substances. They could reduce the risk of HIV infection during vaginal or rectal intercourse. No microbicides are available yet. However, with sufficient funding and demand, microbicides could be available by 2010.

They could be a very important part of global HIV prevention efforts. Currently, male and female condoms are the only tools we have for HIV prevention. However, many men object to wearing condoms. Many women do not feel they can demand, or even ask their male partners to use a condom. Currently, over 50% of new HIV infections worldwide occur in women.

The use of microbicides could be controlled by women. They could be applied before sex. They won't require male cooperation to use, the way male and female condoms do. Some might be products women can use without their partners' knowledge.

They will come in gels, foams, and creams. Some may take the form of a sponge or thin film that can be inserted with the fingers. Rings or diaphragms may also be inserted into the vagina to deliver microbicides. Microbicides can also be put in suppositories, small plugs of medication designed to melt at body temperature when placed in the vagina or rectum.

"Microbicides," Fact Sheet #157, © 2008 AIDS InfoNet. Reprinted with permission. Fact Sheets are regularly updated. Check http://www.aidsinfonet.org for the most recent information.

One study estimated that microbicide use could prevent about 2.5 million HIV infections within three years. This is based on a microbicide that only worked 60% of the time and was used by only 20% of women, in 73 low income countries. Microbicides may also protect women against some other sexually transmitted diseases, in addition to HIV.

Condoms are still the most effective method of preventing infection. Ideally, microbicides would be used along with condoms for added protection. But, for people whose partners won't use condoms, microbicides could offer a way of reducing HIV risk that can be used without a partner's participation.

Microbicides and Vaccines

Vaccines against HIV have gotten much more attention than microbicides in recent years. An effective vaccine would offer important advantages:

- It could be given to a large segment of the population at risk.
- It would be effective for several years.
- It would not depend on people remembering to use it.

Microbicides, on the other hand, depend on people remembering to use them correctly each time they have sex. Once developed, microbicides and vaccines would work together. Microbicides will put the power of prevention directly in women's hands.

After a period of optimism about the development of an HIV vaccine, research has slowed. The virus presents several obstacles to vaccine development. At this point it is not clear when a vaccine might become available. However, it is unlikely to be within the next 10 years.

Microbicide research is further along. But microbicide research has also encountered setbacks. Nonoxynol-9 (N-9) is a spermicide that was tested as a microbicide. Research showed that frequent use of N-9 may actually increase the risk of HIV infection. It can damage the lining of the vagina or rectum, making it easier for HIV to get past the body's defenses. N-9 had to be discarded from the list of potential microbicides.

How Do Microbicides Work?

Microbicides could work in various ways:

- They could immobilize the virus.
- They could create a barrier between the virus and the cells of the vagina or rectum to block infection.
- They could prevent HIV from reproducing and establishing an infection after it has entered the body.

Some potential microbicides work in just one of the ways above and some combine two or more methods, to increase effectiveness.

How Many Microbicides Are near Approval?

No anti-HIV microbicides are currently approved as safe and effective. However, many are being tested. These tests are going on around the world. Large-scale tests are going on mainly in Africa where the HIV rates are highest.

Four microbicides are in Phase III (final) testing. The microbicides closest to approval are Carraguard®, PRO 2000 Gel, BufferGel, and Savvy. Cellulose sulfate gel is also being studied as a contraceptive. However, studies of cellulose sulfate gel (Ushercell) were stopped in 2007.

The Bottom Line

Microbicides are anti-HIV substances designed in various forms to provide additional protection against HIV. They are intended to be used as an additional prevention measure or in cases where a partner is not using condoms.

Dozens of potential microbicides are in various stages of research. Once available, they could help women and men protect themselves. Microbicides may be especially important for women in developing nations who are not always empowered to require partners to wear condoms.

For More Information

The Alliance for Microbicide Development (www.microbicide.org) keeps updated listings on microbicides in various stages of development and information on global clinical trials.

The Global Campaign for Microbicides (www.global-campaign.org) provides information about global microbicide advocacy efforts. It explains how people can become involved in making microbicides a reality as soon as possible.

Chapter 47

Internet Drugs Falsely Claim to Prevent and Treat STDs

The Food and Drug Administration (FDA) is alerting consumers about certain drugs they may have purchased over the internet. The products are sold under the following names:

- Tetrasil
- Genisil
- Aviralex
- OXi-MED
- Imulux
- Beta-mannan
- Micronutrient
- Qina
- SlicPlus

The products falsely claim to prevent or treat the following variety of sexually transmitted diseases:

- Herpes
- Chlamydia
- HIV/AIDS
- Human papillomavirus (HPV)
- Cervical dysplasia

Some of these products falsely claim to have "FDA Approval" and some claim to be "more effective" than conventional medicine. Examples of claims that these products make include:

"Internet Drugs Falsely Claim to Prevent and Treat STDs," U.S. Food and Drug Administration (www.fda.gov), March 12, 2008.

- "Treatment Kills all Herpes Viruses WITHOUT having to use conventional drugs or medications"
- "Greatest STD Protection Without Condoms"
- "The active ingredient in our product is FDA certified to destroy 99.9992 percent of all pathogenic organisms [i.e.] Chlamydia"

Why Consumers Should Be Concerned

"STDs are very serious diseases and these products give consumers a false sense of security that they are protected from STDs," says Janet Woodcock, MD, Director of FDA's Center for Drug Evaluation and Research.

What Consumers Should Do

- Stop using these products immediately.
- Contact your health care professional if you have used any of these products and experienced any bad reactions.
- Notify FDA of any complaints or problems associated with these products through MedWatch, FDA's voluntary reporting program, at 800-FDA-1088 or www.fda.gov/medwatch/report.htm.

What Is FDA Doing?

FDA issued warning letters to six U.S. companies and one foreign individual for marketing these products. The warning letters state that failure to properly resolve violations of the law may cause further enforcement action that can include seizure of illegal products and possible criminal prosecution. Issuing these warning letters is part of FDA's ongoing campaign against fraudulent products marketed on the Internet for serious and life-threatening diseases. The agency also works to educate consumers about the risks and dangers that exist from buying unsafe products.

Chapter 48

Newly Developed Testing Method Catches Nearly Twice as Many Gonorrhea and Chlamydia Infections

A new study shows that a more efficient sexually transmitted disease (STD) screening method—called a nucleic acid amplification test (NAAT)—can detect at least twice as many oropharyngeal (throat) and rectal gonorrhea and chlamydia infections as a bacterial culture test, the standard means of diagnosing gonorrhea and chlamydia infections in extra-genital sites.

Culture testing requires that bacteria be grown in a controlled laboratory setting before the infection can be identified. Because NAATs can detect bacterial DNA directly from a patient sample, they are generally more accurate, easier to use, and provide results faster than culture tests.

Diagnosing and treating infections at all exposed anatomic sites (i.e., genitals, throat, rectum) is essential for preventing the spread of STDs. To date, three NAATs are cleared by the Food and Drug Administration (FDA) to screen for both chlamydia and gonorrhea infections in the urogenital tract. These tests have replaced traditional bacterial culture for those infections in many medical settings. However, none of these NAATs has been cleared by the FDA to screen for infections in the throat or rectum, which are relatively common among men who have sex with men (MSM). FDA clearance of NAATs for use at extra-genital sites would require submission of additional data to verify their effectiveness.

"DNA Testing Method Can Identify Twice as Many Throat and Rectal Gonorrhea and Chlamydia Infections as Traditional Bacterial Culture," 2008 National STD Prevention Conference, Centers for Disease Control and Prevention (www.cdc.gov), April 7, 2008.

To assess whether NAATs already approved for urogenital use are effective in identifying chlamydia and gonorrhea infections in the throat and rectum, researchers from the University of California, San Francisco (UCSF) and the San Francisco Department of Public Health, led by UCSF's Julius Schachter, tested oropharyngeal and rectal swab specimens from 1,110 MSM attending San Francisco's public STD clinic between October 2005 and May 2007. Forty percent of the men had no symptoms for either disease. All collected samples were tested with a traditional culture test, as well as two different NAATs currently FDA-approved for urogenital use.

Among the MSM participating in the study, the tests indicated that chlamydia prevalence was 0.8% in the throat and 6.1% in the rectum; gonorrhea prevalence was 8.3% in the throat and 8.2% in the rectum. Dr. Schachter and colleagues found that both NAATs identified a significantly larger number of chlamydia and gonorrhea infections in the throat and rectum than traditional bacterial culture tests. NAATs were statistically similar in identifying the majority of all chlamydia and gonorrhea infections in the throat and rectum (range: 63%–100%), while culture tests identified significantly fewer proportions of infections in extra-genital sites (range: 27%–44%). Both NAATs also had greater sensitivity (the ability to correctly identify those who are infected) than traditional culture tests, and comparable specificity (the ability to correctly identify those who are not infected).

The authors note that FDA clearance of NAATs to screen for chlamydia and gonorrhea infections in the throat and rectum would clear the way for their widespread use in medical settings, identify more infections, and help stop the continued spread of these diseases—particularly among MSM.

CDC is working with the FDA and test manufacturers to gather, analyze, and coordinate the submission of relevant data to the agency. In the interim, laboratories may use NAATs to test for chlamydia and gonorrhea in the throat or rectum, provided they first perform in-house studies to verify the accuracy of their testing methods in accordance with established federal regulations. The San Francisco Department of Public Health, for example, has performed such a study and now uses NAATs in its laboratory to screen for chlamydia and gonorrhea at all three anatomic sites. CDC encourages dialogue among public health professionals to determine whether their local patient populations are at risk for chlamydia and gonorrhea infections at extra-genital sites, and advises local health departments to work with laboratory directors to ensure the development of diagnostic capacity for such testing if it is needed.

Chapter 49

Human Protein May Offer Novel Target for Blocking HIV Infection

A research group supported by the National Institutes of Health (NIH) has uncovered a new route for attacking the human immunodeficiency virus (HIV) that may offer a way to circumvent problems with drug resistance. In findings published in the online edition of the Proceedings of the National Academy of Sciences, the researchers report that they have blocked HIV infection in the test tube by inactivating a human protein expressed in key immune cells.

Most of the drugs now used to fight HIV, which is the retrovirus that causes acquired immune deficiency syndrome (AIDS), target the virus's own proteins. However, because HIV has a high rate of genetic mutation, those viral targets change quickly and lead to the emergence of drug-resistant viral strains. Doctors have tried to outmaneuver the rapidly mutating virus by prescribing multi-drug regimens or switching drugs. But such strategies can increase the risk of toxic side effects, be difficult for patients to follow, and are not always successful. Recently, interest has grown in attacking HIV on a new front by developing drugs that target proteins of human cells, which are far less prone to mutations than are viral proteins.

In the new study, Pamela Schwartzberg, MD, PhD, a senior investigator at the National Human Genome Research Institute (NHGRI), part of NIH; Andrew J. Henderson, PhD, of Boston University; and

---

"Research Findings Open New Front in Fight against AIDS Virus," National Institutes of Health, U.S. Department of Health and Human Services (www.nih.gov), April 28, 2008.

their colleagues found that when they interfered with a human protein called interleukin-2-inducible T cell kinase (ITK) they inhibited HIV infection of key human immune cells, called T cells. ITK is a signaling protein that activates T cells as part of the body's healthy immune response.

"This new insight represents an important contribution to HIV research," said NHGRI Scientific Director Eric D. Green, MD, PhD. "Finding a cellular target that can be inhibited so as to block HIV validates a novel concept and is an exciting model for deriving potential new HIV therapies."

When HIV enters the body, it infects T cells and takes over the activities of these white blood cells so that the virus can replicate. Eventually, HIV infection compromises the entire immune system and causes AIDS. The new work shows that without active ITK protein, HIV cannot effectively take advantage of many signaling pathways within T cells, which in turn slows or blocks the spread of the virus.

"We were pleased and excited to realize the outcome of our approach," Dr. Schwartzberg said. "Suppression of the ITK protein caused many of the pathways that HIV uses to be less active, thereby inhibiting or slowing HIV replication."

In their laboratory experiments, the researchers used a chemical inhibitor and a type of genetic inhibitor, called RNA interference, to inactivate ITK in human T cells. Then, the T cells were exposed to HIV, and the researchers studied the effects of ITK inactivation upon various stages of HIV's infection and replication cycle. Suppression of ITK reduced HIV's ability to enter T cells and have its genetic material transcribed into new virus particles. However, ITK suppression did not interfere significantly with T cells' normal ability to survive, and mice deficient in ITK were able to ward off other types of viral infection, although antiviral responses were delayed.

"ITK turns out to be a great target to examine," said Dr. Schwartzberg, noting that researchers had been concerned that blocking other human proteins involved in HIV replication might kill or otherwise impair the normal functions of T cells.

According to Dr. Schwartzberg, ITK already is being investigated as a therapeutic target for asthma and other diseases that affect immune response. In people with asthma, ITK is required to activate T cells, triggering lung inflammation and production of excess mucus.

"There are several companies who have published research about ITK inhibitors as part of their target program," Schwartzberg said. "We hope that others will extend our findings and that ITK inhibitors will be pursued as HIV therapies."

NHGRI researchers received support for this work from the NIH Intramural AIDS Targeted Antiviral Program. Chemical compounds used in the research were synthesized at the NIH Chemical Genomics Center, which was established through the NIH Roadmap for Medical Research and is administered by NHGRI. The Boston University group originally participated in the research while at Pennsylvania State University, where they received support from Penn State Tobacco Formula Funds, and where Dr. Henderson received support from the National Institute of Allergy and Infectious Diseases (NIAID).

Chapter 50

New Trials of Pre-Exposure Prophylaxis for HIV Prevention

New approaches to HIV prevention are urgently needed to stem the estimated 2.7 million new HIV infections that occur worldwide each year. While behavior change programs have contributed to dramatic reductions in the number of annual infections in the U.S. and many other nations, far too many individuals remain at high risk. With an effective vaccine years away, there is mounting evidence that antiretroviral drugs may be able to play an important role in reducing the risk of HIV infection. As part of its commitment to developing new HIV prevention strategies, the Centers for Disease Control and Prevention (CDC) is sponsoring three clinical trials of pre-exposure prophylaxis, or PrEP, for HIV prevention, and is participating in a University of Washington–sponsored trial in Kenya and Uganda. The trials test the antiretroviral drug tenofovir disoproxil fumarate (or tenofovir, brand name Viread®) used alone or in combination with emtricitabine (together, known as the brand name Truvada®) taken as a preventative drug.

The CDC-sponsored trials are designed to answer important questions about the safety and efficacy of a tenofovir or tenofovir plus emtricitabine pill taken as a daily oral HIV preventative among three populations at high risk for infection: heterosexuals in Botswana, injection drug users in Thailand, and men who have sex with men (MSM) in the United States. The trials in Botswana and Thailand are safety

---

"CDC Trials of Pre-Exposure Prophylaxis for HIV Prevention," Centers for Disease Control and Prevention (www.cdc.gov), August 3, 2008.

and efficacy trials, while the U.S. trial is an extended safety trial. CDC will also co-manage two trial sites in Uganda as part of the University of Washington Partners PrEP Study, which is examining the safety and efficacy of PrEP among heterosexual couples. All of the trials will also assess the effects of taking a daily pill on HIV risk behaviors, adherence to and acceptability of the regimen, and in cases where participants become HIV-infected, the resistance characteristics of the acquired virus. This information will be critical to guide future studies and HIV prevention programs.

Similar PrEP trials are also being conducted by other agencies. In 2006, Family Health International (FHI), with funding from the Bill and Melinda Gates Foundation, completed a safety trial of tenofovir for HIV prevention among young women in Ghana. The study provided the first data showing PrEP with tenofovir to be both safe and acceptable for use by HIV-negative individuals. The National Institutes of Health (NIH) is currently evaluating the safety and efficacy of PrEP among MSM in Peru, Ecuador, South Africa, and the U.S. and plans to expand its trial to additional countries. Additional trials investigating PrEP among women in Africa are scheduled to be launched by FHI and the Microbicide Trials Network (MTN) within the next year.

Rationale for Trials of Pre-Exposure Prophylaxis for HIV Prevention

Researchers believe that an antiretroviral drug taken as a daily oral preventative is one of the most important new prevention approaches being investigated today. An effective daily preventative treatment could help address the urgent need for female-controlled prevention methods and, when combined with existing prevention measures, could help reduce new HIV infections among men and women at high risk.

The concept of providing a preventative treatment before exposure to an infectious agent is not new. For example, when individuals travel to an area where malaria is common, they are advised to take medication to fight malaria before and during travel to that region. The medicine to prevent illness will then be in their bloodstream if they are exposed to the infectious agent that causes malaria.

Several sources of data suggest that the use of antiretroviral drugs in this manner may be effective in reducing the risk of HIV infection. Theoretically, if HIV replication can be inhibited from the very first moment the virus enters the body, it may not be able to establish a permanent infection. Providing antiretrovirals (ARVs) to HIV-infected women during labor and delivery and to their newborns immediately following birth has been shown to reduce the risk of mother-to-child transmission by about 50%. Additionally, in observational studies, ARV regimens have been associated with an 80% reduction in the risk of HIV infection among health care workers following needle sticks and other accidental exposures, when treatment is initiated promptly and continued for several weeks. Finally, animal studies have shown that tenofovir can reduce the transmission of a virus similar to HIV in monkeys when given before and immediately after a single retroviral exposure. Animal studies have also demonstrated that preexposure administration of tenofovir plus emtricitabine provided significant protection to monkeys exposed repeatedly to an HIV-like virus. These data, combined with the drugs' favorable resistance and safety profiles as HIV treatments, make tenofovir and tenofovir plus emtricitabine ideal candidates for HIV prevention trials.

Tenofovir was approved by the U.S. Food and Drug Administration in 2001 as a treatment for HIV infection, and the tenofovir plus emtricitabine combination pill was approved for use as an HIV treatment in 2004. More than 200,000 HIV-infected people around the world have now used these drugs. As treatments for HIV-infected individuals, tenofovir and tenofovir plus emtricitabine have been shown to be both safe and effective. They have relatively low levels of side effects and slow development of associated drug resistance, compared with other available HIV treatments. Because the therapies are taken orally only once a day, with or without food, they are also among the most convenient-to-use HIV drugs available today. These trials are designed to evaluate the drugs' safety and efficacy among uninfected individuals. Side effects may differ in HIV-negative populations, and it is not yet known if tenofovir or tenofovir plus emtricitabine can prevent HIV infection in humans.

CDC-Sponsored PrEP Trials

Specific Trial Designs and Objectives

All three of CDC's studies are randomized, double-blind, placebo-controlled trials. All participants receive risk-reduction counseling and other prevention services. In addition, half of the participants are randomly assigned to receive one antiretroviral pill daily (either tenofovir or tenofovir plus emtricitabine, depending on the trial), and the other half are randomly assigned to take one daily placebo pill (a similar tablet without active medication). Neither researchers nor participants know an individual's group assignment. In all, the studies will involve 4,000 volunteers. The Thailand and U.S. trials of tenofovir began in 2005 and the Botswana trial of tenofovir plus emtricitabine began in early 2007. The trials are expected to last between four and six years.

To ensure that the studies remain on a solid scientific and ethical foundation, all study procedures and plans are reviewed and approved by scientific and ethical review committees at CDC (called institutional review boards, or IRBs), as well as IRBs established by each host country and research site prior to trial launch. Additionally, data on safety, enrollment, and efficacy will be reviewed regularly by an independent data safety and monitoring board (DSMB) for the Botswana and Thai trials, and by an independent safety review committee for the U.S. trial. These committees review emerging data to ensure that continuing the trial is safe and to determine the point at which the results are conclusive. If scientific questions arise during the course of the research, these committees will meet more frequently.

Botswana and Thailand

The CDC trials in Botswana and Thailand are safety and efficacy trials. The Botswana trial is examining the safety and efficacy of tenofovir plus emtricitabine, and the Thailand trial is examining the safety and efficacy of tenofovir.

- *Botswana:* The Botswana study is being conducted in collaboration with the Botswana government and is enrolling 1,200 HIV-negative heterosexual men and women, ages 18 to 39, in the nation's two largest cities, Gaborone and Francistown. Participants are recruited through a number of venues, including HIV voluntary counseling and testing centers, sexually transmitted disease (STD) and family planning clinics, youth organizations, and community events.
- *Thailand:* The Thailand study is being conducted in collaboration with the Bangkok Metropolitan Administration and the Thailand Ministry of Public Health and is enrolling 2,400 HIV-negative intravenous drug users (IDUs) at 17 drug treatment clinics in Bangkok. Participants are recruited at the drug treatment clinics, at community outreach sites, and through a peer referral program.

The United States

The U.S. trial is designed to assess the clinical and behavioral safety of once-daily tenofovir among HIV-negative MSM. This trial will not be large enough to evaluate the drug's efficacy in reducing HIV transmission. Data from the CDC trial will provide critical information to guide the development of guidelines for use, should efficacy be demonstrated in other trials.

- *United States:* The U.S. study is being conducted at three sites in collaboration with the San Francisco Department of Public Health, the AIDS Research consortium of Atlanta, and Fenway Community Health in Boston. The study has enrolled 400 HIV-negative MSM who reported having had anal intercourse in the prior 12 months. Participants are randomly assigned to one of four study arms. Two arms receive either tenofovir or placebo immediately upon enrollment, while the other two arms receive either tenofovir or placebo after nine months of enrollment. This design will allow researchers to compare risk behaviors among those taking a daily pill and those not taking pills.

Education and Enrollment of Trial Participants

Understanding the potential impact of a daily preventative drug regimen on HIV risk behaviors will be critical, should pre-exposure prophylaxis prove effective in reducing HIV transmission. One of the greatest risks, as efforts progress to identify new biomedical prevention approaches, is that individuals at risk will reduce their use of existing HIV prevention strategies. It will therefore be crucial to reinforce proven behavioral prevention strategies, both within and beyond these trials. All three trials are taking multiple steps to address this issue during the education and enrollment of trial participants and through ongoing participant counseling.

First, it is critical to ensure that participants understand that trial participation may not protect them from HIV infection—either because they may receive a placebo or because they may receive a study drug, the efficacy of which remains unproven. This and other key aspects of the trial, including the potential risks and benefits of participation, are explained to potential volunteers in the language of their choice, prior to their enrollment. To ensure participants fully understand all aspects of their participation, all volunteers are required to pass a comprehension test prior to providing written informed consent. Study participants are also free to withdraw from the trial at any time and for any reason.

Risk-Reduction Counseling and Other Prevention and Treatment Services

To assist participants in eliminating or reducing HIV risk behaviors, extensive counseling is provided at each study visit, and more often if needed. This interactive counseling has proven effective in reducing the risk of HIV and other STDs in multiple populations, including past participants of similar HIV prevention trials. Participants are also offered free condoms and STD testing and treatment to reduce their risk for HIV infection. Additionally, in Thailand, participating IDUs are offered follow-up in a methadone drug treatment program and receive bleach and instructions on how to use it to clean needles. Consistent with Thai government policy, sterile syringes are not provided, but are widely available in Thailand without a prescription and at low cost (one sterile syringe and one needle cost about 5 baht, or about $0.15).

While participants will likely be at lower risk as a result of these prevention services, some individuals will engage in behavior that places them at risk for HIV infection. To ensure that participants who are infected during the trial are quickly referred to the best available medical and psychosocial services, participants receive free rapid HIV testing at every visit. This regular HIV testing will also help guard against the development of drug-resistant virus, as the study drug will be immediately discontinued when infection is detected.

Participants who become infected receive confirmatory testing for infection, post-test risk-reduction and support counseling, and help enrolling in local HIV care programs. Both Thailand and Botswana have antiretroviral treatment and HIV care programs in place at minimal or no cost to patients. In the United States, participants are referred to local health care providers or public health programs for needed medical and social services.

Additionally, to help guide treatment decisions and to determine if prior exposure to tenofovir or tenofovir plus emtricitabine has any effect on the course of disease, initial testing will be provided for viral load, CD4 count, and HIV resistance mutations. Participants will also be followed for an additional 12 months following infection to examine their immune and virologic response. Although study procedures ensure a very low risk of drug-resistant virus emerging, the initial HIV resistance testing will provide important data on the degree to which any resistance does occur.

Monitoring for Side Effects

The health of participants is closely monitored throughout each trial, and participants are linked to any necessary medical care. In addition to scheduled reviews of safety data by the DSMB, both clinical and behavioral safety are closely monitored on an ongoing basis.

Although the drugs being tested have excellent safety profiles, there are potential medical risks. Tenofovir has been associated with minor side effects such as nausea, vomiting, and loss of appetite, as well as rare but more serious effects, such as impaired kidney function or reductions in bone density. Tenofovir plus emtricitabine has similarly been associated with a relatively low level of side effects, including diarrhea, nausea, fatigue, headache, dizziness, and rash, with infrequent reports of more serious side effects, such as impaired kidney function and lactic acidosis (a build-up of lactic acid in the blood). For both drugs, these effects have largely been reversed after use of the drug was discontinued.

Careful monitoring is provided using laboratory testing for any biological abnormalities (such as elevated creatinine or decreased phosphorus), so that the drug being tested can be promptly discontinued if serious concerns are identified. CDC will work with partners in each community to ensure that care is provided if either drug results in any health problems during the trial.

Community Involvement

CDC has and will continue to work closely with community partners at each research site to ensure active community participation during the planning and implementation of these trials.

- **Botswana:** In Botswana, community advisory boards have been established at each site, which include representatives from local governments (elected and traditional), as well as community members and representatives from key stakeholder organizations. Participant advisory boards have also been established. These groups provide input to researchers throughout the trial.
- **Thailand:** In Thailand, a community relations committee, composed of injecting drug users from each of the 17 drug treatment centers, family members, and representatives of local community organizations, meets regularly and provides advice to study staff on all aspects of study design, implementation, and trial conduct.
- **United States:** In the United States, all three sites have established active community advisory boards that are consulted regularly about study procedures and educational materials for potential participants. Members of these boards will provide ongoing advice throughout the trials.

In addition to the regular input received by these established committees, broader outreach and consultations with advocates and community-based organizations representing populations at risk for

HIV are being held, as needed, to address current and future plans for HIV prevention research and programs.

CDC Participation in Partners PrEP Study

The University of Washington is working with collaborators in Kenya and Uganda to conduct the Partners PrEP Study, which is examining the safety and efficacy of two different PrEP regimens—once-daily tenofovir and once-daily tenofovir plus emtricitabine—among heterosexual couples. CDC will co-manage two trial sites in Uganda, in conjunction with The AIDS Support Organization (TASO), the largest indigenous non-governmental organization providing HIV care in Uganda.

This randomized, double-blind, placebo-controlled study will operate at eight trial sites in Kenya and Uganda and include 3,900 serodiscordant couples (couples in which one person is HIV-infected and the other is not). Stable serodiscordant couples are the largest risk group for HIV infection in Africa, and this trial will provide important data on whether PrEP could be used to prevent new HIV infections among this population. HIV-uninfected partners will be assigned to three groups: One group will receive tenofovir, a second group will receive tenofovir plus emtricitabine, and the third group will receive a placebo. All participants will receive ongoing risk-reduction counseling and HIV testing, and their safety will be monitored by the study's DSMB and local IRBs. HIV-infected members of the discordant couples will receive ongoing HIV care.

The trial is the first to test the safety and efficacy of both tenofovir and tenofovir plus emtricitabine in the same population and will allow investigators to simultaneously evaluate the two drugs as candidates for use as PrEP.

Planning for Possible Implementation of PrEP

As we move forward with the search for new HIV prevention strategies, it will be critical to determine how these approaches can best be integrated into existing programs, should they prove effective in reducing risk. Because no strategy is 100% effective in preventing HIV infection, the future impact of PrEP will ultimately be determined by how effectively strategies are used in combination to provide the greatest protection to individuals at risk.

CDC has begun to examine potential implementation strategies with a wide range of stakeholders in the U.S. Experts are examining a number of critical issues including possible funding streams, risk assessment tools, and delivery of PrEP as part of a comprehensive prevention program. Additionally, CDC is conducting research to determine effective models for reaching the populations at greatest risk in the U.S.

At the international level, should efficacy be proven, WHO and UNAIDS would develop normative guidance on PrEP implementation, and individual countries would develop their own programs and policies for integrating PrEP into prevention efforts. As these plans are developed, CDC will provide technical assistance to its international partners and to local countries where CDC trials are being conducted.

Chapter 51

Research Supports Early Treatment for HIV/AIDS

A study recently reported in the journal, *AIDS*, found that people who started taking HIV medicines with higher CD4 cell counts were more likely to have their immune systems restored to near normal levels. This study adds to a growing body of data on the benefits of early anti-HIV treatment.

The Study

The researchers looked at people from the AIDS Therapy Evaluation Project Netherlands (ATHENA) cohort starting HIV drugs for the first time and followed them for seven years. They looked at how likely people were to achieve CD4 counts greater or equal to 800, which is considered normal for an HIV-negative person.

The study participants were 75% male and 63% white. About half were men who have sex with men, 35% heterosexual, and 4% injection drug users. Average CD4 count at the start when starting HIV treatment was 190. Just under 20% started with CD4 counts under 50, while only 7% started with counts above 500.

The Results

Most people in the cohort experienced significant increases in their CD4 counts. Not surprisingly, there was a very strong relationship

---

between a person's CD4 cell count when they started and their likelihood of achieving a count of over 800. Those who started treatment with CD4 counts over 500 were over 23 times more likely to achieve counts of 800 than people who started with counts below 50.

The difference was also significant for groups with much smaller differences in their CD4 counts before starting therapy. Those who started with counts between 350–500 were 2.76 times more likely to achieve counts above 800 than those who started with counts between 200–350.

The same was seen in people with highest and lowest counts when they started. For example, people who started treatment with CD4 counts between 50 and 200 were about twice as likely as those who started below 50 to achieve counts above 800. Likewise, people who started with counts above 500 were 2.4 times more likely than those who started between 200 and 350.

There were several other interesting findings:

- Women were about 26% more likely than men to get to above 800. Injection drug users were about 30% less likely.
- No real differences were seen by ethnic groups.
- The older a person was at the time they started HIV treatment, the less likely they were to see their counts rise above 800.
- People who were over 50 when they started meds were over twice as likely to have their CD4 counts plateau at below 800 as those who started at a younger age.
- Having detectable levels of HIV at any time during the study resulted in a 4.69 times less chance of having CD4 levels above 800.

What Does This All Mean?

Overall, the findings of this study are not surprising. Maybe the most important finding was the big difference in outcomes for people who started treatment with CD4 counts between 350–500 vs. those who started between 200–350. It is relatively uncommon for people to start HIV treatment at either high (over 500) or low (below 200). Many people begin with counts somewhere between 200–500. This study shows they are more likely to achieve high CD4 counts if they start with counts above 350.

The affects of age on treatment outcomes is of growing importance. As we age, our immune systems' ability to recover wanes. This study highlights this fact and argues for earlier treatment for people over 50 living with HIV.

This study will add to the ongoing debate on the best time to start HIV treatment. The current Federal Guidelines recommend starting treatment before your CD4 count falls to 350. It also discusses the possible benefits and risks of starting at higher CD4 counts, but does not make a recommendation.

Without a large, definitive study aimed at determining the best time to start treatments, doctors, activists, and people with HIV have to piece together results from other studies, like this one, to guide them on this important question. If one of the main goals of HIV treatment is to restore a person's immune system to as close to normal as possible, this study strongly supports earlier treatment. This potential benefit must be weighed against the risks and difficulties of HIV treatment. This equation is growing more favorable toward earlier treatment as HIV drugs become more tolerable and convenient.

Part Seven

Additional Help and Information

Chapter 52

Glossary of Terms Related to STDs

acquired immunodeficiency syndrome (AIDS): A deficiency of cellular immunity induced by infection with the human immunodeficiency virus (HIV-1) and characterized by opportunistic diseases, including *Pneumocystis carinii* pneumonia, Kaposi sarcoma, oral hairy leukoplakia, cytomegalovirus disease, tuberculosis, *Mycobacterium avium* complex (MAC) disease, candidal esophagitis, cryptosporidiosis, isosporiasis, cryptococcosis, non-Hodgkin lymphoma, progressive multifocal leukoencephalopathy (PML), herpes zoster, and lymphoma. HIV is transmitted from person to person in cell-rich body fluids (notably blood and semen) through sexual contact, sharing of contaminated needles (as by IV drug abusers), or other contact with contaminated blood (as in accidental needle sticks among health care workers). The primary targets of HIV are cells with the CD4 surface protein, including principally helper T lymphocytes. Antibody to HIV, which appears in the serum six weeks to six months after infection, serves as a reliable diagnostic marker but does not bind or inactivate HIV. Gradual decline in the CD4 lymphocyte count, typically occurring over a period of 10–12 years, culminates in loss of ability to resist opportunistic infections; the appearance of one or more of these defines the onset of AIDS. In some patients, generalized lymphadenopathy, fever, weight

---

This glossary contains terms from *Stedman's Medical Dictionary, 27th Edition*. Lippincott Williams & Wilkins, 2000 (marked with a superscripted 1); terms excerpted from www.aidsinfo.nih.gov, a service of the U.S. Department of Health and Human Services (marked with a superscripted 2); and terms from the Office of Women's Health (www.womenshealth .gov) (marked with a superscripted 3).

loss, dementia, and chronic diarrhea are associated with early stages of the disease. AIDS is uniformly lethal, most patients dying of one or more opportunistic infections or their complications within two to five years of the onset of symptoms. In the U.S., AIDS is the leading cause of death among men 25–44, and the fourth leading cause among women in the same age group. During the past five years, the mortality of the disease and rates of perinatal transmission have declined substantially, as has transmission among homosexual men and intravenous drug users. Meanwhile heterosexual transmission and case rates among blacks and Hispanics have increased. Some 50 million people are estimated to be infected worldwide, with the highest incidence in some Central and East African countries, where as many as 25% of the adult population may be HIV-positive. Besides prophylaxis against opportunistic infection, standard therapy of HIV infection includes use of nucleoside analogs (didanosine, lamivudine, ribavirin, stavudine, zidovudine), nonnucleoside reverse transcriptase inhibitors (delavirdine, efavirenz, nevirapine), and protease inhibitors (Crixivan, indinavir, ritonavir, saquinavir).[1]

bacterial vaginosis: Infection of the human vagina that may be caused by anaerobic bacteria, especially by *Mobiluncus* species or by *Gardnerella vaginalis*. Characterized by excessive, sometimes malodorous, discharge.[1]

bacterium: A microscopic organism consisting of one simple cell. Bacteria occur naturally almost everywhere on earth, including in soil, on skin, in the human gastrointestinal tract, and in many foods. Some bacteria can cause disease in humans.[2]

CD4 cell count: A measurement of the number of CD4 cells in a sample of blood. The CD4 count is one of the most useful indicators of the health of the immune system and the progression of HIV/AIDS. A CD4 cell count is used by health care providers to determine when to begin, interrupt, or halt anti-HIV therapy; when to give preventive treatment for opportunistic infections; and to measure response to treatment. A normal CD4 cell count is between 500 and 1,400 cells/mm^3 of blood, but an individual's CD4 count can vary. In HIV-infected individuals, a CD4 count at or below 200 cells/mm^3 is considered an AIDS-defining condition.[2]

candidiasis: Infection caused by a species of the yeast-like fungus *Candida*, usually *C. albicans*. Candidiasis can affect the skin; nails; and mucous membranes throughout the body, including the mouth (thrush), esophagus, vagina, intestines, and lungs. The infection appears as white patches when in the mouth or any other mucous membrane. Candidiasis is considered an AIDS-defining condition in people with HIV.[2]

cervical cancer: Cervical cancer happens when normal cells in the cervix change into cancer cells. This change normally takes several years to happen, but it can also happen in a very short amount of time. Before the cells turn into cancer, abnormal cells develop on the cervix that can be found by a Pap test. Women generally don't have symptoms of cervical cancer. But when cervical cancer is not found early and spreads deeper into your cervix or to other tissues or organs, you might have pain during sex; bleeding from your vagina after sex, between periods, or after menopause; heavy vaginal discharge that may have a bad odor; heavier bleeding during your period; or a menstrual period that lasts longer than normal. Human papillomavirus (HPV), a group of viruses, can cause abnormal changes on the cervix that can lead to cervical cancer. HPV is very common, and you can get it through sexual contact with another person who has HPV.[3]

chancre: The primary lesion of syphilis, which begins at the site of cutaneous or mucosal infection after an interval of 10–30 days as a papule or area of infiltration, of dull red color, hard, and insensitive; the center usually becomes eroded or breaks down into an ulcer that heals slowly after four to six weeks. Finding *Treponema pallidum* on dark-field examination is diagnostic, except in oral ulcers, in which *T. microdentium* is normally present.[1]

chancroid: A sexually transmitted disease (STD) caused by a bacterium called *Haemophilus ducreyi*. Often causes swollen lymph nodes and painful sores on the penis, vagina, or anus. The lesions appear after an incubation period of three to five days and may facilitate HIV transmission.[2]

chemical barrier: A mechanism that uses chemicals to try to prevent sexually transmitted infections (STIs), including HIV infection. Microbicides are currently being studied as chemical barriers to prevent the transmission of STIs.[2]

chlamydia: A sexually transmitted disease caused by a bacterium called *Chlamydia trachomatis*. The bacteria infect the genital tract and, if left untreated, can cause damage to the female and male reproductive systems, resulting in infertility.[2]

chronic: 1) Referring to a health-related state, lasting a long time. 2) Referring to exposure, prolonged or long-term, sometimes meaning also low intensity. 3) The U.S. National Center for Health Statistics defines a chronic condition as one of three months' duration or longer.[1]

cirrhosis: Endstage liver disease characterized by diffuse damage to hepatic parenchymal cells, with nodular regeneration, fibrosis, and disturbance of normal architecture; associated with failure in the function of hepatic cells and interference with blood flow in the liver, frequently resulting in jaundice, portal hypertension, ascites, and ultimately biochemical and functional signs of hepatic failure.[1]

clinical trial: A research study that uses human volunteers to answer specific health questions. Carefully conducted clinical trials are regarded as the fastest and safest way to find effective treatments for diseases and conditions as well as other ways to improve health. Interventional trials use controlled conditions to determine whether experimental treatments or new ways of using known treatments are safe and effective. Observational trials gather information about health issues from groups of people in their natural settings. Clinical trials may be prospective (studying data from a time point forward) or retrospective (studying data from collected records in the past).[2]

complete blood count (CBC): A general blood test that measures the levels of white and red blood cells, platelets, hematocrit, and hemoglobin in a sample of blood. Changes in the amounts of each of these may indicate infection, anemia, or other health problems.[2]

condom: A barrier method of birth control. There are both male and female condoms. The male condom is a sheath placed over an erect penis before sex that prevents pregnancy by blocking the passage of sperm. A female condom also is a sheath, but is inserted into the vagina to block the passage of sperm.[3]

cytomegalovirus (CMV): A herpesvirus that can cause infections, including pneumonia (infection of the lungs), gastroenteritis (infection of the gastrointestinal tract), encephalitis (inflammation of the brain), or retinitis (infection of the eye), in immunosuppressed people. Although CMV can infect most organs of the body, HIV-infected people are most susceptible to CMV retinitis.[2]

drug resistance: The ability of some micro-organisms, such as bacteria, viruses, and parasites, to adapt so that they can multiply even in the presence of drugs that would normally kill them.[2]

genital warts: Also known as condyloma acuminatum and venereal warts. Growths or bumps that appear in and around the vagina, anus, or cervix in females or on the penis, scrotum, groin, or thigh in males. They can be raised or flat, single or multiple, small or large. Some cluster together to form a cauliflower-like shape. They are caused by the human papillomavirus (HPV) and are usually flesh-colored and painless.[2]

gonorrhea: A contagious catarrhal inflammation of the genital mucous membrane, transmitted chiefly by coitus and due to *Neisseria gonorrhoeae*; may involve the lower or upper genital tract, especially the urethra, endocervix, and uterine tubes, or spread to the peritoneum and rarely to the heart, joints, or other structures by way of the bloodstream.[1]

granuloma inguinale: A specific granuloma, classified as a venereal disease and caused by *Calymmatobacterium granulomatis* observed in macrophages as Donovan bodies; the ulcerating granulomatous lesions occur in the inguinal regions and the genitalia; peripheral extension of the lesions produces extensive destruction.[1]

hepatitis: Inflammation of the liver, due usually to viral infection but sometimes to toxic agents. Previously endemic throughout much of the developing world, viral hepatitis now ranks as a major public health problem in industrialized nations. The three most common types of viral hepatitis (A, B, and C) afflict millions worldwide. Acute viral hepatitis is characterized by varying degrees of fever, malaise, weakness, anorexia, nausea, and abdominal distress. Hepatocellular damage causes bilirubin retention, often with jaundice, and a rise in serum levels of certain enzymes (particularly transaminases). Hepatitis A, caused by an enterovirus, is spread by the fecal-oral route, most often through ingestion of contaminated food or water. The case fatality rate is less than 1%, and recovery is complete. The presence of antibody to hepatitis A virus indicates prior infection, noninfectivity, and immunity to future attacks. Hepatitis B, due to a small DNA virus, is transmitted through sexual contact, sharing of needles by IV drug abusers, needlestick injuries among health care workers, and from mother to fetus. The annual incidence in the U.S. is 300,000 cases. The incubation period is 6–24 weeks. Some patients become carriers, and in some an immune response to the virus induces a chronic phase leading to cirrhosis, hepatic failure, and risk of hepatocellular carcinoma. Hepatitis B surface antigen (HBsAg) is detectable early in serum; its persistence correlates with chronic infection and infectivity. Core antigen (HBcAg) appears later and also indicates infectivity. Hepatitis C is the principal form of transfusion-induced hepatitis; a chronic active form often develops. Acute infection with hepatitis B or C has a higher mortality rate than hepatitis A. Effective vaccines are available for active immunization against hepatitis A and hepatitis B. Interferon-alpha brings about clinical remission in some cases of hepatitis B and hepatitis C. Hepatitis D is due to an RNA virus capable of causing disease only in persons previously infected with hepatitis B. Hepatitis E, which occurs chiefly in the tropics, resembles hepatitis A in that it is transmitted by the fecal-oral route and does not become chronic or lead to a carrier state, but it has a much higher mortality rate.[1]

herpes simplex: A variety of infections caused by herpesvirus types 1 and 2; type 1 infections are marked most commonly by the eruption of one or more groups of vesicles on the vermilion border of the lips or at the external nares, type 2 by such lesions on the genitalia; both types often are recrudescent and reappear during other febrile illnesses or even physiologic states such as menstruation. The viruses frequently become latent and may not be expressed for years.[1]

highly active antiretroviral therapy (HAART): The name given to treatment regimens that aggressively suppress HIV replication and progression of HIV disease. The usual HAART regimen combines three or more anti-HIV drugs from at least two different classes.[2]

horizontal transmission: A term used to describe transmission of a disease from one individual to another, except from parent to offspring. For example, HIV can be spread horizontally through sexual contact or exposure to infected blood. In contrast, spread of disease from parent to offspring is called vertical transmission.[2]

human immunodeficiency virus (HIV): Human T-cell lymphotropic virus type III; a cytopathic retrovirus (genus *Lentivirus*, family *Retroviridae*) that is 100–120 nm in diameter, has a lipid envelope, and has a characteristic dense cylindrical nucleoid containing core proteins and genomic RNA. There are currently two types: HIV-1 infects only human and chimpanzees and is more virulent than HIV-2, which is more closely related to Simian or monkey viruses. HIV-2 is found primarily in West Africa and is not as widespread as HIV-1. In addition to the usual gene associated with retroviruses, this virus has at least six genes that regulate its replication. It is the etiologic agent of acquired immunodeficiency syndrome (AIDS). Formerly or also known as the lymphadenopathy virus (LAV) or the human T-cell lymphotropic virus type III (HTLV-III). Identified in 1984 by Luc Montagnier and colleagues.[1]

human papillomavirus (HPV): A virus that causes various warts, including plantar and genital warts. Some strains of HPV can also cause cervical cancer.[2]

immunization: Protection of susceptible individuals from communicable diseases by administration of a living modified agent (e.g., yellow fever vaccine), a suspension of killed organisms (e.g., pertussis vaccine), or an inactivated toxin (e.g., tetanus).[1]

immunodeficiency: A condition resulting from a defective immune mechanism; may be *primary* (due to a defect in the immune mechanism itself) or *secondary* (dependent upon another disease process), *specific* (due to a defect in either the B-lymphocyte or the T-lymphocyte system, or both) or *nonspecific* (due to a defect in one or another component of the nonspecific immune mechanism: the complement, properdin, or phagocytic system).[1]

liver function tests: Blood tests that measure the levels of liver enzymes (proteins made and used by the liver) to determine if the liver is working properly. The liver enzymes that are routinely measured as part of liver function tests are aspartate aminotransferase (AST)—also called serum glutamic oxaloacetic transaminase (SGOT), alanine aminotransferase (ALT)—also called serum glutamic pyruvic transaminase (SGPT), and gamma-glutamyltransferase (GGT). Increased levels of these enzymes indicate that the liver has been damaged.[2]

lymphogranuloma venereum: A venereal infection usually caused by *Chlamydia trachomatis*, and characterized by a transient genital ulcer and inguinal adenopathy in the male; in the female, perirectal lymph nodes are involved and rectal stricture is a common occurrence.[1]

microbicides: A natural or manmade substance that kills microbes. Researchers are studying the use of microbicides to prevent the transmission of sexually transmitted diseases, including HIV infection.[2]

molluscum contagiosum: A disease of the skin and mucous membranes caused by a virus. The condition causes pearly white or flesh-colored bumps on the face, neck, underarms, hands, and genital region. In people with HIV, molluscum contagiosum can get worse with time and often becomes resistant to treatment.[2]

nongonococcal urethritis: Urethritis not resulting from gonococcal infection; venereally transmitted *Chlamydia trachomatis* is the most common cause.[1]

occupational exposure: Exposure to potentially infectious material, such as blood, tissue, body fluids, medical equipment, or supplies, while at work. The exposure could occur through a needlestick, a cut with an object, contact with the mucous membrane, or contact with skin that has a break in it.[2]

opportunistic infection (OI): An illness caused by any one of various organisms that occur in people with weakened immune systems, including people with HIV/AIDS. OIs that are common in people with AIDS include *Pneumocystis jiroveci* pneumonia (PCP); cryptosporidiosis; histoplasmosis; toxoplasmosis; other parasitic, viral, and fungal infections; and some types of cancers.[2]

Pap smear: A method for the early detection of cancer and other abnormalities of the female genital tract. A Pap smear is done by placing a speculum in the vagina, locating the cervix, and then scraping a thin layer of cells from the cervix. The cells are placed on a slide, sent to a laboratory, and analyzed for abnormalities. HIV-infected women often have abnormal results of Pap smear tests, usually as a result of human papillomavirus (HPV) infection.[2]

pelvic inflammatory disease (PID): Acute or chronic suppurative inflammation of female pelvic structures (endometrium, uterine tubes, pelvic peritoneum) due to infection by *Neisseria gonorrhoeae*, *Chlamydia trachomatis*, or other organisms, typically a complication of sexually transmitted infection of the lower genital tract, may be precipitated by menstruation, parturition, or surgical procedures including abortion; complications include tubo-ovarian abscess, tubal stenosis with resulting infertility or sterility and heightened risk of ectopic pregnancy, and peritoneal adhesions.[1]

perinatal transmission: The passage of HIV from an HIV-infected mother to her infant. The infant may become infected while in the womb, during labor and delivery, or through breastfeeding.[2]

prevalence: The number of people in a population who are affected with a particular disease or condition at a given time. Prevalence can be thought of as a snapshot of all existing cases of a disease or condition at a specified time.[2]

prophylactic treatment: The institution of measures designed to protect a person from an attack of a disease to which the person has been or is liable to be exposed.[1]

retrovirus: A type of virus that stores its genetic information in a single-stranded RNA molecule, and constructs a double-stranded DNA version of its genes using a special enzyme called reverse transcriptase. The DNA copy is then integrated into the host cell's own genetic material. HIV is an example of a retrovirus.[2]

scabies: An eruption due to the mite *Sarcoptes scabiei* var. *hominis*; the female of the species burrows into the skin, producing a vesicular eruption with intense pruritus between the fingers, on the male or female genitalia, buttocks, and elsewhere on the trunk and extremities.[1]

serostatus: The presence or absence of detectable antibodies against an infective agent, such as HIV, in the blood. Seronegativity, or seronegative status, means that the person has no detectable antibodies and is not infected with the agent or has not had the chance to develop antibodies to an early infection. Seropositivity, or seropositive status, means that the person has detectable antibodies and is infected with the agent or had previously been infected with the agent.[2]

spermicides: Chemical jellies, foams, creams, or suppositories, inserted into the vagina prior to intercourse, that kill sperm.[3]

syphilis: A sexually transmitted disease caused by the bacterium *Treponema pallidum*. In the early stage of syphilis, a genital or mouth sore called a chancre develops but eventually disappears on its own. However, if the disease is not treated, the infection can progress over the years to affect the heart and central nervous system. Syphilis can also be transmitted from an infected mother to her fetus during pregnancy, with serious health consequences for the infant.[2]

T cell: A type of lymphocyte (disease-fighting white blood cell). The T stands for the thymus, the organ in which T cells mature. T cells include CD4 cells and CD8 cells, which are both critical components of the body's immune system.[2]

trichomoniasis: A very common STD in both women and men that is caused by a parasite that is passed from one person to another during sexual contact. It also can be passed through contact with damp, moist objects such as towels or wet clothing. Symptoms include yellow, green, or gray vaginal discharge (often foamy) with a strong odor; discomfort during sex and when urinating; irritation and itching of the genital area; or lower abdominal pain (rare).[3]

vaccine: Originally, the live vaccine (vaccinia, cowpox) virus inoculated in the skin as prophylaxis against smallpox and obtained from the skin of calves inoculated with seed virus. Usage has extended the meaning to include essentially any preparation intended for active immunologic prophylaxis; e.g., preparations of killed microbes of virulent strains or living microbes of attenuated (variant or mutant) strains; or microbial, fungal, plant, protozoal, or metazoan derivatives or products. Method of administration varies according to the vaccine, inoculation being the most common, but ingestion is preferred in some instances and nasal spray is used occasionally.[1]

viral load (VL): The amount of HIV RNA in a blood sample, reported as number of HIV RNA copies per milliliter of blood plasma. The VL provides information about the number of cells infected with HIV and is an important indicator of HIV progression and of how well treatment is working. The VL can be measured by different techniques, including branched-chain DNA (bDNA) and reverse transcriptase-polymerase chain reaction (RT-PCR) assays. VL tests are usually done when an individual is diagnosed with HIV infection and at regular intervals after diagnosis.[2]

virus: 1) Formerly, the specific agent of an infectious disease. 2) Specifically, a term for a group of infectious agents, which with few exceptions are capable of passing through fine filters that retain most bacteria, are usually not visible through the light microscope, lack independent metabolism, and are incapable of growth or reproduction apart from living cells. They have a prokaryotic genetic apparatus but differ sharply from bacteria in other respects. The complete particle usually contains either DNA or RNA, not both, and is usually covered by a protein shell or capsid that protects the nucleic acid. They range in size from 15 nanometers up to several hundred nanometers. Classification of viruses depends upon physiochemical characteristics of virions as well as upon mode of transmission, host range, symptomatology, and other factors.[1]

Chapter 53

Directory of STD Organizations and Resources

Organizations That Provide General Information about STDs and Sexual Health

Advocates for Youth
2000 M Street NW, Suite 750
Washington, DC 20036
Phone: 202-419-3420
Fax: 202-419-1448
Website: http://www.advocatesforyouth.org

Alan Guttmacher Institute
125 Maiden Lane, 7th Floor
New York, NY 10038
Phone: 800-355-0244, 212-248-1111
Fax: 212-248-1951
Website: http://www.guttmacher.org

American Academy of Family Physicians
P.O. Box 11210
Shawnee Mission, KS 66207-1210
Phone: 800-274-2237, 913-906-6000 (English and Spanish)
Fax: 913-906-6095
Website: http://www.aafp.org

American College of Obstetricians and Gynecologists
409 12th St., S.W.,
P.O. Box 96920
Washington, DC 20090-6920
Phone: 800-762-2264
Website: http://www.acog.org

The resources in this chapter were compiled from many sources deemed accurate. Inclusion does not constitute endorsement and there is no implication associated with omission. All contact information was verified in January 2009.

American Social Health Association (ASHA)
P. O. Box 13827
Research Triangle Park, NC 27709-3827
Phone: 800-783-9877
Websites: http://www.ashastd.org, www.iwannaknow.org (for teens)

Answer
Center for Applied Psychology at Rutgers University
41 Gordon Road, Suite C
Piscataway, NJ 08854
Phone: 732-445-7929
Fax: 732-445-5333
E-mail: answered@rci.rutgers.edu
Website: http://answer.rutgers.edu, www.sexetc.org (for teens)

AVERT
4 Brighton Road
Horsham
West Sussex
RH13 5BA
UK
E-mail: info@avert.org
Website: http://www.avert.org

CDC Division of STD Prevention (DSTDP)
Centers for Disease Control and Prevention
1600 Clifton Rd.
Atlanta, GA 30333
Phone: 800-CDC-INFO (232-4636)
TTY: 888-232-6348
Website: http://www.cdc.gov/std

CDC National Prevention Information Network (NPIN)
Centers for Disease Control and Prevention
P.O. Box 6003
Rockville, MD 20849-6003
Phone: 800-458-5231
Fax: 888-282-7681
International: 404-679-3860
E-mail: info@cdcnpin.org
Website: http://www.cdcnpin.org/scripts/index.asp

Center for the Advancement of Health
Health Behavior News Service
Phone: 202-387-2829
Website: http://www.hbns.org

Center for Young Women's Health
333 Longwood Avenue
5th Floor
Boston, MA 02115
Phone: 617-355-2994
Fax: 617-730-0186
Website: http://www.youngwomenshealth.org

EngenderHealth
440 Ninth Avenue
New York, NY 10001
Phone: 212-561-8000
Fax: 212-561-8067
Website: http://www.engenderhealth.org

Family Health International
P.O. Box 13950
Research Triangle Park, NC
27709
Phone: 703-516-9779 (DC office),
919-544-7040
Fax: 919-544-7261
Website: http://www.fhi.org/en/
index.htm

Food and Drug Administration
5600 Fishers Lane
Rockville, MD 20857-0001
Phone: 888-INFO-FDA
(463-6332)
Website: http://www.fda.gov

Gay Men's Health Crisis
The Tisch Building
119 West 24 Street
New York, NY 10011
Phone: 212 367-1000
Website: http://www.gmhc.org

Health Initiatives for Youth
235 Montgomery Street
Suite 430
San Francisco, CA 94104
Phone: 415-274-1970
Fax: 415-274-1976
E-mail: info@hify.org
Website: http://www.hify.com

Healthfinder.gov
U.S. Department of Health and
Human Services
P.O. Box 1133
Washington, DC 20013-1133
E-mail: healthfinder@nhic.org
Website: http://
www.healthfinder.gov

Henry J. Kaiser Family Foundation
2400 Sand Hill Road
Menlo Park, CA 94025
Phone: 650-854-9400
Fax: 650-854-4800
Website: http://www.kff.org

Immunization Action Coalition
1573 Selby Avenue
Suite 234
St. Paul, MN 55104
Phone: 651-647-9009
Fax: 651-647-9131
Websites: http://www.immunize
.org,
http://www.vaccineinformation
.org,
http://www.hepprograms.org

Kidshealth.org
Nemours Foundation
Website: http://
www.kidshealth.org

LesbianSTD.com
University of Washington,
Mailstop #359931
Harborview Medical Center
3EC02
Division of Infectious Diseases
325 9th Avenue
Seattle, WA 98104
Phone: 206-731-3679
Fax: 206-731-3693
Website: http://
www.lesbianstd.com

Mayo Foundation for Medical Education and Research
Website: http://www.mayoclinic.com

National Cancer Institute
NCI Public Inquiries Office
6116 Executive Boulevard, Room 3036A
Bethesda, MD 20892-8322
Toll Free: 800-4-CANCER (422-6237), Monday through Friday 9:00 a.m. to 4:30 p.m., EST
Live chat: http://cissecure.nci.nih.gov/livehelp/welcome.asp
Website: http://www.cancer.gov

National Center for Alternative and Complementary Medicine (NCCAM)
National Institutes of Health
9000 Rockville Pike
Bethesda, MD 20892 USA
E-mail: info@nccam.nih.gov
Website: http://nccam.nih.gov

National Digestive Diseases Information Clearinghouse
2 Information Way
Bethesda, MD 20892-3570
Phone: 800-891-5389
TTY: 866-569-1162
Fax: 703-738-4929
E-mail: nddic@info.niddk.nih.gov
Website: http://www.digestive.niddk.nih.gov

National Family Planning and Reproductive Health Association
1627 K Street, NW, 12th Floor
Washington, DC 20006
Phone: 202-293-3114
Fax: 202-293-1990
Website: http://www.nfprha.org

National Institute of Allergy and Infectious Diseases (NIAID)
Office of Communications and Public Liaison
6610 Rockledge Drive, MSC 6612
Bethesda, MD 20892-6612
Phone: 301-496-5717
Website: http://www.niaid.nih.gov

National Institute on Aging
Building 31, Room 5C27
31 Center Drive, MSC 2292
Bethesda, MD 20892
Phone: 301-496-1752
TTY: 800-222-4225
Fax: 301-496-1072
Website: http://www.nia.nih.gov

National Institute on Drug Abuse
6001 Executive Boulevard, Room 5213 (USPS mail only; no FedEx or UPS)
Bethesda, MD 20892-9561
Phone: 301-443-1124
E-mail: information@nida.nih.gov
Website: http://www.drugabuse.gov

National Library of Medicine
Reference and Web Services
8600 Rockville Pike
Bethesda, MD 20894
Phone: 888-FIND-NLM
(346-3656), 301-594-5983
Fax: 301-402-1384
Interlibrary Loan fax:
301-496-2809
TDD access via Maryland Relay
Service: 800-735-2258
Website: http://www.nlm.nih.gov

National Women's Health Information Center
U.S. Department of Health and
Human Services
8270 Willow Oaks Corporate Dr.
Fairfax, VA 22031
Phone: 800-994-9662
TTD: 888-220-5446
Website: http://
www.womenshealth.gov

National Women's Health Network
1413 K St. N.W. 4th Floor
Washington, DC 20005
Phone: 202-347-1140,
202-628-7814 (Health Information)
Fax: 202-347-1168
Website: http://www.nwhn.org

Office of Minority Health
U.S. Department of Health and
Human Services
Phone: 800-444-6472
Fax: 301-251-2160
E-mail: info@omhrc.gov
Website: http://www.omhrc.gov

Parents of Kids with Infectious Diseases (PKIDS)
P.O. Box 5666
Vancouver, WA 98668
Phone: 877-55P-KIDS (557-5437)
E-mail: pkids@pkids.org
Website: http://www.pkids.org

Planned Parenthood Federation of America
NY Office:
434 West 33rd Street
New York, NY 10001
Phone: 212-541-7800
Fax: 212-245-1845
DC Office:
1110 Vermont Ave. NW
Suite 300
Washington, DC 20005
Phone: 202-973-4800
Fax: 202-296-3242
Website: http://
www.plannedparenthood.org

SafeGuards Project
The Family Planning Council
260 South Broad St., 10th Floor
Philadelphia, PA 19102
Phone: 215-985-6873
Fax: 215-985-6824
Website: http://
www.safeguards.org

Senior Action in a Gay Environment (SAGE)
305 7th Avenue, 6th Floor
New York, NY 10001
Phone: 212-741-2247
Website: http://www.sageusa.org

Sexuality Information and Education Council of the United States (SIECUS)
NY Office:
90 John St. Suite 704
New York, NY 10038
Phone: 212-819-9770
Fax: 212-819-9776
DC Office:
1706 R Street, NW
Washington, DC 20009
Phone: 202-265-2405
Fax: 202-462-2340
Website: http://www.siecus.org

Society for Women's Health Research
1025 Connecticut Avenue NW
Suite 701
Washington, DC 20036
Phone: 202-223-8224
Fax: 202-833-3472
Website: http://
www.womenshealthresearch.org

STDresource.com
BC Centre for Disease Control
STD/AIDS Division
655 West 12th Avenue
Vancouver, BC Canada V5Z 4R4
Phone: 604-660-2090
Fax: 604-775-0808
Website: http://
www.stdresource.com

Organizations That Provide Information about HIV/AIDS

AIDS InfoNet
New Mexico AIDS Education and Training Center at the University of New Mexico Health Sciences Center
P.O. Box 810
Arroyo Seco, NM 87514
Website: http://
www.aidsinfonet.org

AIDS Treatment Data Network
611 Broadway, Suite 613
New York, NY 10012
Phone: 800-734-7104,
212-260-8868
Fax: 212-260-8869
Website: http://www.atdn.org

AIDSinfo
U.S. Department of Health and Human Services
P.O. Box 6303
Rockville, MD 20849-6303
Phone: 800-HIV-0440
(800-448-0440), Monday to Friday, 12:00 p.m. to 5:00 p.m. EST
TTY/TTD: 888-480-3739
Website: http://
www.aidsinfo.nih.gov

AIDSmap
NAM
Phone: +44 (0) 20-7840-0050
Fax: +44 (0) 20-7735-5351
E-mail: info@nam.org.uk
Website: http://www.aidsmap.org

The Body
250 West 57 Street
New York, NY 10107
Website: http://www.thebody.com

Center for AIDS Prevention Studies
AIDS Research Institute at the University of California San Francisco
50 Beale Street, Suite 1300
San Francisco, CA 94105
Phone: 415-597-9100
Website: http://www.caps.ucsf.edu

HIV InSite
University of California San Francisco Center for HIV Information
4150 Clement Street, Box 111V
San Francisco, CA 94121
Fax: 415-379-5547
E-mail: info@hivinsite.ucsf.edu
Website: http://hivinsite.ucsf.edu

Latino Commission on AIDS
24 West, 25th Street, 9th Floor
New York, NY 10010
Phone: 212-675-3288, ext. 303–323 (English and Spanish)
Fax: 212-675-3466
Website: http://www.latinoaids.org

National Association of People with AIDS
8401 Colesville Road
Suite 505
Silver Spring, MD 20910
Phone: 240-247-0880
Toll-free: 866-846-9366
Facsimile: 240-247-0574
E-mail: napwa@napwa.org
Website: http://www.napwa.org

National Association on HIV Over Fifty
23 Miner Street
Boston, MA 02215-3318
Website: http://www.hivoverfifty.org

National Minority AIDS Council
1931 13th Street NW
Washington, DC 20009
Phone: 202-483-6622
Fax: 202-483-5387
E-mail: info@nmac.org
Website: http://www.nmac.org

Project Inform
1375 Mission Street
San Francisco, CA 94103-2621
Phone: 415-558-8669
Fax: 415-558-0684
Website: http://www.projectinform.org

Organizations That Provide Information about Specific STDs

American Herpes Foundation
Phone: 201-342-4441, Hotline: 919-361-8488
Fax 978-614-2775
Website: http://www.herpes-foundation.org

American Liver Foundation
75 Maiden Lane, Suite 603
New York, NY 10038-4810
Phone: 800-GO-LIVER (465-4837), 888-4HEP-USA (443-7872), or 212-668-1000
Fax: 212-483-8179
E-mail: info@liverfoundation.org
Website: http://www.liverfoundation.org

Hepatitis B Foundation
3805 Old Easton Road
Doylestown, PA 18902
Phone: 215-489-4900
Fax: 215-489-4313
E-mail: info@hepb.org
Website: http://www.hepb.org

Hepatitis C Support Project
P.O. Box 427037
San Francisco, CA 94142-7037
E-mail: alanfranciscus@hcvadvocate.org
Website: http://www.hcvadvocate.org

Hepatitis Foundation International
504 Blick Drive
Silver Spring, MD 20904-2901
Phone: 800-891-0707 or 301-622-4200
Fax: 301-622-4702
E-mail: hfi@comcast.net
Website: http://www.hepatitisfoundation.org, www.hepfi.org

International Herpes Alliance
Website: http://www.herpesalliance.org

National Cervical Cancer Coalition
6520 Platt Ave. #693
West Hills, CA 91307
Phone: 800-685-5531, 818-909-3849
Fax: 818-780-8199
Website: http://www.nccc-online.org

National Hepatitis C Program
Veteran's Administration
Phone: 800-827-1000
Website: http://www.hepatitis.va.gov

Organizations That Provide Information on Clinical Trials, Research, and STD Testing

Alliance for Microbicide Development
8484 Georgia Avenue, Suite 940
Silver Spring, MD 20910
Phone: 301-587-9690
Fax: 301-588-8390
Website: http://www.microbicide.org

Clinical Trials, U.S. National Institutes of Health
Website: http://www.clinicaltrials.gov

Lab Tests Online
American Association for Physical Chemistry
Website: http://www.labtestsonline.org

National HIV and STD Testing Resources
Centers for Disease Control and Prevention
Website: http://www.hivtest.org

National Institutes of Health HIV vaccine clinical trials
Phone: 866-833-LIFE (866-833-5433)

Hotlines That Provide Assistance on STDs and Sexual Health

AIDS Treatment Data Network
Phone: 800-734-7104, 212-260-8868 (Monday through Friday 9:00 a.m. to 5:00 p.m., EST)
Fax: 212-260-8869

AIDSinfo
Phone: 800-HIV-0440 (448-0440), 301-519-0459 (Monday through Friday 12:00 p.m. to 5:00 p.m., EST)
TTY: 888-480-3739
Fax: 301-519-6616
Chat room: www.aidsinfo.nih.gov/livehelp (Monday through Friday 12:00 p.m. to 4:00 p.m.)
E-mail: contactus@aidsinfo.nih.gov

California HIV/AIDS Hotline
San Francisco AIDS Foundation
995 Market St., Suite 200
San Francisco CA 94103
Phone: 800-367-AIDS (2437)
E-mail: contact-us@aidshotline.org

ChildHelp USA National Child Abuse Hotline
Phone: 800-4-A-CHILD (422-4453), 24 hours a day, 7 days a week

The Gay and Lesbian National Hotline
Phone: 888-THE-GLNH (843-4564), Monday through Friday 4:00 p.m. to 12:00 a.m.; Saturday 12:00 noon to 5:00 p.m. (EST)
E-mail: glnh@glnh.org

National AIDS Hotline
Centers for Disease Control and Prevention
Phone: 800-CDC-INFO (242-4636) (24 hours a day, 7 days a week)

National Association of People with AIDS Hotline
Phone: 240-247-0880 (Monday through Friday 9:00 a.m. to 5:30 p.m., EST)

National Domestic Violence Hotline
Phone: 800-799-7233 (24 hours a day, 7 days a week)
TTY: 800-787-3224

National Herpes Hotline
Phone: 919-361-8488 (Monday through Friday 9:00 a.m. to 6:00 p.m., EST)

National HIV/AIDS Treatment Hotline
Phone: 800-822-7422 (Monday through Friday 10:00 a.m. to 4:00 p.m., PST)

National Sexually Transmitted Diseases Hotline
Phone: 800-227-8922 (24 hours a day, 7 days a week)
Website: http://www.ashastd.org

Women Alive Hotline
800-554-4876 (Monday through Friday 11:00 a.m. to 6:00 p.m., PST)

Chapter 54

Additional Reading about STDs

Magazines and Journals That Publish Information about STDs

A&U: America's AIDS Magazine
http://www.aumag.org

Addiction Journal
http://www.addictionjournal.org

AIDS: Official Journal of the International AIDS Society
http://www.aidsonline.com

Archives of Sexual Behavior
http://www.springer.com/public+health/journal/10508

Clinical Infectious Diseases
http://www.journals.uchicago.edu/CID/home.html

International Journal of STD and AIDS
http://ijsa.rsmjournals.com

Resources listed in this chapter were compiled from many sources deemed accurate. Inclusion does not constitute endorsement and there is no implication associated with omission. All website information was verified in January 2009.

Journal of Acquired Immune Deficiency Syndromes
http://www.jaids.com

Journal of Adolescent Health
http://www.adolescenthealth.org/journal.htm

Journal of Homosexuality
http://www.tandf.co.uk/journals/WJHM

Journal of Infectious Diseases
http://www.journals.uchicago.edu/JID

Journal of Sex Research
http://www.sexscience.org/publications/index.php?category_id=439

Journal of Viral Hepatitis
http://www.blackwellpublishing.com/journal.asp?ref=1352-0504

Liver Health Today
http://www.liverhealthtoday.org

Morbidity and Mortality Weekly Report
http://www.cdc.gov/mmwr

Perspectives on Sexual and Reproductive Health
http://www.blackwellpublishing.com/journal.asp?ref=1538-6341&site=1

POZ Magazine
http://www.poz.com

Sex, etc. *(for teens)*
http://www.sexetc.org/page/subscribe

Sexually Transmitted Diseases
http://www.stdjournal.com

Sexually Transmitted Infections
http://sti.bmj.com

Topics in HIV Medicine
http://www.iasusa.org/pub

Virology Journal
http://virologyj.com

Books about STDs

Barnett, Tony; Whiteside, Alan. *AIDS in the Twenty-First Century, Fully Revised and Updated Edition: Disease and Globalization, Second Edition.* Palgrave Macmillan, 2006. ISBN 1403997683.

Bartlett, John G.; Finkbeiner, Ann K. *The Guide to Living with HIV Infection: Developed at the Johns Hopkins AIDS Clinic, Sixth Edition.* Johns Hopkins University Press, 2006. ISBN 0801884853.

Ebel, Charles; Wald, Anna. *Managing Herpes: Living and Loving with HSV.* American Social Health Association, 2007. ISBN 1885833083.

Engel, Jonathan. *The Epidemic: A Global History of AIDS*. Collins, 2006. ISBN 0061144886.

Everson, Gregory T.; Weinberg, Hedy. *Living with Hepatitis B: A Survivor's Guide*. Hatherleigh Press, 2001. ISBN 1578260841.

Everson, Gregory T.; Weinberg, Hedy. *Living with Hepatitis C: A Survivor's Guide, Fourth Edition.* Hatherleigh Press, 2006. ISBN 1578262259.

Gifford, Allen; Lorig, Kate; Laurent, Diana; Gonzalez, Virginia. *Living Well with HIV & AIDS, Third Edition.* Bull Publishing Company, 2005. ISBN 0923521860.

Grimes, Jill. *Seductive Delusions: How Everyday People Catch STDs.* The Johns Hopkins University Press, 2008. ISBN 0801890675.

Grodeck, Brett. *The First Year: HIV: An Essential Guide for the Newly Diagnosed, Revised Edition.* Da Capo Press, 2007. ISBN 1600940137.

Hunter, Susan. *AIDS in America*. Palgrave Macmillan, 2006. ISBN 1403971994.

Krishnan, Shobha S. *The HPV Vaccine Controversy: Sex, Cancer, God, and Politics: A Guide for Parents, Women, Men, and Teenagers*. Praeger Publishers, 2008. ISBN 0313350116.

Marr, Lisa. *Sexually Transmitted Diseases: A Physician Tells You What You Need to Know, Second Edition.* The Johns Hopkins University Press, 2007. ISBN 0801886597.

Moore, Elaine A.; Moore, Lisa Marie. *Encyclopedia of Sexually Transmitted Diseases*. McFarland & Company, 2008. ISBN 0786443170.

Nack, Adina. *Damaged Goods?: Women Living with Incurable Sexually Transmitted Diseases*. Temple University Press, 2008. ISBN 1592137083.

Palmer, Melissa. *Dr. Melissa Palmer's Guide to Hepatitis and Liver Disease, Revised Edition.* Avery, 2004. ISBN 1583331883.

Westheimer, Ruth. *Dr. Ruth's Guide to Talking about Herpes*. Grove Press, 2004. ISBN 080214120X.

Index

Index

Page numbers followed by 'n' indicate a footnote. Page numbers in *italics* indicate a table or illustration.

A

B

C

D

E

F

H

I

N

O

P

Q

R

S

T

V

W

Y

Z

Health Reference Series

Complete Catalog

List price $93 per volume. School and library price $84 per volume.

Adolescent Health Sourcebook, 2nd Edition

Basic Consumer Health Information about the Physical, Mental, and Emotional Growth and Development of Adolescents, Including Medical Care, Nutritional and Physical Activity Requirements, Puberty, Sexual Activity, Acne, Tanning, Body Piercing, Common Physical Illnesses and Disorders, Eating Disorders, Attention Deficit Hyperactivity Disorder, Depression, Bullying, Hazing, and Adolescent Injuries Related to Sports, Driving, and Work

Along with Substance Abuse Information about Nicotine, Alcohol, and Drug Use, a Glossary, and Directory of Additional Resources

Edited by Joyce Brennfleck Shannon. 655 pages. 2007. 978-0-7808-0943-7.

"A particularly good resource for both parents and teens. The concise presentation of the material in brief and well-organized chapters creates an easy volume to browse."

—*School Library Journal, Jun '07*

"I don't believe there are any other books written in such easy to understand language that encompass such a breadth of topics. This is a complete revision of the book and is an excellent resource for parents and teens."

—*Doody's Review Service, 2007*

Adult Health Concerns Sourcebook

Basic Consumer Health Information about Medical and Mental Concerns of Adults, Including Facts about Choosing Healthcare Providers, Navigating Insurance Options, Maintaining Wellness, Preventing Cancer, Heart Disease, Stroke, Diabetes, and Osteoporosis, and Understanding Aging-Related Health Concerns, Including Menopause, Cognitive Changes, and Changes in the Coronary and Vascular Systems

Along with Tips on Caring for Aging Parents and Dealing with Health-Related Work and Travel Issues, a Glossary, and a Directory of Resources for Additional Help and Information

Edited by Sandra J. Judd. 648 pages. 2008. 978-0-7808-0999-4.

"Provides a thorough list of topics that are important to adult health and for caregivers."

—*CHOICE, Nov '08*

"Written in easy-to-understand language . . . the content is well-organized and is intended to aid adults in making health care-related decisions."

—*AORN Journal, Dec '08*

AIDS Sourcebook, 4th Edition

Basic Consumer Health Information about Human Immunodeficiency Virus (HIV) and Acquired Immunodeficiency Syndrome (AIDS), Featuring Updated Statistics and Facts about Risks, Prevention, Screening, Diagnosis, Treatments, Side Effects, and Complications, and Including a Section about the Impact of HIV/AIDS on the Health of Women, Children, and Adolescents

Along with Tips on Managing Life with AIDS, Reports on Current Research Initiatives and Clinical Trials, a Glossary of Related Terms, and Resource Directories for Further Help and Information

Edited by Ivy L. Alexander. 680 pages. 2008. 978-0-7808-0997-0.

SEE ALSO *Contagious Diseases Sourcebook, 2nd Edition*

Alcoholism Sourcebook, 2nd Edition

Basic Consumer Health Information about Alcohol Use, Abuse, and Dependence, Featuring Facts about the Physical, Mental, and Social Health Effects of Alcohol Addiction, Including Alcoholic Liver Disease, Pancreatic Disease, Cardiovascular Disease, Neurological Disorders, and the Effects of Drinking during Pregnancy

Along with Information about Alcohol Treatment, Medications, and Recovery Programs, in Addition to Tips for Reducing the Prevalence of Underage Drinking, Statistics about Alcohol Use, a Glossary of Related Terms, and Directories of Resources for More Help and Information

Edited by Amy L. Sutton. 625 pages. 2007. 978-0-7808-0942-0.

"A comprehensive look at the adverse effects of alcohol on people of all ages . . . It serves to whet the reader's appetite to continue learning using other resources. It is practical, easy to read, and enlightening, and is the first book a lay person should consult to learn about alcoholism."

—*Doody's Review Service, 2007*

"Should be a basic acquisition for any serious public or college-level library including health reference titles for general-interest readers."

—*California Bookwatch, Feb '07*

SEE ALSO *Drug Abuse Sourcebook, 2nd Edition*

Allergies Sourcebook, 3rd Edition

Basic Consumer Health Information about Allergic Disorders, Such as Anaphylaxis, Hives, Eczema, Rhinitis, Sinusitis, and Conjunctivitis, and Their Triggers, Including Pollen, Mold, Dust Mites, Animal Dander, Insects, Chemicals, Food, Food Additives, and Medications

Along with Advice about the Diagnosis and Treatment of Allergy Symptoms, a Glossary of Related Terms, a Directory of Resources for Help and Information, and Suggestions for Additional Reading

Edited by Amy L. Sutton. 588 pages. 2007. 978-0-7808-0950-5.

SEE ALSO *Asthma Sourcebook, 2nd Edition*

Alzheimer Disease Sourcebook, 4th Edition

Basic Consumer Health Information about Alzheimer Disease, Other Dementias, and Related Disorders, Including Multi-Infarct Dementia, Dementia with Lewy Bodies, Frontotemporal Dementia (Pick Disease), Wernicke-Korsakoff Syndrome (Alcohol-Related Dementia), AIDS Dementia Complex, Huntington Disease, Creutzfeldt-Jacob Disease, and Delirium

Along with Information about Coping with Memory Loss and Forgetfulness, Maintaining Skills, and Long-Term Planning for People with Dementia, and Suggestions Addressing Common Caregiver Concerns, Updated Information about Current Research Efforts, a Glossary of Related Terms, and Directories of Sources for Additional Help and Information

Edited by Karen Bellenir. 603 pages. 2008. 978-0-7808-1001-3.

"An invaluable resource for persons who have received a diagnosis, for caregivers, and for family members dealing with this insidious disease. It is recommended for public, community college, and ready-reference sections in academic libraries."

—*ARBAonline, Jul '08*

SEE ALSO *Brain Disorders Sourcebook, 2nd Edition*

Arthritis Sourcebook, 2nd Edition

Basic Consumer Health Information about Osteoarthritis, Rheumatoid Arthritis, Other Rheumatic Disorders, Infectious Forms of Arthritis, and Diseases with Symptoms Linked to Arthritis, Featuring Facts about Diagnosis, Pain Management, and Surgical Therapies

Along with Coping Strategies, Research Updates, a Glossary, and Resources for Additional Help and Information

Edited by Amy L. Sutton. 567 pages. 2004. 978-0-7808-0667-2.

"This easy-to-read volume is recommended for consumer health collections within public or academic libraries."

—*E-Streams, May '05*

"As expected, this updated edition continues the excellent reputation of this series in providing sound, usable health information. . . . Highly recommended."

—*American Reference Books Annual, 2005*

Asthma Sourcebook, 2nd Edition

Basic Consumer Health Information about the Causes, Symptoms, Diagnosis, and Treatment of Asthma in Infants, Children, Teenagers, and Adults, Including Facts about Different Types of Asthma, Common Co-Occurring Conditions, Asthma Management Plans, Triggers, Medications, and Medication Delivery Devices

Along with Asthma Statistics, Research Updates, a Glossary, a Directory of Asthma-Related Resources, and More

Edited by Karen Bellenir. 581 pages. 2006. 978-0-7808-0866-9.

Attention Deficit Disorder Sourcebook

Basic Consumer Health Information about Attention Deficit/Hyperactivity Disorder in Children and Adults, Including Facts about Causes, Symptoms, Diagnostic Criteria, and Treatment Options Such as Medications, Behavior Therapy, Coaching, and Homeopathy

Along with Reports on Current Research Initiatives, Legal Issues, and Government Regulations, and Featuring a Glossary of Related Terms, Internet Resources, and a List of Additional Reading Material

Edited by Dawn D. Matthews. 447 pages. 2002. 978-0-7808-0624-5.

"Recommended reference source."

—*Booklist, Jan '03*

SEE ALSO *Learning Disabilities Sourcebook, 3rd Edition*

Autism and Pervasive Developmental Disorders Sourcebook

Basic Consumer Health Information about Autism Spectrum and Pervasive Developmental Disorders, Such as Classical Autism, Asperger Syndrome, Rett Syndrome, and Childhood Disintegrative Disorder, Including Information about Related Genetic Disorders and Medical Problems and Facts about Causes, Screening Methods, Diagnostic Criteria, Treatments and Interventions, and Family and Education Issues

Along with a Glossary of Related Terms, Tips for Evaluating the Validity of Health Claims, and a Directory of Resources for Additional Help and Information

Edited by Sandra J. Judd. 603 pages. 2007. 978-0-7808-0953-6.

"Recommended for public libraries"

—*SciTech Book News, Mar '08*

SEE ALSO *Learning Disabilities Sourcebook, 3rd Edition*

Back and Neck Disorders Sourcebook, 2nd Edition

Basic Consumer Health Information about Spinal Pain, Spinal Cord Injuries, and Related Disorders, Such as Degenerative Disk Disease, Osteoarthritis, Scoliosis, Sciatica, Spina Bifida, and Spinal Stenosis, and Featuring Facts about Maintaining Spinal Health, Self-Care, Pain Management, Rehabilitative Care, Chiropractic Care, Spinal Surgeries, and Complementary Therapies

Along with Suggestions for Preventing Back and Neck Pain, a Glossary of Related Terms, and a Directory of Resources

Edited by Amy L. Sutton. 607 pages. 2004. 978-0-7808-0738-9.

"Recommended. ...An easy to use, comprehensive medical reference book."

—*E-Streams, Sep '05*

"For anyone who has back or neck problems, this book is ideal. Its easy-to-understand language and variety of topics makes this sourcebook a worthwhile read. The price...is reasonable for the amount of information contained in the book"

—*Occupational Therapy in Health Care, 2007*

Blood and Circulatory Disorders Sourcebook, 2nd Edition

Basic Consumer Health Information about the Blood and Circulatory System and Related Disorders, Such as Anemia and Other Hemoglobin Diseases, Cancer of the Blood and Associated Bone Marrow Disorders, Clotting and Bleeding Problems, and Conditions That Affect the Veins, Blood Vessels, and Arteries, Including Facts about the Donation and Transplantation of Bone Marrow, Stem Cells, and Blood and Tips for Keeping the Blood and Circulatory System Healthy

Along with a Glossary of Related Terms and Resources for Additional Help and Information

Edited by Amy L. Sutton. 634 pages. 2005. 978-0-7808-0746-4.

"Highly recommended pick for basic consumer health reference holdings at all levels."

—*The Bookwatch, Aug '05*

Brain Disorders Sourcebook, 2nd Edition

Basic Consumer Health Information about Acquired and Traumatic Brain Injuries, Infections of the Brain, Epilepsy and Seizure Disorders, Cerebral Palsy, and Degenerative Neurological Disorders, Including Amyotrophic Lateral Sclerosis (ALS), Dementias, Multiple Sclerosis, and More

Along with Information on the Brain's Structure and Function, Treatment and Rehabilitation Options, Reports on Current Research Initiatives, a Glossary of Terms Related to Brain Disorders and Injuries, and a Directory of Sources for Further Help and Information

Edited by Sandra J. Judd. 600 pages. 2005. 978-0-7808-0744-0.

"This easy-to-read volume provides up-to-date health information... Recommended for consumer health collections within public or academic libraries."

—E-Streams, Feb '06

SEE ALSO *Alzheimer Disease Sourcebook, 4th Edition*

Breast Cancer Sourcebook, 3rd Edition

Basic Consumer Health Information about Breast Health and Breast Cancer, Including Facts about Environmental, Genetic, and Other Risk Factors, Prevention Efforts, Screening and Diagnostic Methods, Surgical Treatment Options and Other Care Choices, Complementary and Alternative Therapies, and Post-Treatment Concerns

Along with Statistical Data, News about Research Advances, a Glossary of Related Terms, and Directories of Resources for Additional Information and Support

Edited by Karen Bellenir. 606 pages. 2009. 978-0-7808-1030-3.

SEE ALSO *Cancer Sourcebook for Women, 3rd Edition, Women's Health Concerns Sourcebook, 3rd Edition*

Breastfeeding Sourcebook

Basic Consumer Health Information about the Benefits of Breastmilk, Preparing to Breastfeed, Breastfeeding as a Baby Grows, Nutrition, and More, Including Information on Special Situations and Concerns Such as Mastitis, Illness, Medications, Allergies, Multiple Births, Prematurity, Special Needs, and Adoption

Along with a Glossary and Resources for Additional Help and Information

Edited by Jenni Lynn Colson. 367 pages. 2002. 978-0-7808-0332-9.

SEE ALSO *Pregnancy and Birth Sourcebook, 2nd Edition*

Burns Sourcebook

Basic Consumer Health Information about Various Types of Burns and Scalds, Including Flame, Heat, Cold, Electrical, Chemical, and Sun Burns

Along with Information on Short-Term and Long-Term Treatments, Tissue Reconstruction, Plastic Surgery, Prevention Suggestions, and First Aid

Edited by Allan R. Cook. 604 pages. 1999. 978-0-7808-0204-9.

"This is an exceptional addition to the series and is highly recommended for all consumer health collections, hospital libraries, and academic medical centers."

—E-Streams, Mar '00

"This key reference guide is an invaluable addition to all health care and public libraries in confronting this ongoing health issue."

—American Reference Books Annual, 2000

SEE ALSO *Dermatological Disorders Sourcebook, 2nd Edition*

Cancer Sourcebook, 5th Edition

Basic Consumer Health Information about Major Forms and Stages of Cancer, Featuring Facts about Head and Neck Cancers, Lung Cancers, Gastrointestinal Cancers, Genitourinary Cancers, Lymphomas, Blood Cell Cancers, Endocrine Cancers, Skin Cancers, Bone Cancers, Metastatic Cancers, and More

Along with Facts about Cancer Treatments, Cancer Risks and Prevention, a Glossary of Related Terms, Statistical Data, and a Directory of Resources for Additional Information

Edited by Karen Bellenir. 1105 pages. 2007. 978-0-7808-0947-5.

"The 5th, updated edition of *Cancer Sourcebook* should be in every public and health lending library collection... An unparalleled discussion essential for any health collections considering an all-in-one basic general reference."

—*California Bookwatch, Aug '07*

SEE ALSO *Breast Cancer Sourcebook, 3rd Edition, Cancer Sourcebook for Women, 3rd Edition, Cancer Survivorship Sourcebook, Leukemia Sourcebook*

Cancer Sourcebook for Women, 3rd Edition

Basic Consumer Health Information about Leading Causes of Cancer in Women, Featuring Facts about Gynecologic Cancers and Related Concerns, Such as Breast Cancer, Cervical Cancer, Endometrial Cancer, Uterine Sarcoma, Vaginal Cancer, Vulvar Cancer, and Common Non-Cancerous Gynecologic Conditions, in Addition to Facts about Lung Cancer, Colorectal Cancer, and Thyroid Cancer in Women

Along with Information about Cancer Risk Factors, Screening and Prevention, Treatment Options, and Tips on Coping with Life after Cancer Treatment, a Glossary of Cancer Terms, and a Directory of Resources for Additional Help and Information

Edited by Amy L. Sutton. 687 pages. 2006. 978-0-7808-0867-6.

"This excellent book provides the general public with information compiled in a way that will help them to gain the knowledge they need. 4 Stars!"

—*Doody's Review Service, Dec '06*

"An indispensable reference for health consumers and cancer patients. Recommended for public libraries and academic libraries with a medical department."

—*E-Streams, Sep '08*

Cancer Survivorship Sourcebook

Basic Consumer Health Information about the Physical, Educational, Emotional, Social, and Financial Needs of Cancer Patients from Diagnosis, through Cancer Treatment, and Beyond, Including Facts about Researching Specific Types of Cancer and Learning about Clinical Trials and Treatment Options, and Featuring Tips for Coping with the Side Effects of Cancer Treatments and Adjusting to Life after Cancer Treatment Concludes

Along with Suggestions for Caregivers, Friends, and Family Members of Cancer Patients, a Glossary of Cancer Care Terms, and Directories of Related Resources

Edited by Karen Bellenir. 633 pages. 2007. 978-0-7808-0985-7.

"Well organized and comprehensive in coverage, the book speaks to issues encountered both during and after cancer treatment. Recommended for consumer health and public libraries."

—*Library Journal, Aug 1 '07*

"*Cancer Survivorship Sourcebook* will be useful to anyone who has a friend or loved one with a cancer diagnosis."

—*American Reference Books Annual, 2008*

SEE ALSO *Cancer Sourcebook, 5th Edition*

Cardiovascular Diseases and Disorders Sourcebook, 3rd Edition

Basic Consumer Health Information about Heart and Vascular Diseases and Disorders, Such as Angina, Heart Attacks, Arrhythmias, Cardiomyopathy, Valve Disease, Atherosclerosis, and Aneurysms, with Information about Managing Cardiovascular Risk Factors and Maintaining Heart Health, Medications and Procedures Used to Treat Cardiovascular Disorders, and Concerns of Special Significance to Women

Along with Reports on Current Research Initiatives, a Glossary of Related Medical Terms, and a Directory of Sources for Further Help and Information

Edited by Sandra J. Judd. 687 pages. 2005. 978-0-7808-0739-6.

"This updated sourcebook is still the best first stop for comprehensive introductory information on cardiovascular diseases."

—*American Reference Books Annual, 2006*

"Recommended for public libraries and libraries supporting health care professionals."

—*E-Streams, Sep '05*

Caregiving Sourcebook

Basic Consumer Health Information for Caregivers, Including a Profile of Caregivers, Caregiving Responsibilities and Concerns, Tips for Specific Conditions, Care Environments, and the Effects of Caregiving

Along with Facts about Legal Issues, Financial Information, and Future Planning, a Glossary, and a Listing of Additional Resources

Edited by Joyce Brennfleck Shannon. 583 pages. 2001. 978-0-7808-0331-2.

"Essential for most collections."

—*Library Journal, Apr 1 '02*

"An ideal addition to the reference collection of any public library. Health sciences information professionals may also want to acquire the *Caregiving Sourcebook* for their hospital or academic library for use as a ready reference tool by health care workers interested in aging and caregiving."

—*E-Streams, Jan '02*

Child Abuse Sourcebook, 2nd Edition

Basic Consumer Health Information about the Physical, Sexual, and Emotional Abuse of Children, Neglect, Münchhausen Syndrome by Proxy (MSBP), and Shaken Baby Syndrome, and Featuring Facts about Withholding Medical Care, Corporal Punishment, Child Maltreatment in Youth Sports, and Parental Substance Abuse

Along with Information about Child Protective Services, Foster Care, Adoption, Parenting Challenges, Abuse Prevention Programs, and Intervention, Treatment, and Recovery Guidelines, a Glossary of Related Terms, and Resources for Additional Help and Information

Edited by Joyce Brennfleck Shannon. 600 pages. 2009. 978-0-7808-1037-2.

SEE ALSO *Domestic Violence Sourcebook, 3rd Edition*

Childhood Diseases and Disorders Sourcebook, 2nd Edition

Basic Consumer Health Information about the Physical, Mental, and Developmental Health of Pre-Adolescent Children, Including Facts about Infectious Diseases, Asthma, Allergies, Diabetes, and Other Acute and Chronic Conditions Affecting the Gastrointestinal Tract, Ears, Nose, Throat, Liver, Kidneys, Heart, Blood, Brain, Muscles, Bones, and Skin

Along with Reports on Recommended Childhood Vaccinations, Wellness Guidelines, a Glossary of Related Medical Terms, and a List of Resources for Parents

Edited by Sandra J. Judd. 694 pages. 2009. 978-0-7808-1031-0.

SEE ALSO *Healthy Children Sourcebook*

Colds, Flu and Other Common Ailments Sourcebook

Basic Consumer Health Information about Common Ailments and Injuries, Including Colds, Coughs, the Flu, Sinus Problems, Headaches, Fever, Nausea and Vomiting, Menstrual Cramps, Diarrhea, Constipation, Hemorrhoids, Back Pain, Dandruff, Dry and Itchy Skin, Cuts, Scrapes, Sprains, Bruises, and More

Along with Information about Prevention, Self-Care, Choosing a Doctor, Over-the-Counter Medications, Folk Remedies, and Alternative Therapies, and Including a Glossary of Important Terms and a Directory of Resources for Further Help and Information

Edited by Chad T. Kimball. 622 pages. 2001. 978-0-7808-0435-7.

"A good starting point for research on common illnesses. It will be a useful addition to public and consumer health library collections."

—*American Reference Books Annual, 2002*

"Will prove valuable to any library seeking to maintain a current, comprehensive reference collection of health resources. . . Excellent reference."

—*The Bookwatch, Aug '01*

Communication Disorders Sourcebook

Basic Information about Deafness and Hearing Loss, Speech and Language Disorders, Voice Disorders, Balance and Vestibular Disorders, and Disorders of Smell, Taste, and Touch

Edited by Linda M. Ross. 533 pages. 1996. 978-0-7808-0077-9.

"This is skillfully edited and is a welcome resource for the layperson. It should be found in every public and medical library."

—Booklist Health Sciences Supplement, Oct '97

Complementary and Alternative Medicine Sourcebook, 3rd Edition

Basic Consumer Health Information about Complementary and Alternative Medical Therapies, Including Acupuncture, Ayurveda, Traditional Chinese Medicine, Herbal Medicine, Homeopathy, Naturopathy, Biofeedback, Hypnotherapy, Yoga, Art Therapy, Aromatherapy, Clinical Nutrition, Vitamin and Mineral Supplements, Chiropractic, Massage, Reflexology, Crystal Therapy, Therapeutic Touch, and More

Along with Facts about Alternative and Complementary Treatments for Specific Conditions Such as Cancer, Diabetes, Osteoarthritis, Chronic Pain, Menopause, Gastrointestinal Disorders, Headaches, and Mental Illness, a Glossary, and a Resource List for Additional Help and Information

Edited by Sandra J. Judd. 630 pages. 2006. 978-0-7808-0864-5.

"A 'must' reference for any serious healthcare collection. Public library holdings, too, will welcome it as a popular reference."

—California Bookwatch, Oct '06

"Both basic and informative at the same time. . . a useful resource for health care professionals as well as consumers interested in learning more information about CAM therapies."

—AORN Journal, Jan '08

"A quality, indexed, referenced guideline for many alternative practices that are quite popular around the world...It is neatly organized to find facts quickly, is peer-reviewed, and stays current with the most recent advances."

—Journal of Dental Hygiene, Jul '07

Congenital Disorders Sourcebook, 2nd Edition

Basic Consumer Health Information about Nonhereditary Birth Defects and Disorders Related to Prematurity, Gestational Injuries, Congenital Infections, and Birth Complications, Including Heart Defects, Hydrocephalus, Spina Bifida, Cleft Lip and Palate, Cerebral Palsy, and More

Along with Facts about the Prevention of Birth Defects, Fetal Surgery and Other Treatment Options, Research Initiatives, a Glossary of Related Terms, and Resources for Additional Information and Support

Edited by Sandra J. Judd. 619 pages. 2007. 978-0-7808-0945-1.

"Congenital Disorders Sourcebook provides an excellent, non-technical overview of many aspects of pregnancy with the focus on congenital disorders."

—American Reference Books Annual, 2008

"An excellent readable reference aimed at the lay public for difficult to understand medical problems. An excellent starting point for the interested parent or family member who may then be motivated to seek more information."

—Doody's Review Service, 2007

SEE ALSO *Pregnancy and Birth Sourcebook, 2nd Edition*

Contagious Diseases Sourcebook, 2nd Edition

Basic Consumer Health Information about Diseases Spread from Person to Person through Direct Physical Contact, Airborne Transmissions, Sexual Contact, or Contact with Blood or Other Body Fluids, Including Pneumococcal, Staphylococcal, and Streptococcal Diseases, Colds, Influenza, Lice, Measles, Mumps, Tuberculosis, and Others

Along with Facts about Self-Care and Over-the-Counter Medications, Antibiotics and Drug Resistance, Disease Prevention, Vaccines, and Bioterrorism, a Glossary, and a Directory of Resources for More Information

Edited by Joyce Brennfleck Shannon. 600 pages. 2009. 978-0-7808-1075-4.

SEE ALSO *AIDS Sourcebook, 4th Edition, Hepatitis Sourcebook*

Cosmetic and Reconstructive Surgery Sourcebook, 2nd Edition

Basic Consumer Information about Plastic Surgery and Non-Surgical Appearance-Enhancing Procedures, Including Facts about Botulinum Toxin, Collagen Replacement, Dermabrasion,

Chemical Peels, Eyelid Surgery, Nose Reshaping, Lip Augmentation, Liposuction, Breast Enlargement and Reduction, Tummy Tucking, and Other Skin, Hair, Facial, and Body Shaping Procedures

Along with Information about Reconstructive Procedures for Congenital Disorders, Disfiguring Diseases, Burns, and Traumatic Injuries, a Glossary of Related Terms, and a Directory of Additional Resources

Edited by Karen Bellenir. 483 pages. 2007. 978-0-7808-0951-2.

"A practical guide for health care consumers and health care workers. . . . This easy-to-read reference guide would be useful for novice and veteran health care consumers, surgical technology students, nursing students, and perioperative nurses new to plastic and reconstructive surgery. It also may be helpful for medical-surgical nurses as a guide for patient teaching in their practices."

—*AORN Journal, Aug '08*

SEE ALSO *Surgery Sourcebook, 2nd Edition*

Death and Dying Sourcebook, 2nd Edition

Basic Consumer Health Information about End-of-Life Care and Related Perspectives and Ethical Issues, Including End-of-Life Symptoms and Treatments, Pain Management, Quality-of-Life Concerns, the Use of Life Support, Patients' Rights and Privacy Issues, Advance Directives, Physician-Assisted Suicide, Caregiving, Organ and Tissue Donation, Autopsies, Funeral Arrangements, and Grief

Along with Statistical Data, Information about the Leading Causes of Death, a Glossary, and Directories of Support Groups and Other Resources

Edited by Joyce Brennfleck Shannon. 626 pages. 2006. 978-0-7808-0871-3.

Dental Care and Oral Health Sourcebook, 3rd Edition

Basic Consumer Health Information about Dental Care and Oral Health Throughout the Lifespan, Including Facts about Cavities, Bad Breath, Cold and Canker Sores, Dry Mouth, Toothaches, Gum Disease, Malocclusion, Temporomandibular Joint and Muscle Disorders, Oral Cancers, and Dental Emergencies

Along with Information about Mouth Hygiene, Crowns, Bridges, Implants, and Fillings, Surgical, Orthodontic, and Cosmetic Dental Procedures, Pain Management, Health Conditions that Impact Oral Care, a Glossary of Related Terms, and a Directory of Additional Resources

Edited by Amy L. Sutton. 619 pages. 2008. 978-0-7808-1032-7.

Depression Sourcebook, 2nd Edition

Basic Consumer Health Information about Unipolar Depression, Bipolar Disorder, Dysthymia, Seasonal Affective Disorder, Postpartum Depression, and Other Depressive Disorders, Including Facts about Populations at Special Risk, Coexisting Medical Conditions, Symptoms, Treatment Options, and Suicide Prevention

Along with Statistical Data, a Glossary of Related Terms, and a Directory of Resources for Additional Help and Information

Edited by Sandra J. Judd. 646 pages. 2008. 978-0-7808-1003-7.

"Recommended for public libraries."

—*ARBAonline, Nov '08*

SEE ALSO *Mental Health Disorders Sourcebook, 4th Edition*

Dermatological Disorders Sourcebook, 2nd Edition

Basic Consumer Health Information about Conditions and Disorders Affecting the Skin, Hair, and Nails, Such as Acne, Rosacea, Rashes, Dermatitis, Pigmentation Disorders, Birthmarks, Skin Cancer, Skin Injuries, Psoriasis, Scleroderma, and Hair Loss, Including Facts about Medications and Treatments for Dermatological Disorders and Tips for Maintaining Healthy Skin, Hair, and Nails

Along with Information about How Aging Affects the Skin, a Glossary of Related Terms, and a Directory of Resources for Additional Help and Information

Edited by Amy L. Sutton. 617 pages. 2006. 978-0-7808-0795-2.

"Helpfully brings together. . . sources in one convenient place, saving the user hours of research time."
—*American Reference Books Annual, 2006*

SEE ALSO *Burns Sourcebook*

Diabetes Sourcebook, 4th Edition

Basic Consumer Health Information about Type 1 and Type 2 Diabetes Mellitus, Gestational Diabetes, Monogenic Forms of Diabetes, and Insulin Resistance, with Guidelines for Lifestyle Modifications and the Medical Management of Diabetes, Including Facts about Insulin, Insulin Delivery Devices, Oral Diabetes Medications, Self-Monitoring of Blood Glucose, Meal Planning, Physical Activity Recommendations, Foot Care, and Treatment Options for People with Kidney Failure

Along with a Section about Diabetes Complications and Co-Occurring Conditions, a Glossary of Related Terms, and Directories of Resources for Additional Help and Information

Edited by Karen Bellenir. 627 pages. 2008. 978-0-7808-1005-1.

"Completely and comprehensively covering almost everything a student or physician would need to know.... well worth the investment."
—*Internet Bookwatch, Dec '08*

SEE ALSO *Endocrine and Metabolic Disorders Sourcebook, 2nd Edition*

Diet and Nutrition Sourcebook, 3rd Edition

Basic Consumer Health Information about Dietary Guidelines and the Food Guidance System, Recommended Daily Nutrient Intakes, Serving Proportions, Weight Control, Vitamins and Supplements, Nutrition Issues for Different Life Stages and Lifestyles, and the Needs of People with Specific Medical Concerns, Including Cancer, Celiac Disease, Diabetes, Eating Disorders, Food Allergies, and Cardiovascular Disease

Along with Facts about Federal Nutrition Support Programs, a Glossary of Nutrition and Dietary Terms, and Directories of Additional Resources for More Information about Nutrition

Edited by Joyce Brennfleck Shannon. 605 pages. 2006. 978-0-7808-0800-3.

"A valuable resource tool for any individual."
—*Journal of Dental Hygiene, Apr '07*

"From different recommended eating habits to reduce disease and common ailments to nutrition advice for those with specific conditions, *Diet and Nutrition Sourcebook* is especially important because so much is changing in this area, and so rapidly."
—*California Bookwatch, Jun '06*

SEE ALSO *Digestive Diseases and Disorders Sourcebook, Eating Disorders Sourcebook, 2nd Edition, Gastrointestinal Diseases and Disorders Sourcebook, 2nd Edition, Vegetarian Sourcebook*

Digestive Diseases and Disorders Sourcebook

Basic Consumer Health Information about Diseases and Disorders that Impact the Upper and Lower Digestive System, Including Celiac Disease, Constipation, Crohn's Disease, Cyclic Vomiting Syndrome, Diarrhea, Diverticulosis and Diverticulitis, Gallstones, Heartburn, Hemorrhoids, Hernias, Indigestion (Dyspepsia), Irritable Bowel Syndrome, Lactose Intolerance, Ulcers, and More

Along with Information about Medications and Other Treatments, Tips for Maintaining a Healthy Digestive Tract, a Glossary, and Directory of Digestive Diseases Organizations

Edited by Karen Bellenir. 323 pages. 2000. 978-0-7808-0327-5.

"An excellent addition to all public or patient-research libraries."
—*American Reference Books Annual, 2001*

"Recommended reference source."
—*Booklist, May '00*

SEE ALSO *Diet and Nutrition Sourcebook, 3rd Edition, Gastrointestinal Diseases and Disorders Sourcebook, 2nd Edition*

Disabilities Sourcebook

Basic Consumer Health Information about Physical and Psychiatric Disabilities, Including Descriptions of Major Causes of Disability, Assistive and Adaptive Aids, Workplace Issues, and Accessibility Concerns

Along with Information about the Americans with Disabilities Act, a Glossary, and Resources for Additional Help and Information

Edited by Dawn D. Matthews. 602 pages. 2000. 978-0-7808-0389-3.

"A must for libraries with a consumer health section."

—*American Reference Books Annual, 2002*

"A much needed addition to the Omnigraphics *Health Reference Series*. A current reference work to provide people with disabilities, their families, caregivers or those who work with them, a broad range of information in one volume, has not been available until now. . . . It is recommended for all public and academic library reference collections."

—*E-Streams, May '01*

"An excellent source book in easy-to-read format covering many current topics; highly recommended for all libraries."

—*CHOICE, Jan '01*

Disease Management Sourcebook

Basic Consumer Health Information about Coping with Chronic and Serious Illnesses, Navigating the Health Care System, Communicating with Health Care Providers, Assessing Health Care Quality, and Making Informed Health Care Decisions, Including Facts about Second Opinions, Hospitalization, Surgery, and Medications

Along with a Section about Children with Chronic Conditions, Information about Legal, Financial, and Insurance Issues, a Glossary of Related Terms, and Directories of Additional Resources

Edited by Joyce Brennfleck Shannon. 621 pages. 2008. 978-0-7808-1002-0.

"Consumers need to know how to manage their health care the same way they manage anything else in their lives. The text is very readable and is written for the layperson and consumer. The cost is not prohibitive. This book should be in all collections of health care libraries and public libraries."

—*ARBAonline, Jul '08*

"The information is very current, and the selection of font and layout make the book easy to read. A hardback that will stand up to much usage, this is an excellent resource for consumers. . . . Recommended. General readers."

—*CHOICE, Nov '08*

"Intended for lay readers, this resource clarifies the many confusing and overwhelming details associated with chronic disease care. Meticulous and clearly explained, the book even includes diagrams intended to ease comprehension of over-the-counter medication labels. An essential guide to navigating the health-care rapids."

—*Library Journal, Aug '08*

Domestic Violence Sourcebook, 3rd Edition

Basic Consumer Health Information about Warning Signs, Risk Factors, and Health Consequences of Intimate Partner Violence, Sexual Violence and Rape, Stalking, Human Trafficking, Child Maltreatment, Teen Dating Violence, and Elder Abuse

Along with Facts about Victims and Perpetrators, Strategies for Violence Prevention, and Emergency Interventions, Safety Plans, and Financial and Legal Tips for Victims, a Glossary of Related Terms, and Directories of Resources for Additional Information and Support

Edited by Joyce Brennfleck Shannon. 600 pages. 2009. 978-0-7808-1038-9.

SEE ALSO *Child Abuse Sourcebook, 2nd Edition*

Drug Abuse Sourcebook, 2nd Edition

Basic Consumer Health Information about Illicit Substances of Abuse and the Misuse of Prescription and Over-the-Counter Medications, Including Depressants, Hallucinogens, Inhalants, Marijuana, Stimulants, and Anabolic Steroids

Along with Facts about Related Health Risks, Treatment Programs, Prevention Programs, a Glossary of Abuse and Addiction Terms, a Glossary of Drug-Related Street Terms, and a Directory of Resources for More Information

Edited by Catherine Ginther. 581 pages. 2004. 978-0-7808-0740-2.

"Commendable for organizing useful, normally scattered government and association-produced data into a logical sequence."

—*American Reference Books Annual, 2006*

"An excellent library reference."
—*The Bookwatch, May '05*

SEE ALSO *Alcoholism Sourcebook, 2nd Edition*

Ear, Nose, and Throat Disorders Sourcebook, 2nd Edition

Basic Consumer Health Information about Disorders of the Ears, Hearing Loss, Vestibular Disorders, Nasal and Sinus Problems, Throat and Vocal Cord Disorders, and Otolaryngologic Cancers, Including Facts about Ear Infections and Injuries, Genetic and Congenital Deafness, Sensorineural Hearing Disorders, Tinnitus, Vertigo, Ménière Disease, Rhinitis, Sinusitis, Snoring, Sore Throats, Hoarseness, and More

Along with Reports on Current Research Initiatives, a Glossary of Related Medical Terms, and a Directory of Sources for Further Help and Information

Edited by Sandra J. Judd. 631 pages. 2007. 978-0-7808-0872-0.

"A resource book for the general public that provides comprehensive coverage of basic up-to-date medical information about the causes, symptoms, diagnosis, and treatment of diseases and disorders that affect the ears, nose, sinuses, throat, and voice. . . . The majority of information is presented in question and answer format, much like questions a patient might ask of a health care provider. An extensive index facilitates the reader's ability to easily access information on any specific topic."
—*Journal of Dental Hygiene, Oct '07*

"A handy compilation of information on common and some not so common ailments of the ears, nose, and throat."
—*Doody's Review Service, 2007*

Eating Disorders Sourcebook, 2nd Edition

Basic Consumer Health Information about Anorexia Nervosa, Bulimia, Binge Eating, Compulsive Exercise, Female Athlete Triad, and Other Eating Disorders, Including Facts about Body Image and Other Cultural and Age-Related Risk Factors, Prevention Efforts, Adverse Health Effects, Treatment Options, and the Recovery Process

Along with Guidelines for Healthy Weight Control, a Glossary, and Directories of Additional Resources

Edited by Joyce Brennfleck Shannon. 557 pages. 2007. 978-0-7808-0948-2.

"Recommended for the reference collection of large public libraries."
—*American Reference Books Annual, 2008*

"A basic health reference any health or general library needs."
—*Internet Bookwatch, Jun '07*

SEE ALSO *Diet and Nutrition Sourcebook, 3rd Edition, Mental Health Disorders Sourcebook, 4th Edition*

Emergency Medical Services Sourcebook

Basic Consumer Health Information about Preventing, Preparing for, and Managing Emergency Situations, When and Who to Call for Help, What to Expect in the Emergency Room, the Emergency Medical Team, Patient Issues, and Current Topics in Emergency Medicine

Along with Statistical Data, a Glossary, and Sources of Additional Help and Information

Edited by Jenni Lynn Colson. 472 pages. 2002. 978-0-7808-0420-3.

"Handy and convenient for home, public, school, and college libraries. Recommended."
—*CHOICE, Apr '03*

"This reference can provide the consumer with answers to most questions about emergency care in the United States, or it will direct them to a resource where the answer can be found."
—*American Reference Books Annual, 2003*

SEE ALSO *Injury and Trauma Sourcebook*

Endocrine and Metabolic Disorders Sourcebook, 2nd Edition

Basic Consumer Health Information about Hormonal and Metabolic Disorders that Affect the Body's Growth, Development, and Functioning, Including Disorders of the Pancreas, Ovaries and Testes, and Pituitary, Thyroid, Parathyroid, and Adrenal Glands, with Facts about Growth Disorders, Addison Disease, Cushing Syndrome, Conn Syndrome, Diabetic Disorders, Multiple Endocrine Neoplasia, Inborn Errors of Metabolism, and More

Along with Information about Endocrine Functioning, Diagnostic and Screening Tests, a Glossary of Related Terms, and Directories of Additional Resources

Edited by Joyce Brennfleck Shannon. 597 pages. 2007. 978-0-7808-0952-9.

SEE ALSO *Diabetes Sourcebook, 4th Edition*

Environmental Health Sourcebook, 2nd Edition

Basic Consumer Health Information about the Environment and Its Effect on Human Health, Including the Effects of Air Pollution, Water Pollution, Hazardous Chemicals, Food Hazards, Radiation Hazards, Biological Agents, Household Hazards, Such as Radon, Asbestos, Carbon Monoxide, and Mold, and Information about Associated Diseases and Disorders, Including Cancer, Allergies, Respiratory Problems, and Skin Disorders

Along with Information about Environmental Concerns for Specific Populations, a Glossary of Related Terms, and Resources for Further Help and Information

Edited by Dawn D. Matthews. 650 pages. 2003. 978-0-7808-0632-0.

"Recommended for teenage and adult students and readers, and for public and academic libraries, as well as any library focusing on consumer health."

—*E-Streams, May '04*

"This recently updated edition continues the level of quality and the reputation of the numerous other volumes in Omnigraphics' *Health Reference Series.*"

—*American Reference Books Annual, 2004*

Ethnic Diseases Sourcebook

Basic Consumer Health Information for Ethnic and Racial Minority Groups in the United States, Including General Health Indicators and Behaviors, Ethnic Diseases, Genetic Testing, the Impact of Chronic Diseases, Women's Health, Mental Health Issues, and Preventive Health Care Services

Along with a Glossary and a Listing of Additional Resources

Edited by Joyce Brennfleck Shannon. 648 pages. 2001. 978-0-7808-0336-7.

"Not many books have been written on this topic to date, and the *Ethnic Diseases Sourcebook* is a strong addition to the list. It will be an important introductory resource for health consumers, students, health care personnel, and social scientists. It is recommended for public, academic, and large hospital libraries."

—*American Reference Books Annual, 2002*

"Will prove valuable to any library seeking to maintain a current, comprehensive reference collection of health resources. . . . An excellent source of health information about genetic disorders which affect particular ethnic and racial minorities in the U.S."

—*The Bookwatch, Aug '01*

Eye Care Sourcebook, 3rd Edition

Basic Consumer Health Information about Eye Care and Eye Disorders, Including Facts about the Diagnosis, Prevention, and Treatment of Refractive Disorders, Cataracts, Glaucoma, Macular Degeneration, and Problems Affecting the Cornea, Retina, and Lacrimal Glands

Along with Advice about Preventing Eye Injuries and Tips for Living with Low Vision or Blindness, a Glossary of Related Terms, and Directories of Resources for More Help and Information

Edited by Amy L. Sutton. 646 pages. 2008. 978-0-7808-1000-6.

Family Planning Sourcebook

Basic Consumer Health Information about Planning for Pregnancy and Contraception, Including Traditional Methods, Barrier Methods, Hormonal Methods, Permanent Methods, Future Methods, Emergency Contraception, and Birth Control Choices for Women at Each Stage of Life

Along with Statistics, a Glossary, and Sources of Additional Information

Edited by Amy Marcaccio Keyzer. 503 pages. 2001. 978-0-7808-0379-4.

"Recommended for public, health, and undergraduate libraries as part of the circulating collection."

—*E-Streams, Mar '02*

"Will prove valuable to any library seeking to maintain a current, comprehensive reference collection of health resources. . . . Excellent reference."

—*The Bookwatch, Aug '01*

SEE ALSO *Pregnancy and Birth Sourcebook, 2nd Edition*

Fitness and Exercise Sourcebook, 3rd Edition

Basic Consumer Health Information about the Physical and Mental Benefits of Fitness, Including Cardiorespiratory Endurance, Muscular Strength, Muscular Endurance, and Flexibility, with Facts about Sports Nutrition and Exercise-Related Injuries and Tips about Physical Activity and Exercises for People of All Ages and for People with Health Concerns

Along with Advice on Selecting and Using Exercise Equipment, Maintaining Exercise Motivation, a Glossary of Related Terms, and a Directory of Resources for More Help and Information

Edited by Amy L. Sutton. 635 pages. 2007. 978-0-7808-0946-8.

"Updates the consumer information on the physical and mental benefits of physical activity throughout the lifespan offered in earlier editions. . . . Recommended. All readers; all levels."

—*CHOICE, Oct '07*

"An exceptionally well-rounded coverage perfect for any concerned about developing and understanding a fitness program."

—*California Bookwatch, Jun '07*

SEE ALSO *Sports Injuries Sourcebook, 3rd Edition*

Food Safety Sourcebook

Basic Consumer Health Information about the Safe Handling of Meat, Poultry, Seafood, Eggs, Fruit Juices, and Other Food Items, and Facts about Pesticides, Drinking Water, Food Safety Overseas, and the Onset, Duration, and Symptoms of Foodborne Illnesses, Including Types of Pathogenic Bacteria, Parasitic Protozoa, Worms, Viruses, and Natural Toxins

Along with the Role of the Consumer, the Food Handler, and the Government in Food Safety; a Glossary, and Resources for Additional Help and Information

Edited by Dawn D. Matthews. 327 pages. 1999. 978-0-7808-0326-8.

"Recommended reference source."

—*Booklist, May '00*

"This book takes the complex issues of food safety and foodborne pathogens and presents them in an easily understood manner. [It does] an excellent job of covering a large and often confusing topic."

— *American Reference Books Annual, 2000*

Forensic Medicine Sourcebook

Basic Consumer Information for the Layperson about Forensic Medicine, Including Crime Scene Investigation, Evidence Collection and Analysis, Expert Testimony, Computer-Aided Criminal Identification, Digital Imaging in the Courtroom, DNA Profiling, Accident Reconstruction, Autopsies, Ballistics, Drugs and Explosives Detection, Latent Fingerprints, Product Tampering, and Questioned Document Examination

Along with Statistical Data, a Glossary of Forensics Terminology, and Listings of Sources for Further Help and Information

Edited by Annemarie S. Muth. 574 pages. 1999. 978-0-7808-0232-2.

"Given the expected widespread interest in its content and its easy to read style, this book is recommended for most public and all college and university libraries."

—*E-Streams, Feb '01*

"A wealth of information, useful statistics, references are up-to-date and extremely complete. This wonderful collection of data will help students who are interested in a career in any type of forensic field. It is a great resource for attorneys who need information about types of expert witnesses needed in a particular case. It also offers useful information for fiction and nonfiction writers whose work involves a crime. A fascinating compilation. All levels."

—*CHOICE, Jan '00*

"There are several items that make this book attractive to consumers who are seeking certain forensic data. . . . This is a useful current

source for those seeking general forensic medical answers."

—*American Reference Books Annual, 2000*

Gastrointestinal Diseases and Disorders Sourcebook, 2nd Edition

Basic Consumer Health Information about the Upper and Lower Gastrointestinal (GI) Tract, Including the Esophagus, Stomach, Intestines, Rectum, Liver, and Pancreas, with Facts about Gastroesophageal Reflux Disease, Gastritis, Hernias, Ulcers, Celiac Disease, Diverticulitis, Irritable Bowel Syndrome, Hemorrhoids, Gastrointestinal Cancers, and Other Diseases and Disorders Related to the Digestive Process

Along with Information about Commonly Used Diagnostic and Surgical Procedures, Statistics, Reports on Current Research Initiatives and Clinical Trials, a Glossary, and Resources for Additional Help and Information

Edited by Sandra J. Judd. 654 pages. 2006. 978-0-7808-0798-3.

"The text is designed for the general reader seeking information on prevention, disease warning signs, diagnostic and therapeutic questions. . . . It is an excellent resource for the general reader to conveniently locate credible, coordinated and indexed information. . . . The sourcebook will prove very helpful for patients, caregivers and should be available in every physician waiting room."

—*Doody's Review Service, 2006*

SEE ALSO *Diet and Nutrition Sourcebook, 3rd Edition, Digestive Diseases and Disorders Sourcebook*

Genetic Disorders Sourcebook, 4th Edition

Basic Consumer Health Information about Hereditary Diseases and Disorders, Including Facts about the Human Genome, Genetic Inheritance Patterns, Disorders Associated with Specific Genes, Such as Sickle Cell Disease, Hemophilia, and Cystic Fibrosis, Chromosome Disorders, Such as Down Syndrome, Fragile X Syndrome, and Turner Syndrome, and Complex Diseases and Disorders Resulting from the Interaction of Environmental and Genetic Factors, Such as Allergies, Cancer, and Obesity

Along with Facts about Genetic Testing, Suggestions for Parents of Children with Special Needs, Reports on Current Research Initiatives, a Glossary of Genetic Terminology, and Resources for Additional Help and Information

Edited by Sandra J. Judd. 600 pages. 2009. 978-0-7808-1076-1.

Head Trauma Sourcebook

Basic Information for the Layperson about Open-Head and Closed-Head Injuries, Treatment Advances, Recovery, and Rehabilitation

Along with Reports on Current Research Initiatives

Edited by Karen Bellenir. 414 pages. 1997. 978-0-7808-0208-7.

Headache Sourcebook

Basic Consumer Health Information about Migraine, Tension, Cluster, Rebound and Other Types of Headaches, with Facts about the Cause and Prevention of Headaches, the Effects of Stress and the Environment, Headaches during Pregnancy and Menopause, and Childhood Headaches

Along with a Glossary and Other Resources for Additional Help and Information

Edited by Dawn D. Matthews. 342 pages. 2002. 978-0-7808-0337-4.

"Highly recommended for academic and medical reference collections."

—*Library Bookwatch, Sep '02*

SEE ALSO *Pain Sourcebook, 3rd Edition*

Healthy Aging Sourcebook

Basic Consumer Health Information about Maintaining Health through the Aging Process, Including Advice on Nutrition, Exercise, and Sleep, Help in Making Decisions about Midlife Issues and Retirement, and Guidance Concerning Practical and Informed Choices in Health Consumerism

Along with Data Concerning the Theories of Aging, Different Experiences in Aging by Minority Groups, and Facts about Aging Now and Aging in the Future; and Featuring a Glossary, a Guide to Consumer Help, Additional Suggested Reading, and Practical Resource Directory

Edited by Jenifer Swanson. 537 pages. 1999. 978-0-7808-0390-9.

"Recommended reference source."

—*Booklist, Feb '00*

SEE ALSO *Physical and Mental Issues in Aging Sourcebook*

Healthy Children Sourcebook

Basic Consumer Health Information about the Physical and Mental Development of Children between the Ages of 3 and 12, Including Routine Health Care, Preventative Health Services, Safety and First Aid, Healthy Sleep, Dental Care, Nutrition, and Fitness, and Featuring Parenting Tips on Such Topics as Bedwetting, Choosing Day Care, Monitoring TV and Other Media, and Establishing a Foundation for Substance Abuse Prevention

Along with a Glossary of Commonly Used Pediatric Terms and Resources for Additional Help and Information.

Edited by Chad T. Kimball. 624 pages. 2003. 978-0-7808-0247-6.

"Should be required reading for parents and teachers."

—*E-Streams, Jun '04*

"It is hard to imagine that any other single resource exists that would provide such a comprehensive guide of timely information on health promotion and disease prevention for children aged 3 to 12."

—*American Reference Books Annual, 2004*

"This easy-to-read volume is a tremendous resource."

—*AORN Journal, May '05*

SEE ALSO *Childhood Diseases and Disorders Sourcebook, 2nd Edition*

Healthy Heart Sourcebook for Women

Basic Consumer Health Information about Cardiac Issues Specific to Women, Including Facts about Major Risk Factors and Prevention, Treatment and Control Strategies, and Important Dietary Issues

Along with a Special Section Regarding the Pros and Cons of Hormone Replacement Therapy and Its Impact on Heart Health, and Additional Help, Including Recipes, a Glossary, and a Directory of Resources

Edited by Dawn D. Matthews. 321 pages. 2000. 978-0-7808-0329-9.

"A good reference source and recommended for all public, academic, medical, and hospital libraries."

—*Medical Reference Services Quarterly, Summer '01*

"Contains very important information about coronary artery disease that all women should know. The information is current and presented in an easy-to-read format. The book will make a good addition to any library."

—*American Medical Writers Association Journal, Summer '00*

SEE ALSO *Cardiovascular Diseases and Disorders Sourcebook, 3rd Edition, Women's Health Concerns Sourcebook, 3rd Edition*

Hepatitis Sourcebook

Basic Consumer Health Information about Hepatitis A, Hepatitis B, Hepatitis C, and Other Forms of Hepatitis, Including Autoimmune Hepatitis, Alcoholic Hepatitis, Nonalcoholic Steatohepatitis, and Toxic Hepatitis, with Facts about Risk Factors, Screening Methods, Diagnostic Tests, and Treatment Options

Along with Information on Liver Health, Tips for People Living with Chronic Hepatitis, Reports on Current Research Initiatives, a Glossary of Terms Related to Hepatitis, and a Directory of Sources for Further Help and Information

Edited by Sandra J. Judd. 570 pages. 2006. 978-0-7808-0749-5.

"The breadth of information found in this one book would not be readily found in another source. Highly recommended."

—*American Reference Books Annual, 2006*

SEE ALSO *Contagious Diseases Sourcebook*

Household Safety Sourcebook

Basic Consumer Health Information about Household Safety, Including Information about Poisons, Chemicals, Fire, and Water Hazards in the Home

Along with Advice about the Safe Use of Home Maintenance Equipment, Choosing Toys and Nursery Furniture, Holiday and Recreation Safety, a Glossary, and Resources for Further Help and Information

Edited by Dawn D. Matthews. 587 pages. 2002. 978-0-7808-0338-1.

"As a sourcebook on household safety this book meets its mark. It is encyclopedic in scope and covers a wide range of safety issues that are commonly seen in the home."

—*E-Streams, Jul '02*

Hypertension Sourcebook

Basic Consumer Health Information about the Causes, Diagnosis, and Treatment of High Blood Pressure, with Facts about Consequences, Complications, and Co-Occurring Disorders, Such as Coronary Heart Disease, Diabetes, Stroke, Kidney Disease, and Hypertensive Retinopathy, and Issues in Blood Pressure Control, Including Dietary Choices, Stress Management, and Medications

Along with Reports on Current Research Initiatives and Clinical Trials, a Glossary, and Resources for Additional Help and Information

Edited by Dawn D. Matthews and Karen Bellenir. 588 pages. 2004. 978-0-7808-0674-0.

"Academic, public, and medical libraries will want to add the *Hypertension Sourcebook* to their collections."

—*E-Streams, Aug '05*

"The strength of this source is the wide range of information given about hypertension."

—*American Reference Books Annual, 2005*

SEE ALSO *Stroke Sourcebook, 2nd Edition*

Immune System Disorders Sourcebook, 2nd Edition

Basic Consumer Health Information about Disorders of the Immune System, Including Immune System Function and Response, Diagnosis of Immune Disorders, Information about Inherited Immune Disease, Acquired Immune Disease, and Autoimmune Diseases, Including Primary Immune Deficiency, Acquired Immunodeficiency Syndrome (AIDS), Lupus, Multiple Sclerosis, Type 1 Diabetes, Rheumatoid Arthritis, and Graves' Disease

Along with Treatments, Tips for Coping with Immune Disorders, a Glossary, and a Directory of Additional Resources

Edited by Joyce Brennfleck Shannon. 643 pages. 2005. 978-0-7808-0748-8.

"Highly recommended for academic and public libraries."

—*American Reference Books Annual, 2006*

"The updated second edition is a 'must' for any consumer health library seeking a solid resource covering the treatments, symptoms, and options for immune disorder sufferers. . . . An excellent guide."

—*MBR Bookwatch, Jan '06*

SEE ALSO *AIDS Sourcebook, 4th Edition, Arthritis Sourcebook, 2nd Edition*

Infant and Toddler Health Sourcebook

Basic Consumer Health Information about the Physical and Mental Development of Newborns, Infants, and Toddlers, Including Neonatal Concerns, Nutrition Recommendations, Immunization Schedules, Common Pediatric Disorders, Assessments and Milestones, Safety Tips, and Advice for Parents and Other Caregivers

Along with a Glossary of Terms and Resource Listings for Additional Help

Edited by Jenifer Swanson. 570 pages. 2000. 978-0-7808-0246-9.

"As a reference for the general public, this would be useful in any library."

—*E-Streams, May '01*

"Recommended reference source."

—*Booklist, Feb '01*

Infectious Diseases Sourcebook

Basic Consumer Health Information about Non-Contagious Bacterial, Viral, Prion, Fungal, and Parasitic Diseases Spread by Food and Water, Insects and Animals, or Environmental Contact, Including Botulism, E. Coli, Encephalitis, Legionnaires' Disease, Lyme Disease, Malaria, Plague, Rabies, Salmonella, Tetanus, and Others, and Facts about Newly Emerging Diseases, Such as Hantavirus, Mad Cow Disease, Monkeypox, and West Nile Virus

Along with Information about Preventing Disease Transmission, the Threat of Bioterrorism, and Current Research Initiatives, with a Glossary and Directory of Resources for More Information

Edited by Karen Bellenir. 610 pages. 2004. 978-0-7808-0675-7.

"This reference continues the excellent tradition of the *Health Reference Series* in consolidating a wealth of information on a selected topic into a format that is easy to use and accessible to the general public."

—*American Reference Books Annual, 2005*

"Recommended for public and academic libraries."

—*E-Streams, Jan '05*

Injury and Trauma Sourcebook

Basic Consumer Health Information about the Impact of Injury, the Diagnosis and Treatment of Common and Traumatic Injuries, Emergency Care, and Specific Injuries Related to Home, Community, Workplace, Transportation, and Recreation

Along with Guidelines for Injury Prevention, a Glossary, and a Directory of Additional Resources

Edited by Joyce Brennfleck Shannon. 675 pages. 2002. 978-0-7808-0421-0.

"Practitioners should be aware of guides such as this in order to facilitate their use by patients and their families."

—*Doody's Health Sciences Book Review Journal, Sep-Oct '02*

"Recommended reference source."

—*Booklist, Sep '02*

"Highly recommended for academic and medical reference collections."

—*Library Bookwatch, Sep '02*

SEE ALSO *Emergency Medical Services Sourcebook, Sports Injuries Sourcebook, 3rd Edition*

Learning Disabilities Sourcebook, 3rd Edition

Basic Consumer Health Information about Dyslexia, Auditory and Visual Processing Disorders, Communication Disorders, Dyscalculia, Dysgraphia, and Other Conditions That Impede Learning, Including Attention Deficit/Hyperactivity Disorder, Autism Spectrum Disorders, Hearing and Visual Impairments, Chromosome-Based Disorders, and Brain Injury

Along with Facts about Brain Function, Assessment, Therapy and Remediation, Accommodations, Assistive Technology, Legal Protections, and Tips about Family Life, School Transitions, and Employment Strategies, a Glossary of Related Terms, and Directories of Additional Resources

Edited by Joyce Brennfleck Shannon. 613 pages. 2009. 978-0-7808-1039-6.

SEE ALSO *Attention Deficit Disorder Sourcebook, Autism and Pervasive Developmental Disorders Sourcebook*

Leukemia Sourcebook

Basic Consumer Health Information about Adult and Childhood Leukemias, Including Acute Lymphocytic Leukemia (ALL), Chronic Lymphocytic Leukemia (CLL), Acute Myelogenous Leukemia (AML), Chronic Myelogenous Leukemia (CML), and Hairy Cell Leukemia, and Treatments Such as Chemotherapy, Radiation Therapy, Peripheral Blood Stem Cell and Marrow Transplantation, and Immunotherapy

Along with Tips for Life During and After Treatment, a Glossary, and Directories of Additional Resources

Edited by Joyce Brennfleck Shannon. 564 pages. 2003. 978-0-7808-0627-6.

"Unlike other medical books for the layperson, . . . the language does not talk down to the reader. . . . This volume is highly recommended for all libraries."

—*American Reference Books Annual, 2004*

"A fine title which ranges from diagnosis to alternative treatments, staging, and tips for life during and after diagnosis."

—*The Bookwatch, Dec '03*

SEE ALSO *Cancer Sourcebook, 5th Edition*

Liver Disorders Sourcebook

Basic Consumer Health Information about the Liver and How It Works; Liver Diseases, Including Cancer, Cirrhosis, Hepatitis, and Toxic and Drug Related Diseases; Tips for Maintaining a Healthy Liver; Laboratory Tests, Radiology Tests, and Facts about Liver Transplantation

Along with a Section on Support Groups, a Glossary, and Resource Listings

Edited by Joyce Brennfleck Shannon. 580 pages. 2000. 978-0-7808-0383-1.

"This title is recommended for health sciences and public libraries with consumer health collections."

—*E-Streams, Oct '00*

"Recommended reference source."

—*Booklist, Jun '00*

SEE ALSO *Gastrointestinal Diseases and Disorders Sourcebook, 2nd Edition, Hepatitis Sourcebook*

Lung Disorders Sourcebook

Basic Consumer Health Information about Emphysema, Pneumonia, Tuberculosis, Asthma, Cystic Fibrosis, and Other Lung Disorders, Including Facts about Diagnostic Procedures, Treatment Strategies, Disease Prevention Efforts, and Such Risk Factors as Smoking, Air Pollution, and Exposure to Asbestos, Radon, and Other Agents

Along with a Glossary and Resources for Additional Help and Information

Edited by Dawn D. Matthews. 657 pages. 2002. 978-0-7808-0339-8.

"Highly recommended for academic and medical reference collections."

—*Library Bookwatch, Sep '02*

SEE ALSO *Respiratory Disorders Sourcebook, 2nd Edition*

Medical Tests Sourcebook, 3rd Edition

Basic Consumer Health Information about X-Rays, Blood Tests, Stool and Urine Tests, Biopsies, Mammography, Endoscopic Procedures, Ultrasound Exams, Computed Tomography, Magnetic Resonance Imaging (MRI), Nuclear Medicine, Genetic Testing, Home-Use Tests, and More

Along with Facts about Preventive Care and Screening Test Guidelines, Screening and Assessment Tests Associated with Such Specific Concerns as Cancer, Heart Disease, Allergies, Diabetes, Thyroid Disfunction, and Infertility, a Glossary of Related Terms, and a Directory of Resources for Additional Help and Information

Edited by Karen Bellenir. 627 pages. 2008. 978-0-7808-1040-2

"This volume has a wide scope that makes it useful . . . Can be a valuable reference guide."

—*ARBAonline, Nov '08*

Men's Health Concerns Sourcebook, 3rd Edition

Basic Consumer Health Information about Wellness in Men and Gender-Related Differences in Health, With Facts about Heart Disease, Cancer, Traumatic Injury, and Other Leading Causes of Death in Men, Reproductive Concerns, Sexual Dysfunction, Disorders of the Prostate, Penis, and Testes, Sex-Linked Genetic Disorders, and Other Medical and Mental Concerns of Men

Along with Statistical Data, a Glossary of Related Terms, and a Directory of Resources for Additional Information

Edited by Sandra J. Judd. 600 pages. 2009. 978-0-7808-1033-4.

SEE ALSO *Prostate and Urological Disorders Sourcebook*

Mental Health Disorders Sourcebook, 4th Edition

Basic Consumer Health Information about the Causes and Symptoms of Mental Health Problems, Including Depression, Bipolar Disorder, Anxiety Disorders, Posttraumatic Stress Disorder, Obsessive-Compulsive Disorder, Eating Disorders, Addictions, and Personality and Psychotic Disorders

Along with Information about Medications and Treatments, Mental Health Concerns in Children, Adolescents, and Adults, Tips on Living with Mental Health Disorders, a Glossary of Related Terms, and a Directory of Resources for Additional Help and Information

Edited by Amy L. Sutton. 600 pages. 2009. 978-0-7808-1041-9.

SEE ALSO *Depression Sourcebook, 2nd Edition, Stress-Related Disorders Sourcebook, 2nd Edition*

Mental Retardation Sourcebook

Basic Consumer Health Information about Mental Retardation and Its Causes, Including

Down Syndrome, Fetal Alcohol Syndrome, Fragile X Syndrome, Genetic Conditions, Injury, and Environmental Sources

Along with Preventive Strategies, Parenting Issues, Educational Implications, Health Care Needs, Employment and Economic Matters, Legal Issues, a Glossary, and a Resource Listing for Additional Help and Information

Edited by Joyce Brennfleck Shannon. 627 pages. 2000. 978-0-7808-0377-0.

"Public libraries will find the book useful for reference and as a beginning research point for students, parents, and caregivers."
—*American Reference Books Annual, 2001*

"The strength of this work is that it compiles many basic fact sheets and addresses for further information in one volume. It is intended and suitable for the general public."
—*E-Streams, Nov '00*

"An invaluable overview."
—*Reviewer's Bookwatch, Jul '00*

Movement Disorders Sourcebook, 2nd Edition

Basic Consumer Health Information about the Symptoms and Causes of Movement Disorders, Including Parkinson Disease, Amyotrophic Lateral Sclerosis, Cerebral Palsy, Muscular Dystrophy, Multiple Sclerosis, Myasthenia, Myoclonus, Spina Bifida, Dystonia, Essential Tremor, Choreatic Disorders, Huntington Disease, Tourette Syndrome, and Other Disorders That Cause Slowed, Absent, or Excessive Movements

Along with Information about Surgical and Nonsurgical Interventions, Physical Therapies, Strategies for Independent Living, a Glossary of Related Terms, and a Directory of Resources for Additional Help and Information

Edited by Amy L. Sutton. 600 pages. 2009. 978-0-7808-1034-1.

SEE ALSO *Multiple Sclerosis Sourcebook, Muscular Dystrophy Sourcebook*

Multiple Sclerosis Sourcebook

Basic Consumer Health Information about Multiple Sclerosis (MS) and Its Effects on Mobility, Vision, Bladder Function, Speech, Swallowing, and Cognition, Including Facts about Risk Factors, Causes, Diagnostic Procedures, Pain Management, Drug Treatments, and Physical and Occupational Therapies

Along with Guidelines for Nutrition and Exercise, Tips on Choosing Assistive Equipment, Information about Disability, Work, Financial, and Legal Issues, a Glossary of Related Terms, and a Directory of Additional Resources

Edited by Joyce Brennfleck Shannon. 553 pages. 2007. 978-0-7808-0998-7.

SEE ALSO *Movement Disorders Sourcebook, 2nd Edition*

Muscular Dystrophy Sourcebook

Basic Consumer Health Information about Congenital, Childhood-Onset, and Adult-Onset Forms of Muscular Dystrophy, Such as Duchenne, Becker, Emery-Dreifuss, Distal, Limb-Girdle, Facioscapulohumeral (FSHD), Myotonic, and Ophthalmoplegic Muscular Dystrophies, Including Facts about Diagnostic Tests, Medical and Physical Therapies, Management of Co-Occurring Conditions, and Parenting Guidelines

Along with Practical Tips for Home Care, a Glossary, and Directories of Additional Resources

Edited by Joyce Brennfleck Shannon. 552 pages. 2004. 978-0-7808-0676-4.

"This book is highly recommended for public and academic libraries as well as health care offices that support the information needs of patients and their families."
—*E-Streams, Apr '05*

"Excellent reference."
—*The Bookwatch, Jan '05*

SEE ALSO *Movement Disorders Sourcebook, 2nd Edition*

Obesity Sourcebook

Basic Consumer Health Information about Diseases and Other Problems Associated with Obesity, and Including Facts about Risk Factors, Prevention Issues, and Management Approaches

Along with Statistical and Demographic Data, Information about Special Populations,

Research Updates, a Glossary, and Source Listings for Further Help and Information

Edited by Wilma Caldwell and Chad T. Kimball. 360 pages. 2001. 978-0-7808-0333-6.

"The book synthesizes the reliable medical literature on obesity into one easy-to-read and useful resource for the general public."

—*American Reference Books Annual, 2002*

"Well suited for the health reference collection of a public library or an academic health science library that serves the general population."

—*E-Streams, Sep '01*

Osteoporosis Sourcebook

Basic Consumer Health Information about Primary and Secondary Osteoporosis and Juvenile Osteoporosis and Related Conditions, Including Fibrous Dysplasia, Gaucher Disease, Hyperthyroidism, Hypophosphatasia, Myeloma, Osteopetrosis, Osteogenesis Imperfecta, and Paget's Disease

Along with Information about Risk Factors, Treatments, Traditional and Non-Traditional Pain Management, a Glossary of Related Terms, and a Directory of Resources

Edited by Allan R. Cook. 568 pages. 2001. 978-0-7808-0239-1.

"This resource is recommended as a great reference source for public, health, and academic libraries, and is another triumph for the editors of Omnigraphics."

—*American Reference Books Annual, 2002*

"Will prove valuable to any library seeking to maintain a current, comprehensive reference collection of health resources. . . . From prevention to treatment and associated conditions, this provides an excellent survey."

—*The Bookwatch, Aug '01*

SEE ALSO *Healthy Aging Sourcebook, Women's Health Concerns Sourcebook, 3rd Edition*

Pain Sourcebook, 3rd Edition

Basic Consumer Health Information about Acute and Chronic Pain, Including Nerve Pain, Bone Pain, Muscle Pain, Cancer Pain, and Disorders Characterized by Pain, Such as Arthritis, Temporomandibular Muscle and Joint (TMJ) Disorder, Carpal Tunnel Syndrome, Headaches, Heartburn, Sciatica, and Shingles, and Facts about Diagnostic Tests and Treatment Options for Pain, Including Over-the-Counter and Prescription Drugs, Physical Rehabilitation, Injection and Infusion Therapies, Implantable Technologies, and Complementary Medicine

Along with Tips for Living with Pain, a Glossary of Related Terms, and a Directory of Additional Resources

Edited by Joyce Brennfleck Shannon. 644 pages. 2008. 978-0-7808-1006-8.

"Excellent for ready-reference users and can be used for beginning students in health fields . . . appropriate for the consumer health collection in both public and academic libraries."

—*ARBAonline, Nov '08*

Pediatric Cancer Sourcebook

Basic Consumer Health Information about Leukemias, Brain Tumors, Sarcomas, Lymphomas, and Other Cancers in Infants, Children, and Adolescents, Including Descriptions of Cancers, Treatments, and Coping Strategies

Along with Suggestions for Parents, Caregivers, and Concerned Relatives, a Glossary of Cancer Terms, and Resource Listings

Edited by Edward J. Prucha. 575 pages. 1999. 978-0-7808-0245-2.

"An excellent source of information. Recommended for public, hospital, and health science libraries with consumer health collections."

—*E-Streams, Jun '00*

"A valuable addition to all libraries specializing in health services and many public libraries."

—*American Reference Books Annual, 2000*

SEE ALSO *Childhood Diseases and Disorders Sourcebook, 2nd Edition, Healthy Children Sourcebook*

Physical and Mental Issues in Aging Sourcebook

Basic Consumer Health Information on Physical and Mental Disorders Associated with the Aging Process, Including Concerns about Cardiovascular Disease, Pulmonary Disease, Oral Health, Digestive Disorders, Musculoskeletal and Skin Disorders, Metabolic

Changes, Sexual and Reproductive Issues, and Changes in Vision, Hearing, and Other Senses

Along with Data about Longevity and Causes of Death, Information on Acute and Chronic Pain, Descriptions of Mental Concerns, a Glossary of Terms, and Resource Listings for Additional Help

Edited by Jenifer Swanson. 660 pages. 1999. 978-0-7808-0233-9.

"This is a treasure of health information for the layperson."

—*CHOICE Health Sciences Supplement, May '00*

"Recommended for public libraries."

—*American Reference Books Annual, 2000*

SEE ALSO *Healthy Aging Sourcebook*

Podiatry Sourcebook, 2nd Edition

Basic Consumer Health Information about Disorders, Diseases, and Deformities that Affect the Foot and Ankle, Including Sprains, Corns, Calluses, Bunions, Plantar Warts, Plantar Fasciitis, Neuromas, Clubfoot, Flat Feet, Achilles Tendonitis, and Much More

Along with Information about Selecting a Foot Care Specialist, Foot Fitness, Shoes and Socks, Diagnostic Tests and Corrective Procedures, Financial Assistance for Corrective Devices, a Glossary of Related Terms, and a Directory of Resources for Additional Help and Information

Edited by Ivy L. Alexander. 516 pages. 2007. 978-0-7808-0944-4.

"An excellent resource. . . . Although there have been various types of 'foot books' published in the past, none are as comprehensive as this one. 5 Stars (out of 5)!"

—*Doody's Review Service, 2007*

"Perfect for both health libraries and general-interest lending collections."

—*Internet Bookwatch, Jul '07*

Pregnancy and Birth Sourcebook, 3rd Edition

Basic Consumer Health Information about Pregnancy and Fetal Development, Including Facts about Fertility and Conception, Physical and Emotional Changes during Pregnancy, Prenatal Care and Diagnostic Tests, High-Risk Pregnancies and Complications, Labor, Delivery, and the Postpartum Period

Along with Tips on Maintaining Health and Wellness during Pregnancy and Caring for Newborn Infants, a Glossary of Related Terms, and Directories of Resources for Additional Help and Information

Edited by Amy L. Sutton. 600 pages. 2009. 978-0-7808-1074-7.

SEE ALSO *Breastfeeding Sourcebook, Congenital Disorders Sourcebook, 2nd Edition, Family Planning Sourcebook, Women's Health Concerns Sourcebook, 3rd Edition*

Prostate and Urological Disorders Sourcebook

Basic Consumer Health Information about Urogenital and Sexual Disorders in Men, Including Prostate and Other Andrological Cancers, Prostatitis, Benign Prostatic Hyperplasia, Testicular and Penile Trauma, Cryptorchidism, Peyronie Disease, Erectile Dysfunction, and Male Factor Infertility, and Facts about Commonly Used Tests and Procedures, Such as Prostatectomy, Vasectomy, Vasectomy Reversal, Penile Implants, and Semen Analysis

Along with a Glossary of Andrological Terms and a Directory of Resources for Additional Information

Edited by Karen Bellenir. 604 pages. 2006. 978-0-7808-0797-6.

"Certain to be a popular pick among library reference holdings. . . . No prior knowledge is assumed for any of the conditions or terms herein, making it a most accessible general-interest reference."

—*California Bookwatch, Apr '06*

SEE ALSO *Men's Health Concerns Sourcebook, 3rd Edition, Urinary Tract and Kidney Diseases and Disorders Sourcebook, 2nd Edition*

Prostate Cancer Sourcebook

Basic Consumer Health Information about Prostate Cancer, Including Information about the Associated Risk Factors, Detection, Diagnosis, and Treatment of Prostate Cancer

Along with Information on Non-Malignant Prostate Conditions, and Featuring a Section

Listing Support and Treatment Centers and a Glossary of Related Terms

Edited by Dawn D. Matthews. 340 pages. 2001. 978-0-7808-0324-4.

"Recommended reference source."
—*Booklist, Jan '02*

"A valuable resource for health care consumers seeking information on the subject. . . . All text is written in a clear, easy-to-understand language that avoids technical jargon. Any library that collects consumer health resources would strengthen their collection with the addition of the *Prostate Cancer Sourcebook*."
—*American Reference Books Annual, 2002*

SEE ALSO *Cancer Sourcebook, 5th Edition, Men's Health Concerns Sourcebook, 3rd Edition*

Rehabilitation Sourcebook

Basic Consumer Health Information about Rehabilitation for People Recovering from Heart Surgery, Spinal Cord Injury, Stroke, Orthopedic Impairments, Amputation, Pulmonary Impairments, Traumatic Injury, and More, Including Physical Therapy, Occupational Therapy, Speech/Language Therapy, Massage Therapy, Dance Therapy, Art Therapy, and Recreational Therapy

Along with Information on Assistive and Adaptive Devices, a Glossary, and Resources for Additional Help and Information

Edited by Dawn D. Matthews. 519 pages. 2000. 978-0-7808-0236-0.

"This is an excellent resource for public library reference and health collections."
—*American Reference Books Annual, 2001*

"Recommended reference source."
—*Booklist, May '00*

Respiratory Disorders Sourcebook, 2nd Edition

Basic Consumer Health Information about Infectious, Inflammatory, and Chronic Conditions Affecting the Lungs and Respiratory System, Including Pneumonia, Bronchitis, Influenza, Tuberculosis, Sarcoidosis, Asthma, Cystic Fibrosis, Chronic Obstructive Pulmonary Disease, Lung Abscesses, Pulmonary Embolism, Occupational Lung Diseases, and Other Bacterial, Viral, and Fungal Infections

Along with Facts about the Structure and Function of the Lungs and Airways, Methods of Diagnosing Respiratory Disorders, and Treatment and Rehabilitation Options, a Glossary of Related Terms, and a Directory of Resources for Additional Help and Information

Edited by Sandra L. Judd. 638 pages. 2008. 978-0-7808-1007-5.

"A great addition for public and school libraries because it provides concise health information . . . readers can start with this reference source and get satisfactory answers before proceeding to other medical reference tools for more in depth information . . . A good guide for health education on lung disorders."
—*ARBAonline, Nov '08*

SEE ALSO *Lung Disorders Sourcebook*

Sexually Transmitted Diseases Sourcebook, 4th Edition

Basic Consumer Health Information about Chlamydial Infections, Gonorrhea, Hepatitis, Herpes, HIV/AIDS, Human Papillomavirus, Pubic Lice, Scabies, Syphilis, Trichomoniasis, Vaginal Infections, and Other Sexually Transmitted Diseases, Including Facts about Risk Factors, Symptoms, Diagnosis, Treatment, and the Prevention of Sexually Transmitted Infections

Along with Updates on Current Research Initiatives, a Glossary of Related Terms, and Resources for Additional Help and Information

Edited by Laura Larsen. 600 pages. 2009. 978-0-7808-1073-0.

SEE ALSO *AIDS Sourcebook, 4th Edition, Contagious Diseases Sourcebook, 2nd Edition, Men's Health Concerns Sourcebook, 3rd Edition, Women's Health Concerns Sourcebook, 3rd Edition*

Sleep Disorders Sourcebook, 2nd Edition

Basic Consumer Health Information about Sleep and Sleep Disorders, Including Insomnia, Sleep Apnea, Restless Legs Syndrome, Narcolepsy, Parasomnias, and Other Health Problems That Affect Sleep, Plus Facts about Diagnostic Procedures, Treatment Strategies,

Sleep Medications, and Tips for Improving Sleep Quality

Along with a Glossary of Related Terms and Resources for Additional Help and Information

Edited by Amy L. Sutton. 567 pages. 2005. 978-0-7808-0743-3.

"This book will be useful for just about everybody, especially the 40 million Americans with sleep disorders."

—*American Reference Books Annual, 2006*

"A welcome addition to public libraries and consumer health libraries."

—*Medical Reference Services Quarterly, Summer '06*

Smoking Concerns Sourcebook

Basic Consumer Health Information about Nicotine Addiction and Smoking Cessation, Featuring Facts about the Health Effects of Tobacco Use, Including Lung and Other Cancers, Heart Disease, Stroke, and Respiratory Disorders, Such as Emphysema and Chronic Bronchitis

Along with Information about Smoking Prevention Programs, Suggestions for Achieving and Maintaining a Smoke-Free Lifestyle, Statistics about Tobacco Use, Reports on Current Research Initiatives, a Glossary of Related Terms, and Directories of Resources for Additional Help and Information

Edited by Karen Bellenir. 595 pages. 2004. 978-0-7808-0323-7.

"Provides everything needed for the student or general reader seeking practical details on the effects of tobacco use."

—*The Bookwatch, Mar '05*

"Public libraries and consumer health care libraries will find this work useful."

—*American Reference Books Annual, 2005*

SEE ALSO *Respiratory Disorders Sourcebook, 2nd Edition*

Sports Injuries Sourcebook, 3rd Edition

Basic Consumer Health Information about Sprains and Strains, Fractures, Growth Plate Injuries, Overtraining Injuries, and Injuries to the Head, Face, Shoulders, Elbows, Hands, Spinal Column, Knees, Ankles, and Feet, and with Facts about Heat-Related Illness, Steroids and Sport Supplements, Protective Equipment, Diagnostic Procedures, Treatment Options, and Rehabilitation

Along with a Glossary of Related Terms and a Directory of Resources for Additional Help and Information

Edited by Sandra J. Judd. 623 pages. 2007. 978-0-7808-0949-9.

SEE ALSO *Fitness and Exercise Sourcebook, 3rd Edition*

Stress-Related Disorders Sourcebook, 2nd Edition

Basic Consumer Health Information about Stress and Stress-Related Disorders, Including Types of Stress, Sources of Acute and Chronic Stress, the Impact of Stress on the Body's Systems, and Mental and Emotional Health Problems Associated with Stress, Such as Depression, Anxiety Disorders, Substance Abuse, Posttraumatic Stress Disorder, and Suicide

Along with Advice about Getting Help for Stress-Related Disorders, Information about Stress Management Techniques, a Glossary of Stress-Related Terms, and a Directory of Resources for Additional Help and Information

Edited by Amy L. Sutton. 608 pages. 2007. 978-0-7808-0996-3.

"Accessible to the lay reader. Highly recommended for medical and psychiatric collections."

—*Library Journal, Mar '08*

"Well-written for a general readership, the 2nd Edition of *Stress-Related Disorders Sourcebook* is a useful addition to the health reference literature."

—*American Reference Books Annual, 2008*

SEE ALSO *Mental Health Disorders Sourcebook, 4th Edition*

Stroke Sourcebook, 2nd Edition

Basic Consumer Health Information about Stroke, Including Ischemic, Hemorrhagic, and Mini Strokes, as Well as Risk Factors, Prevention Guidelines, Diagnostic Tests, Medications and

Surgical Treatments, and Complications of Stroke

Along with Rehabilitation Techniques and Innovations, Tips on Staying Healthy and Maintaining Independence after Stroke, a Glossary of Related Terms, and a Directory of Resources for Stroke Survivors and Their Families

Edited by Amy L. Sutton. 626 pages. 2008. 978-0-7808-1035-8.

"An encyclopedic handbook on stroke that is written in a language the layperson can understand. . . . This is one of the most helpful, readable books on stroke. This volume is highly recommended and should be in every medical, hospital and public library; in addition, every family practitioner should have a copy in his or her office."

—*ARBAonline Dec '08*

SEE ALSO *Hypertension Sourcebook*

Surgery Sourcebook, 2nd Edition

Basic Consumer Health Information about Common Inpatient and Outpatient Surgeries, Including Critical Care and Trauma, Gastrointestinal, Gynecologic and Obstetric, Cardiac and Vascular, Neurologic, Ophthalmologic, Orthopedic, Reconstructive and Cosmetic, and Other Major and Minor Surgeries

Along with Information about Anesthesia and Pain Relief Options, Risks and Complications, Postoperative Recovery Concerns, and Innovative Surgical Techniques and Tools, a Glossary of Related Terms, and a Directory of Additional Resources

Edited by Amy L. Sutton. 645 pages. 2008. 978-0-7808-1004-4.

"Large public libraries and medical libraries would benefit from this material in their reference collections."

—*ARBAonline Aug '08*

SEE ALSO *Cosmetic and Reconstructive Surgery Sourcebook, 2nd Edition*

Thyroid Disorders Sourcebook

Basic Consumer Health Information about Disorders of the Thyroid and Parathyroid Glands, Including Hypothyroidism, Hyperthyroidism, Graves Disease, Hashimoto Thyroiditis, Thyroid Cancer, and Parathyroid Disorders, Featuring Facts about Symptoms, Risk Factors, Tests, and Treatments

Along with Information about the Effects of Thyroid Imbalance on Other Body Systems, Environmental Factors That Affect the Thyroid Gland, a Glossary, and a Directory of Additional Resources

Edited by Joyce Brennfleck Shannon. 573 pages. 2005. 978-0-7808-0745-7.

"Recommended for consumer health collections."

—*American Reference Books Annual, 2006*

"Highly recommended pick for basic consumer health reference holdings at all levels."

—*The Bookwatch, Aug '05*

SEE ALSO *Endocrine and Metabolic Disorders Sourcebook, 2nd Edition*

Transplantation Sourcebook

Basic Consumer Health Information about Organ and Tissue Transplantation, Including Physical and Financial Preparations, Procedures and Issues Relating to Specific Solid Organ and Tissue Transplants, Rehabilitation, Pediatric Transplant Information, the Future of Transplantation, and Organ and Tissue Donation

Along with a Glossary and Listings of Additional Resources

Edited by Joyce Brennfleck Shannon. 610 pages. 2002. 978-0-7808-0322-0.

"Recommended for libraries with an interest in offering consumer health information."

—*E-Streams, Jul '02*

"This is a unique and valuable resource for patients facing transplantation and their families."

—*Doody's Review Service, Jun '02*

Traveler's Health Sourcebook

Basic Consumer Health Information for Travelers, Including Physical and Medical Preparations, Transportation Health and Safety, Essential Information about Food and Water, Sun Exposure, Insect and Snake Bites, Camping and Wilderness Medicine, and Travel with Physical or Medical Disabilities

Along with International Travel Tips, Vaccination Recommendations, Geographical Health Issues, Disease Risks, a Glossary, and a Listing of Additional Resources

Edited by Joyce Brennfleck Shannon. 619 pages. 2000. 978-0-7808-0384-8.

"Recommended reference source."
—*Booklist, Feb '01*

"This book is recommended for any public library, any travel collection, and especially any collection for the physically disabled."
—*American Reference Books Annual, 2001*

SEE ALSO *Worldwide Health Sourcebook*

Urinary Tract and Kidney Diseases and Disorders Sourcebook, 2nd Edition

Basic Consumer Health Information about the Urinary System, Including the Bladder, Urethra, Ureters, and Kidneys, with Facts about Urinary Tract Infections, Incontinence, Congenital Disorders, Kidney Stones, Cancers of the Urinary Tract and Kidneys, Kidney Failure, Dialysis, and Kidney Transplantation

Along with Statistical and Demographic Information, Reports on Current Research in Kidney and Urologic Health, a Summary of Commonly Used Diagnostic Tests, a Glossary of Related Terms, and a Directory of Resources for Additional Help and Information

Edited by Ivy L. Alexander. 621 pages. 2005. 978-0-7808-0750-1.

"A good choice for a consumer health information library or for a medical library needing information to refer to their patients."
—*American Reference Books Annual, 2006*

SEE ALSO *Prostate and Urological Disorders Sourcebook*

Vegetarian Sourcebook

Basic Consumer Health Information about Vegetarian Diets, Lifestyle, and Philosophy, Including Definitions of Vegetarianism and Veganism, Tips about Adopting Vegetarianism, Creating a Vegetarian Pantry, and Meeting Nutritional Needs of Vegetarians, with Facts Regarding Vegetarianism's Effect on Pregnant and Lactating Women, Children, Athletes, and Senior Citizens

Along with a Glossary of Commonly Used Vegetarian Terms and Resources for Additional Help and Information

Edited by Chad T. Kimball. 337 pages. 2002. 978-0-7808-0439-5.

"Organizes into one concise volume the answers to the most common questions concerning vegetarian diets and lifestyles. This title is recommended for public and secondary school libraries."
—*E-Streams, Apr '03*

"Invaluable reference for public and school library collections alike."
—*Library Bookwatch, Apr '03*

"The articles in this volume are easy to read and come from authoritative sources. The book does not necessarily support the vegetarian diet but instead provides the pros and cons of this important decision. . . . Recommended for public libraries and consumer health libraries."
—*American Reference Books Annual, 2003*

SEE ALSO *Diet and Nutrition Sourcebook, 3rd Edition*

Women's Health Concerns Sourcebook, 3rd Edition

Basic Consumer Health Information about Issues and Trends in Women's Health and Health Conditions of Special Concern to Women, Including Endometriosis, Uterine Fibroids, Menstrual Irregularities, Menopause, Sexual Dysfunction, Infertility, Cancer in Women, and Other Such Chronic Disorders as Lupus, Fibromyalgia, and Thyroid Disease

Along with Statistical Data, Tips for Maintaining Wellness, a Glossary, and a Directory of Resources for Further Help and Information

Edited by Sandra J. Judd. 600 pages. 2009. 978-0-7808-1036-5.

SEE ALSO *Breast Cancer Sourcebook, 3rd Edition, Cancer Sourcebook for Women, 3rd Edition, Healthy Heart Sourcebook for Women, Osteoporosis Sourcebook*

Workplace Health and Safety Sourcebook

Basic Consumer Health Information about Workplace Health and Safety, Including the Effect of Workplace Hazards on the Lungs,

Skin, Heart, Ears, Eyes, Brain, Reproductive Organs, Musculoskeletal System, and Other Organs and Body Parts

Along with Information about Occupational Cancer, Personal Protective Equipment, Toxic and Hazardous Chemicals, Child Labor, Stress, and Workplace Violence

Edited by Chad T. Kimball. 610 pages. 2000. 978-0-7808-0231-5.

"As a reference for the general public, this would be useful in any library."

—*E-Streams, Jun '01*

"Provides helpful information for primary care physicians and other caregivers interested in occupational medicine. . . . General readers; professionals."

—*CHOICE, May '01*

Worldwide Health Sourcebook

Basic Information about Global Health Issues, Including Malnutrition, Reproductive Health, Disease Dispersion and Prevention, Emerging Diseases, Risky Health Behaviors, and the Leading Causes of Death

Along with Global Health Concerns for Children, Women, and the Elderly, Mental Health Issues, Research and Technology Advancements, and Economic, Environmental, and Political Health Implications, a Glossary, and a Resource Listing for Additional Help and Information

Edited by Joyce Brennfleck Shannon. 597 pages. 2001. 978-0-7808-0330-5.

"Named an Outstanding Academic Title."

—*CHOICE, Jan '02*

"Yet another handy but also unique compilation in the extensive *Health Reference Series*, this is a useful work because many of the international publications reprinted or excerpted are not readily available. Highly recommended."

—*CHOICE, Nov '01*

SEE ALSO *Traveler's Health Sourcebook*

Teen Health Series

Complete Catalog

List price $69 per volume. School and library price $62 per volume.

Abuse and Violence Information for Teens

Health Tips about the Causes and Consequences of Abusive and Violent Behavior

Including Facts about the Types of Abuse and Violence, the Warning Signs of Abusive and Violent Behavior, Health Concerns of Victims, and Getting Help and Staying Safe

Edited by Sandra Augustyn Lawton. 411 pages. 2008. 978-0-7808-1008-2.

"A useful resource for schools and organizations providing services to teens and may also be a starting point in research projects."
—*Reference and Research Book News, Aug '08*

"Violence is a serious problem for teens. . . . This resource gives teens the information they need to face potential threats and get help—either for themselves or for their friends."
—*ARBAonline, Aug '08*

Accident and Safety Information for Teens

Health Tips about Medical Emergencies, Traumatic Injuries, and Disaster Preparedness

Including Facts about Motor Vehicle Accidents, Burns, Poisoning, Firearms, Natural Disasters, National Security Threats, and More

Edited by Karen Bellenir. 420 pages. 2008. 978-0-7808-1046-4.

SEE ALSO *Sports Injuries Information for Teens, 2nd Edition*

Alcohol Information for Teens, 2nd Edition

Health Tips about Alcohol and Alcoholism

Including Facts about Alcohol's Effects on the Body, Brain, and Behavior, the Consequences of Underage Drinking, Alcohol Abuse Prevention and Treatment, and Coping with Alcoholic Parents

Edited by Lisa Bakewell. 400 pages. 2009. 978-0-7808-1043-3.

SEE ALSO *Drug Information for Teens, 2nd Edition*

Allergy Information for Teens

Health Tips about Allergic Reactions Such as Anaphylaxis, Respiratory Problems, and Rashes

Including Facts about Identifying and Managing Allergies to Food, Pollen, Mold, Animals, Chemicals, Drugs, and Other Substances

Edited by Karen Bellenir. 410 pages. 2006. 978-0-7808-0799-0.

"This is a comprehensive, readable text on the subject of allergic diseases in teenagers. 5 Stars (out of 5)!"
—*Doody's Review Service, Jun '06*

"This authoritative and useful self-help title is a solid addition to YA collections, whether for personal interest or reports."
—*School Library Journal, Jul '06*

Asthma Information for Teens

Health Tips about Managing Asthma and Related Concerns

Including Facts about Asthma Causes, Triggers, Symptoms, Diagnosis, and Treatment

Edited by Karen Bellenir. 386 pages. 2005. 978-0-7808-0770-9.

"Highly recommended for medical libraries, public school libraries, and public libraries."
—*American Reference Books Annual, 2006*

"Although this volume is nearly 400 pages long, it is so clearly written and well organized that even hesitant readers will be able to find the facts they need, whether for reports or personal information. . . . A succinct but complete resource."
—*School Library Journal, Sep '05*

Body Information for Teens

Health Tips about Maintaining Well-Being for a Lifetime

Including Facts about the Development and Functioning of the Body's Systems, Organs, and Structures and the Health Impact of Lifestyle Choices

Edited by Sandra Augustyn Lawton. 458 pages. 2007. 978-0-7808-0443-2.

Cancer Information for Teens, 2nd Edition

Health Tips about Cancer Awareness, Symptoms, Prevention, Diagnosis, and Treatment

Including Facts about Common Cancers Affecting Teens, Causes, Detection, Coping Strategies, Clinical Trials, Nutrition and Exercise, Cancer in Friends or Family, and More

Edited by Karen Bellenir and Lisa Bakewell. 400 pages. 2009. 978-0-7808-1085-3.

Complementary and Alternative Medicine Information for Teens

Health Tips about Non-Traditional and Non-Western Medical Practices

Including Information about Acupuncture, Chiropractic Medicine, Dietary and Herbal Supplements, Hypnosis, Massage Therapy, Prayer and Spirituality, Reflexology, Yoga, and More

Edited by Sandra Augustyn Lawton. 407 pages. 2007. 978-0-7808-0966-6.

"This volume covers CAM specifically for teenagers but of general use also. It should be a welcome addition to both public and academic libraries."

—*American Reference Books Annual, 2008*

"This volume provides a solid foundation for further investigation of the subject, making it useful for both public and high school libraries."

—*VOYA: Voice of Youth Advocates, Jun '07*

Diabetes Information for Teens

Health Tips about Managing Diabetes and Preventing Related Complications

Including Information about Insulin, Glucose Control, Healthy Eating, Physical Activity, and Learning to Live with Diabetes

Edited by Sandra Augustyn Lawton. 410 pages. 2006. 978-0-7808-0811-9.

"A comprehensive instructional guide for teens. . . . some of the material may also be directed towards parents or teachers. 5 stars (out of 5)!"

—*Doody's Review Service, 2006*

"Students dealing with their own diabetes or that of a friend or family member or those writing reports on the topic will find this a valuable resource."

—*School Library Journal, Aug '06*

"This text is directed to the teen population and would be an excellent library resource for a health class or for the teacher as a reference for class preparation. It can, however, serve a much wider audience. The clinical educator on diabetes may find it valuable to educate the newly diagnosed client regardless of age. It also would be an excellent reference and education tool for a preventive medicine seminar on diabetes."

—*Physical Therapy, Mar '07*

Diet Information for Teens, 2nd Edition

Health Tips about Diet and Nutrition

Including Facts about Dietary Guidelines, Food Groups, Nutrients, Healthy Meals, Snacks, Weight Control, Medical Concerns Related to Diet, and More

Edited by Karen Bellenir. 432 pages. 2006. 978-0-7808-0820-1.

"A very quick and pleasant read in spite of the fact that it is very detailed in the information it gives. . . . A book for anyone concerned about diet and nutrition."

—*American Reference Books Annual, 2007*

SEE ALSO *Eating Disorders Information for Teens, 2nd Edition*

Drug Information for Teens, 2nd Edition

Health Tips about the Physical and Mental Effects of Substance Abuse

Including Information about Marijuana, Inhalants, Club Drugs, Stimulants, Hallucinogens,

Opiates, Prescription and Over-the-Counter Drugs, Herbal Products, Tobacco, Alcohol, and More

Edited by Sandra Augustyn Lawton. 468 pages. 2006. 978-0-7808-0862-1.

"As with earlier installments in Omnigraphics' *Teen Health Series, Drug Information for Teens* is designed specifically to meet the needs and interests of middle and high school students. . . . Strongly recommended for both academic and public libraries."

—*American Reference Books Annual, 2007*

"Solid thoughtful advice is given about how to handle peer pressure, drug-related health concerns, and treatment strategies."

—*School Library Journal, Dec '06*

SEE ALSO *Alcohol Information for Teens, 2nd Edition, Tobacco Information for Teens*

Eating Disorders Information for Teens, 2nd Edition

Health Tips about Anorexia, Bulimia, Binge Eating, And Other Eating Disorders

Including Information about Risk Factors, Diagnosis and Treatment, Prevention, Related Health Concerns, and Other Issues

Edited by Sandra Augustyn Lawton. 377 pages. 2009. 978-0-7808-1044-0.

SEE ALSO *Diet Information for Teens, 2nd Edition*

Fitness Information for Teens, 2nd Edition

Health Tips about Exercise, Physical Well-Being, and Health Maintenance

Including Facts about Conditioning, Stretching, Strength Training, Body Shape and Body Image, Sports Nutrition, and Specific Activities for Athletes and Non-Athletes

Edited by Lisa Bakewell. 432 pages. 2009. 978-0-7808-1045-7.

SEE ALSO *Diet Information for Teens, 2nd Edition, Sports Injuries Information for Teens, 2nd Edition*

Learning Disabilities Information for Teens

Health Tips about Academic Skills Disorders and Other Disabilities That Affect Learning

Including Information about Common Signs of Learning Disabilities, School Issues, Learning to Live with a Learning Disability, and Other Related Issues

Edited by Sandra Augustyn Lawton. 400 pages. 2006. 978-0-7808-0796-9.

"This book provides a wealth of information for any reader interested in the signs, causes, and consequences of learning disabilities, as well as related legal rights and educational interventions. . . . Public and academic libraries should want this title for both students and general readers."

—*American Reference Books Annual, 2006*

Mental Health Information for Teens, 2nd Edition

Health Tips about Mental Wellness and Mental Illness

Including Facts about Mental and Emotional Health, Depression and Other Mood Disorders, Anxiety Disorders, Conduct Disorder, Self-Injury, Psychosis, Schizophrenia, and More

Edited by Karen Bellenir. 424 pages. 2006. 978-0-7808-0863-8.

"This excellent overview of the psychological disorders that affect teens provides clear definitions and descriptions, and discusses resources, therapies, coping mechanisms, and medications."

—*School Library Journal Curriculum Connections, Fall '07*

"A well done reference for a specific, often under-represented group."

—*Doody's Review Service, 2006*

SEE ALSO *Stress Information for Teens*

Pregnancy Information for Teens

Health Tips about Teen Pregnancy and Teen Parenting

Including Facts about Prenatal Care, Pregnancy Complications, Labor and Delivery,

Postpartum Care, Pregnancy-Related Lifestyle Concerns, and More

Edited by Sandra Augustyn Lawton. 434 pages. 2007. 978-0-7808-0984-0.

SEE ALSO *Sexual Health Information for Teens, 2nd Edition*

Sexual Health Information for Teens, 2nd Edition

Health Tips about Sexual Development, Reproduction, Contraception, and Sexually Transmitted Infections

Including Facts about Puberty, Sexuality, Birth Control, Chlamydia, Gonorrhea, Herpes, Human Papillomavirus, Syphilis, and More

Edited by Sandra Augustyn Lawton. 430 pages. 2008. 978-0-7808-1010-5.

"This offering represents the most up-to-date information available on an array of topics including abstinence-only sexual education and pregnancy-prevention methods. . . . The range of coverage—from puberty and anatomy to sexually transmitted diseases—is thorough and extensive. Each chapter includes a bibliographic citation, and the three back sections containing additional resources, further reading, and the index are all first-rate. . . . This volume will be well used by students in need of the facts, whether for educational or personal reasons."

—*School Library Journal, Nov '08*

SEE ALSO *Pregnancy Information for Teens*

Skin Health Information for Teens, 2nd Edition

Health Tips about Dermatological Concerns and Skin Cancer Risks

Including Facts about Acne, Warts, Allergies, and Other Conditions and Lifestyle Choices, Such as Tanning, Tattooing, and Piercing, That Affect the Skin, Nails, Scalp, and Hair

Edited by Edited by Kim Wohlenhaus. 400 pages. 2009. 978-0-7808-1042-6.

Sleep Information for Teens

Health Tips about Adolescent Sleep Requirements, Sleep Disorders, and the Effects of Sleep Deprivation

Including Facts about Why People Need Sleep, Sleep Patterns, Circadian Rhythms, Dreaming, Insomnia, Sleep Apnea, Narcolepsy, and More

Edited by Karen Bellenir. 355 pages. 2008. 978-0-7808-1009-9.

SEE ALSO *Body Information for Teens*

Sports Injuries Information for Teens, 2nd Edition

Health Tips about Acute, Traumatic, and Chronic Injuries in Adolescent Athletes

Including Facts about Sprains, Fractures, and Overuse Injuries, Treatment, Rehabilitation, Sport-Specific Safety Guidelines, Fitness Suggestions, and More

Edited by Karen Bellenir. 429 pages. 2008. 978-0-7808-1011-2.

"An engaging selection of informative articles about the prevention and treatment of sports injuries. . . The value of this book is that the articles have been vetted and are often augmented with inserts of useful facts, definitions of technical terms, and quick tips. Sensitive topics like injuries to genitalia are discussed openly and responsibly. This revised edition contains updated articles and defines sport more broadly than the first edition."

—*School Library Journal, Nov '08*

"This work will be useful in the young adult collections of public libraries as well as high school libraries. . . . A useful resource for student research."

—*ARBAonline, Aug '08*

SEE ALSO *Accident and Safety Information for Teens*

Stress Information for Teens

Health Tips about the Mental and Physical Consequences of Stress

Including Information about the Different Kinds of Stress, Symptoms of Stress, Frequent Causes of Stress, Stress Management Techniques, and More

Edited by Sandra Augustyn Lawton. 392 pages. 2008. 978-0-7808-1012-9.

"Understanding what stress is, what causes it, how the body and the mind are impacted by it,

and what teens can do are the general categories addressed here. . . . The chapters are brief but informative, and the list of community-help organizations is exhaustive. Report writers will find information quickly and easily, as will those who have personal concerns. The print is clear and the format is readable, making this an accessible resource for struggling readers and researchers."

—*School Library Journal, Dec '08*

"The articles selected will specifically appeal to young adults and are designed to answer their most common questions."

—*ARBAonline, Aug '08*

SEE ALSO *Mental Health Information for Teens, 2nd Edition*

Suicide Information for Teens

Health Tips about Suicide Causes and Prevention

Including Facts about Depression, Risk Factors, Getting Help, Survivor Support, and More

Edited by Joyce Brennfleck Shannon. 368 pages. 2005. 978-0-7808-0737-2.

"Highly Recommended for libraries serving teenagers as well as those who work with them."

—*E-Streams, Apr '06*

SEE ALSO *Mental Health Information for Teens, 2nd Edition*

Tobacco Information for Teens

Health Tips about the Hazards of Using Cigarettes, Smokeless Tobacco, and Other Nicotine Products

Including Facts about Nicotine Addiction, Immediate and Long-Term Health Effects of Tobacco Use, Related Cancers, Smoking Cessation, Tobacco Use Prevention, and Tobacco Use Statistics

Edited by Karen Bellenir. 440 pages. 2007. 978-0-7808-0976-5.

"A comprehensive resource. Each chapter is written to stand alone, so students can dip in and use the information in each section for reports or to answer personal questions without having to read the entire book. . . . The book is packed full of statistics, with sources to help students look up more."

—*School Library Journal, Sep '07*

"Pulls together a wide variety of authoritative sources to provide a comprehensive overview of tobacco use for this age group. . . . This reasonably priced reference title should be considered a necessary purchase for all public libraries and school media centers, along with academic libraries supporting teacher education."

—*American Reference Books Annual, 2008*

SEE ALSO *Drug Information for Teens, 2nd Edition*

Health Reference Series

Adolescent Health Sourcebook, 2nd Edition
Adult Health Concerns Sourcebook
AIDS Sourcebook, 4th Edition
Alcoholism Sourcebook, 2nd Edition
Allergies Sourcebook, 3rd Edition
Alzheimer Disease Sourcebook, 4th Edition
Arthritis Sourcebook, 2nd Edition
Asthma Sourcebook, 2nd Edition
Attention Deficit Disorder Sourcebook
Autism & Pervasive Developmental Disorders Sourcebook
Back & Neck Sourcebook, 2nd Edition
Blood & Circulatory Disorders Sourcebook, 2nd Edition
Brain Disorders Sourcebook, 2nd Edition
Breast Cancer Sourcebook, 3rd Edition
Breastfeeding Sourcebook
Burns Sourcebook
Cancer Sourcebook, 5th Edition
Cancer Sourcebook for Women, 3rd Edition
Cancer Survivorship Sourcebook
Cardiovascular Diseases & Disorders Sourcebook, 3rd Edition
Caregiving Sourcebook
Child Abuse Sourcebook
Childhood Diseases & Disorders Sourcebook, 2nd Edition
Colds, Flu & Other Common Ailments Sourcebook
Communication Disorders Sourcebook
Complementary & Alternative Medicine Sourcebook, 3rd Edition
Congenital Disorders Sourcebook, 2nd Edition
Contagious Diseases Sourcebook
Cosmetic & Reconstructive Surgery Sourcebook, 2nd Edition
Death & Dying Sourcebook, 2nd Edition
Dental Care & Oral Health Sourcebook, 3rd Edition
Depression Sourcebook, 2nd Edition
Dermatological Disorders Sourcebook, 2nd Edition
Diabetes Sourcebook, 4th Edition
Diet & Nutrition Sourcebook, 3rd Edition
Digestive Diseases & Disorder Sourcebook
Disabilities Sourcebook
Disease Management Sourcebook
Domestic Violence Sourcebook, 3rd Edition
Drug Abuse Sourcebook, 2nd Edition
Ear, Nose & Throat Disorders Sourcebook, 2nd Edition
Eating Disorders Sourcebook, 2nd Edition
Emergency Medical Services Sourcebook
Endocrine & Metabolic Disorders Sourcebook, 2nd Edition
Environmental Health Sourcebook, 2nd Edition
Ethnic Diseases Sourcebook
Eye Care Sourcebook, 3rd Edition
Family Planning Sourcebook
Fitness & Exercise Sourcebook, 3rd Edition
Food Safety Sourcebook
Forensic Medicine Sourcebook
Gastrointestinal Diseases & Disorders Sourcebook, 2nd Edition
Genetic Disorders Sourcebook, 3rd Edition
Head Trauma Sourcebook
Headache Sourcebook
Health Insurance Sourcebook
Healthy Aging Sourcebook
Healthy Children Sourcebook
Healthy Heart Sourcebook for Women
Hepatitis Sourcebook
Household Safety Sourcebook
Hypertension Sourcebook
Immune System Disorders Sourcebook, 2nd Edition
Infant & Toddler Health Sourcebook
Infectious Diseases Sourcebook
Injury & Trauma Sourcebook